Computer Intelligence Against Pandemics

Intelligent Biomedical Data Analysis (IBDA)

Edited by
Deepak Gupta, Nhu Gia Nguyen,
Ashish Khanna and Siddhartha Bhattacharyya

Volume 9

Computer Intelligence Against Pandemics

Tools and Methods to Face New Strains of COVID-19

Edited by
Siddhartha Bhattacharyya, Jyoti Sekhar Banerjee,
Sergey Gorbachev, Khan Muhammad and Mario Koeppen

DE GRUYTER

Editors
Prof. Dr. Siddhartha Bhattacharyya
Algebra University College
Zagreb
Croatia
and
Rajnagar Mahavidyalaya
Rajnagar, Birbhum 713130
West Bengal
India
dr.siddhartha.bhattacharyya@gmail.com

Dr. Jyoti Sekhar Banerjee
Department of Computer Science and Engineering (AI & ML)
Bengal Institute of Technology
1 Tech Town, Hadia, Government Colony
700150 Kolkata
West Bengal
India
tojyoti2001@yahoo.co.in

Dr. Sergey Gorbachev
School of Mathematics and Information Engineering
Chongqing University of Education
1 Chongjiao Road, Nanshan Street
400065 Chongqing
Nan'an District
Republic of China
spp03@sibmail.com

Dr. Khan Muhammad
Department of Applied Artificial Intelligence
Sungkyunkwan University
03063 Seoul
Republic of Korea
khan.muhammad@ieee.org

Prof. Dr. Mario Koeppen
Department of Computer Science and Electronics
Graduate School of Creative Informatics
Kyushu Institute of Technology
680-4 Kawazu, Iizuka
820 8502 Fukuoka
Japan
mkoeppen@ieee.org

ISBN 978-3-11-076766-7
e-ISBN (PDF) 978-3-11-076768-1
e-ISBN (EPUB) 978-3-11-076775-9
ISSN 2629-7140

Library of Congress Control Number: 2023934966

Bibliographic information published by the Deutsche Nationalbibliothek
The Deutsche Nationalbibliothek lists this publication in the Deutsche Nationalbibliografie; detailed bibliographic data are available on the Internet at http://dnb.dnb.de.

Cover image: gettyimages/thinkstockphotos, Abalone Shell
Typesetting: Integra Software Services Pvt. Ltd.
Printing and binding: CPI books GmbH, Leck

www.degruyter.com

The editors would like to dedicate this volume to the departed souls during the COVID-19 pandemic.

Preface

The global pandemic COVID-19 operates its devastation for more than 2 years globally. As of October 5, 2022, more than 624 million people were infected with this disease, and more than 6.5 million lost their lives worldwide. This novel coronavirus is not only a threat to life but also diminishing the economy of the world. Different medical institutes, virology, and pharmacology research centers strive to develop vaccines, antidotes, and antibiotics to eliminate the virus and mitigate its effects on patients. Now, different newly invented vaccines are applied through the scheduled vaccination process, which is continuing globally to eliminate this deadly virus.

However, we have experienced different waves of COVID-19 caused by some new strains of COVID-19. Since December 2020, several coronavirus variants have been identified and are under investigation. Each new variant raises questions: Are people more at risk of getting sick? Will the COVID-19 vaccines still work? Are there new or different things we should do now to stay safe? So, an exciting area of research is that the invented vaccines, whether effective to mitigate the new strains or some modifications, must be ensured. Hence, again, the entire COVID-19 research is under scrutiny in every aspect whenever a new strain is identified.

This volume introduces the most recent research and innovative developments regarding the new strains of COVID-19. While the subfields of medical and natural sciences have been working instantly on deriving solutions and trying to protect humankind against such virus types, there is also a great focus on technological developments for improving the mechanism – momentum of science for effective and efficient solutions. At this point, computer intelligence is the most powerful tool for researchers to fight against COVID-19. Thanks to instant data analysis and predictive techniques by computer intelligence, it is possible to get positive results and introduce revolutionary solutions against related medical diseases. By running capabilities – resources for rising computational intelligence, technological fields like artificial intelligence (AI) (with machine learning (ML)/deep learning (DL)), data mining, and applied mathematics are essential components for processing data, recognizing patterns, modeling new techniques, and improving the advantages of computational intelligence. Nowadays, there is a great interest in the application potentials of computer intelligence to be an effective approach for taking humankind one step away, after COVID-19 and before pandemics similar to COVID-19 may appear. The need to guarantee that newly developed vaccinations are successful in preventing the spread of new strains of viruses, is an intriguing field of study. In this context, the book aims to inform the target audience about the latest findings – results regarding a wide variety of computer intelligence applications for fighting against the new strains of COVID-19.

This volume presents the most recent research and innovative developments regarding the new strains of COVID-19. This volume also focuses on the instant data analysis and predictive techniques by computer intelligence, discussion to get positive results, and

https://doi.org/10.1515/9783110767681-202

the introduction of revolutionary solutions against related medical diseases. The volume comprises 15 contributory chapters to report the latest developments in this direction.

The COVID-19 pandemic is one of the biggest catastrophes of this century. Since January 2020, global COVID-19-induced mortality has attained a new record every day and continues its hegemony even in 2022. Nations are fighting wave after wave of the attacks of this pandemic. The humiliating devastation, non-guaranteed preventive option, and zero-guaranteed treatments have left human beings in extreme despair. An inestimable escalation in victimization has already created a mismatch between the current rate of occupancy in clinical establishments, quarantine centers, and skilled care demand. The emergence of such a pandemic is not new but uncommon. History has evidenced the outbreaks of major diseases like cholera, plague, swineflu, AIDS, SARS-Cov, and Mars-Cov. Each pandemic has challenged the very fundamental existence of mankind. The mutual relationship between the causes and effects of infection is heterogeneous and complex. It has been observed that epidemics, endemics, and pandemics are caused by zoonotic pathogens, that is, bacteria, viruses, or parasites, that are transmitted to humans through the environment or direct contact with food, water, or animals. Regardless of the various speculative theories, investigating the proper mechanism of transmission and developing methods to control and prevent incidents are essential. Vaccination is the only path to salvation from such a pandemic. Rather, a fusion of treatment and prevention has the ability to escape such an attack. During any pandemic, survival instincts have driven the human community into a behavioral shift. But, every pandemic leaves the same question, are we ready to face the next one?

Chapter 1 has summarized and fundamentally addressed the historical emergence of different pandemics in the human community of the world. Moreover, a brief outcome of the management of the COVID-19 pandemic has also been observed.

AI is the precise simulation of human intelligence by machines. AI and computer-aided diagnosis are routinely used in medical imaging. In the context of the COVID-19 pandemic, early and accurate diagnosis of COVID-19 cases reduces the spread and mortality caused by SARS-CoV-2, the causative agent of COVID-19. AI has been used to improve the precise detection of COVID-19 cases. The gold standard for the detection of SARS-CoV-2 is RT-PCR. However, RT-PCR is a time-consuming process that can give false-negative results and requires skilled laboratory technicians, which may not be possible in some resource-constrained regions. Contrastingly, AI-based screening and detection of specific changes in X-ray and CT scan images of suspected COVID-19 patients can offer a cost-effective, speedy, and accurate diagnosis of clinical cases. The convolutional neural network (CNN), a DL algorithm, can improve the accuracy and reliability of the diagnosis of COVID-19 from chest X-rays. An enormous amount of training data is required to make accurate predictions of clinical cases via CNN. Several pretrained models such as GoogLeNet, AlexNet, VGG, and open databases such as GitHub can help with the training of DL networks. In Chapter 2, we look at how AI, ML, and DL can be used to improve the specificity, sensitivity, and accuracy of SARS-CoV-2 diagnosis.

Depression, stress, and anxiety are major issues affecting society among many age groups over a period of time. Of late, the COVID-19 pandemic has brought a jump in a phenomenal increase in cases among the younger age group population. In Chapter 3, the authors attempt to explore various DASS-21 variables among millennials and Gen-Z adults due to COVID-19. A strong association between DASS-21 variables and COVID-19 was established among Gen-Z and millennials. Based on the survey, various factors were ranked to understand the COVID-19 effect on DASS-21 variables. It is found that gender and educational qualifications played no role in the effect of COVID-19 on Gen-Z and millennials. Uncertainty in job and business emerges to be a major cause of depression, anxiety, and stress. The results obtained could help psychologists and government bodies to take appropriate steps to improve the mental health conditions of Gen-Z and millennials in society.

COVID-19 has cost 5 million lives worldwide and destabilized the economic and healthcare systems in just two years. An important strategy to combat COVID-19 is to propose a fast and accurate method of screening infected persons. One such efficient technique of screening is doing radiology examinations using chest X-rays. It was found in earlier studies that people affected with COVID-19 display abnormalities in chest radiography images. A large number of works detecting COVID-19 are presently available however; the works do not give a high accuracy of detection. Motivated by this drawback, a deep network-based solution to determine COVID-19 from X-rays of the chest has been proposed in Chapter 4. With the advent of the different variants of the COVID-19 virus determining whether a patient is affected by COVID-19 is not enough. The variant of COVID-19 also needs to be determined. The proposed work also provides an efficient algorithm for variant detection, that is, delta, omicron, or alpha variant. The proposed algorithm is split into two stages. Detection of COVID-19 is undertaken in the first stage, and in the next stage, the variant detection of COVID-19 is done for patients whose test results are COVID-19 positive. The proposed CNN model is inspired by the residual network model ResNet50. The suggested CNN model is inspired by the residual network model ResNet50. The model proposed is efficient and produces a high accuracy of 99.47% for stage 1 of the algorithm, that is, COVID-19 detection, and an accuracy of 98.46% for stage 2, that is, COVID-19 variant detection on the used dataset obtained from images of patients of Eastern India.

The coronavirus disease that caused the novel severe acute respiratory syndrome coronavirus 2 (SARS-CoV-2) affected a bulk population worldwide. Understanding the evolution and pathogenesis of the virus is a key to the control of COVID-19 that can be accomplished by computational genome sequencing. The genome sequence of SARS-CoV-2 was instantly discovered and distributed on GenBank (MN908947.3). Many strains are evaluated because of the mutations in the genome of the virus. However, most of the exposed strain (alpha, beta, gamma, delta, epsilon, zeta, eta, lambda, kappa, theta, omicron, and lota) sequences and lineages of concerned resources have rapidly been determined by next-generation sequencing (NGS) and shared on bioinformatics databases like BV-BRC BETA. Illumina NGS sequencing consists of four major steps such as sample preparation, cluster generation, sequencing, and data analysis. NGS presents an efficient and unbiased way to classify the new strains of COVID-19 as well as provides an opportunity for the tracking of the global transmission route of the virus, detection of mutations to prevent the spread of new strains, reduce the use of molecular diagnostics assays, target screening for possible therapeutics, and characterization of coinfections, potent phenotype, therapeutic strategy, and genetic relatedness. In Chapter 5, the authors have covered advancements in technical aspects and platforms for SARS-CoV-2 computational genome sequencing.

Chapter 6 provides a comprehensive review of different existing epidemiological models proposed for analyzing the impact of COVID-19. Since December 2019, COVID-19 emerged as an alarming threat to mankind. To mitigate the impact of the pandemic several preventive measures have been practiced by nations. But due to the mutation of the virus, the pandemic prevails. This review provides a vivid description of the contributions of different existing epidemiological models on COVID-19. A comparative analysis of SIR, ESIR, SEPIR, SEIR, SEIJR, SEIAR, SEIR-P, SIRD, SEIRD, RSEIRD, SEIRDH, SEIQARDT, SIDARTHE, theta-SEIHRD, and SIRDV models has been highlighted. The effects of important parameters like infection rate and recovery rate on different epidemiological models have been addressed. Model parameters, assumptions about the model, techniques used, contributions, and drawbacks of the respective models have also been discussed. Apart from epidemical models, this chapter aims to focus on the precise illustration of multiple strains of SARSCoV-2. A comprehensive analysis of the impact of vaccination on multiple strains has also been reported.

SARS-CoV-2, a lineage of beta coronavirus, is the causative agent of COVID-19, which has caused millions of deaths and crippled economies around the world. Early detection and treatment of COVID-19 cases are crucial for the containment and reduction of disease transmission. During an emergency such as a pandemic like COVID-19, when there is a lack of available treatment against a new disease, drug repurposing or repositioning can be an effective strategy to control the disease. Drug repositioning is cost-effective, minimizes failure in clinical trials, and obtains relatively speedy approval from regulatory authorities. AI-mediated drug repositioning treatment of COVID-19 patients can speed up the management and medical care for the patients. AI, which includes cognitive computing, DL, CNNs, and ML, can identify potential antiviral drugs for treating a disease. The time frame for extracting essential facts, statistics, and evaluation of the existing preapproved and approved drugs using molecular descriptors can be reduced by AI technology. Based on experimental data, different supervised ML and DL algorithms are implemented as part of AI strategies to identify the repurposable drug effectively. Screening of presently available drugs and the existing library of natural compounds or novel drug candidates for the treatments against COVID-19 can be based on protein-ligand or protein–peptide interactions, which are facilitated through ML and DL. Such screening reduces the frequency of failures that might occur in clinical trials. In Chapter 7, the authors focus on repurposing existing drugs using AI strategies, particularly in the context of SARS-CoV-2.

Biological databases are a treasure trove of authentic information for healthcare and allied field. Biomedical data can be accessed and made into customized training sets for algorithms to generate healthcare informatics-based solutions. In this preliminary work, two such databases were reviewed to identify the most significant subtypes of psychological disorders (NCBI-PUBMED database) reported most frequently in scientific studies during and before the COVID pandemic. To identify the root cause of these disorders RSB-PDB database was explored that contains data on structurally identified bio-molecules related to diseases, determined by experimental methods like X-ray crystallography. There has been a disastrous impact of the pandemic and prolonged lockdown on general psychological well-being in all societies. Recent studies reported that understanding the key issues related to mental health care during and beyond the COVID crisis would play a major role to palliate the psychological calamity. This simple data mining strategy identified the 22 most significant subtypes of psychological disorders that have been reported during and immediately after the pandemic. The hydrolases (a class of biological enzymes) have been identified as a major entity that may be linked with most of these psychological disorders. To reduce bias towards some handful of scientific reports and to eliminate chances of false-positive or false-negative entries the robustness of the whole database was utilized. Chapter 8 aims to ascertain the role of health informatics to provide insightful medical information in a cost-effective manner.

Technology revolution 4.0 has brought e-banking financial products and services to development because it helps to increase transparency, ensure privacy, and speed-up transaction processing, thereby creating trust and maintaining loyalty to the customers. Financial inclusion has made important contributions to economic growth in many countries. In the context of the COVID-19 pandemic, countries that have continuously maintained a state of social distancing have changed the consumption habits of people and businesses. Through empirical research of an emerging country in Southeast Asia, the research results show that financial inclusion has greatly supported basic financial products and services such as mobilizing and lending capital at a reasonable cost. In addition, the research results also confirm that Internet banking, Mobile banking, and Fintech services are most commonly used while other services such as securities investment and technology insurance are not yet developed. In addition, Chapter 9 also stated that the COVID-19 pandemic could lead to faster development of financial inclusion due to people's changing habits and the increasing use of financial technology in transactions.

Pandemics have affected our world every once in a while. In 1918, the influenza pandemic, also known as the Spanish flu, took about 500 million lives. In 1957, the Asian flu emerged in East Asia, and more than 1.1 million people lost their lives. In 1968, the H3N2 virus caused the Hong Kong flu, which took around 4 million lives. And in the most recent coronavirus (COVID-19) more than 5.4 million people lost their lives. It is quite clear that, even after being in the modern age, people are not safe. Technologies and innovations are at a high, but still we are not able to protect ourselves from these disasters. Prevention is better than cure; therefore, we need to be prepared for such drastic events. With the advancement in technologies like AI, ML, the IoT, and IoD we have the leverage to come up with measures to counter these pandemics in the future with minimum loss of life and property. In Chapter 10, the authors discuss how the technologies like AI, IoT, and IoD can help us overcome or minimize the effect of such pandemics.

Between April 1 and May 14, 2020, the daily COVID-19 infection rate in India was regularly between 20.64% and 30.81% of patients who are actually sick. India is now coping with the epidemic issue. In India, the number of patients who have become infected since May 14 has roughly followed an exponential trajectory. If this pattern continues for another week, there will be between 1 and 13 lakh infected persons, by the middle of March, and India will face a grave situation. By mid-March 2020, there will be a demand for up to 710,761 hospital isolation beds since intensive care units will then be at capacity. In Chapter 11, the authors have covered the COVID-19 preparations and their effects on the world's second-most populous nation. A prognostication model is suggested as a contribution to accurately predict COVID-19 corroborated instances. Their study could help political leading lights and health-conscious organizations allocate the necessary employees, beds, and intensive care facilities to handle the issue over the coming days and weeks.

The key hurdles in COVID-19 mitigation include effective immunization, treatment, and adaptable containment techniques. The promise of AI in COVID-19 tracking, diagnostics, and prognosis, medication discovery, vaccine development, and therapy of COVID-19 surveillance is the subject of Chapter 12. AI attempts to emulate the cognitive powers of the human brain, such as problem-solving and learning capacities, using massive data. ML, a subtype of AI, has particular potential for solving issues based on data-curated experiences. Advances in AI approaches have offered a previously unheard-of potential for constructing agile surveillance systems based on a flood of data gathered in a short period of time. Many publications in course of the COVID-19 pandemic highlighted the AI techniques in prioritizing, distribution, surveillance, and medications, vaccines, and non-pharmaceutical therapies. This review will go over the clinical efficacy of AI-based models as well as the constraints and problems that AI systems face such as model generalizability, explainability, and trust as pillars for real-world deployment in healthcare.

Currently, when the entire world is reeling from the effects of the second wave of the pandemic, the third wave is in its beginning and expected to be more deadly than earlier. Since the first COVID case was detected, the virus has undergone several mutations with the delta plus variant, the delta variant, and the lambda variant being a few of the worst COVID-19 variants detected so far. During the last few months, there has been an exponential rise in the number of omicron cases all over the world. Proper identification and detection of these new variants are vital in recent times. In Chapter 13, various DL and transfer learning models like CNN, Resnet50, VGGNet, and InceptionV3 have been explored that can help to forecast the spread and further mutations of the virus. The objective of Chapter 13 is to study the performance details of all those algorithms comprehensively for COVID case prediction. As DL models are powerful in extracting complex features automatically without human effort, these models can formulate prevention strategies for the new strains of COVID.

Intelligent computing complemented by the adoption of technology has been the key to minimizing the pandemic's rippling effect by manifolds. At a time when the pandemic has affected millions of lives, it is essential for humankind to keep investing in technologies such as IoT and Drones to combat the newer strains and future pandemics. IoT has helped smart frameworks and intelligent systems in place to respond to ever-increasing COVID-19 cases in a much better way, whereas Drones gave critical stakeholders an advantage over time and management constraints. During COVID-19 certain countries utilized drone services for disinfection, increased testing rates, speedy medical deliveries, etc. Chapter 14 aims to discuss the role of IoT and Drones to tackle COVID-19 from a global perspective. It highlights various use cases of leveraging drones and IoT in tackling COVID-19 effectively. An insight into this Chapter 14 will help tackle future pandemics or epidemics in a much more convenient way. It will provide the readers with a brief of the scenarios when technologies were leveraged and spark a field for future researchers to understand the gap and improve on the existing system.

Finally, the authors of Chapter 15 provide a possible solution through a mobile application to integrate multiple features required by people to make themselves habitual in this "New Normal" condition. The primary reason is the social distancing constraints that have been imposed on cab bookings, local shops, and restaurants. The application provides the perfect solution for organizations like the Airport Authority of India or any similar organization to resume their business and thrive in this period. All the said facilities are separately provided by many companies and gain a huge profit while the Airport Authority does not profit. To trade off all these things, the authors of Chapter 15 have deployed such a solution that can give all the required supports that are required by the commuters while traveling via airplane and at the same time, Airport Authority also gets due profit through providing facilities to the commuters maintaining social distancing and COVID-19 risk prediction.

This volume explains the need for computer intelligence against ongoing pandemics to face new strains of COVID-19. Though the concept of this book is aimed at the advanced level and can be considered as a research monograph, the book still covers chapters at the medium level (verbally and technically) as it tries to target a wide audience including beginner, medium, and upper level readers. The book can be used in computational intelligence, medical, biomedical, AI, ML, DL, and even data (i.e., image and signal) processing-oriented courses given at especially health, biology, biomedical engineering, or similar programs of universities and institutions.

The editors

Contents

Brief Biography of the Editors

Dr. Siddhartha Bhattacharyya [FRSA (UK), FIET (UK), FIE (I), FIETE, LFOSI, SMIEEE, SMACM, SMAAIA, SMIETI] did his Bachelors in Physics, Bachelors in Optics and Optoelectronics, and Masters in Optics and Optoelectronics from the University of Calcutta, India in 1995, 1998, and 2000 respectively. He completed his Ph.D. in Computer Science and Engineering from Jadavpur University, India in 2008. He is the recipient of the University Gold Medal from the University of Calcutta for his Masters. He is the recipient of several coveted awards including the Distinguished HoD Award and Distinguished Professor Award conferred by the Computer Society of India, Mumbai Chapter, India in 2017, the Honorary Doctorate Award (D. Litt.) from The University of South America, and the South East Asian Regional Computing Confederation (SEARCC) International Digital Award ICT Educator of the Year in 2017. He has been appointed as the ACM Distinguished Speaker for the tenure of 2018–2020. He has been inducted into the People of ACM hall of fame by ACM, the USA in 2020. He has been appointed as the IEEE Computer Society Distinguished Visitor for the tenure of 2021–2023. He has been elected as a full foreign member of the Russian Academy of Natural Sciences and the Russian Academy of Engineering. He has been elected a full fellow of The Royal Society for Arts, Manufacturers and Commerce (RSA), London, UK.

He is currently serving as the Principal of Rajnagar Mahavidyalaya, Rajnagar, Birbhum. He is also serving as a scientific advisor in Algebra University College, Zagreb, Croatia. He served as a Professor in the Department of Computer Science and Engineering of Christ University, Bangalore. He served as the Principal of RCC Institute of Information Technology, Kolkata, India during 2017–2019. He has also served as a Senior Research Scientist in the Faculty of Electrical Engineering and Computer Science of VSB Technical University of Ostrava, Czech Republic (2018–2019). Prior to this, he was the Professor of Information Technology at RCC Institute of Information Technology, Kolkata, India. He served as the Head of the Department from March 2014 to December 2016. Prior to this, he was an Associate Professor of Information Technology at RCC Institute of Information Technology, Kolkata, India from 2011–2014. Before that, he served as an Assistant Professor in Computer Science and Information Technology at the University Institute of Technology, The University of Burdwan, India from 2005–2011. He was a Lecturer in Information Technology at Kalyani Government Engineering College, India during 2001-2005. He is a co-author of 6 books and the co-editor of 98 books and has more than 400 research publications in international journals and conference proceedings to his credit. He has got two PCTs and 19 patents to his credit. He has been a member of the organizing and technical program committees of several national and international conferences. He is the founding Chair of ICCICN 2014, ICRCICN (2015, 2016, 2017, 2018), and ISSIP (2017, 2018) (Kolkata, India). He was the General Chair of several international conferences like WCNSSP 2016 (Chiang Mai, Thailand), ICACCP (2017, 2019) (Sikkim, India) and (ICICC 2018 (New Delhi, India), and ICICC 2019 (Ostrava, Czech Republic).

He is the Associate Editor of several reputed journals including Applied Soft Computing, IEEE Access, Evolutionary Intelligence, and IET Quantum Communications. He is the editor of the International Journal of Pattern Recognition Research and the founding Editor in Chief of the International Journal of Hybrid Intelligence, Inderscience. He has guest-edited several issues with several international journals. He is serving as the Series Editor of IGI Global Book Series Advances in Information Quality and Management (AIQM), De Gruyter Book Series(s) Frontiers in Computational Intelligence (FCI) and Intelligent Biomedical Data Analysis (IBDA), CRC Press Book Series(s) Computational Intelligence and Applications & Quantum Machine Intelligence, Wiley Book Series Intelligent Signal and Data Processing, Elsevier Book Series Hybrid Computational Intelligence for Pattern Analysis and Understanding and Springer Tracts on Human Centered Computing.

https://doi.org/10.1515/9783110767681-204

His research interests include hybrid intelligence, pattern recognition, multimedia data processing, social networks, and quantum computing.

He is a life fellow of the Optical Society of India (OSI), India, a life fellow of the International Society of Research and Development (ISRD), UK, a fellow of the Institution of Engineering and Technology (IET), UK, a fellow of Institute of Electronics and Telecommunication Engineers (IETE), India and a fellow of Institution of Engineers (IEI), India. He is also a senior member of the Institute of Electrical and Electronics Engineers (IEEE), USA, International Institute of Engineering and Technology (IETI), Hong Kong, and the Association for Computing Machinery (ACM), USA.

He is a life member of the Cryptology Research Society of India (CRSI), Computer Society of India (CSI), Indian Society for Technical Education (ISTE), Indian Unit for Pattern Recognition and Artificial Intelligence (IUPRAI), Center for Education Growth and Research (CEGR), Integrated Chambers of Commerce and Industry (ICCI), and Association of Leaders and Industries (ALI). He is a member of the Institution of Engineering and Technology (IET), UK, International Rough Set Society, International Association for Engineers (IAENG), Hong Kong, Computer Science Teachers Association (CSTA), USA, International Association of Academicians, Scholars, Scientists and Engineers (IAASSE), USA, Institute of Doctors Engineers and Scientists (IDES), India, The International Society of Service Innovation Professionals (ISSIP) and The Society of Digital Information and Wireless Communications (SDIWC). He is also a certified Chartered Engineer of the Institution of Engineers (IEI), India. He is on the Board of Directors of the International Institute of Engineering and Technology (IETI), Hong Kong.

Dr. Jyoti Sekhar Banerjee, B.Tech, M.E, Ph.D. (Engg.), is currently serving as the Head of the Department in the Computer Science and Engineering (AI & ML) Department at the Bengal Institute of Technology, Kolkata, India. Additionally, He is also the professor-in-charge, R & D and Consultancy Cell & Nodal Officer of the IPR Cell of BIT. Dr. Banerjee did his Post-Doctoral Fellowship at Nottingham Trent University, UK, in the Department of Computer Science. He also completed the Post Graduate Diploma in IPR & TBM from MAKAUT, WB. He has teaching and research experience spanning 18 years and completed one IEI funded project. He is a member of the CSI, IEEE, ISTE, IEI, ISOC, IAENG and fellow of IETE. He is the present honorary Secretary-cum-Treasurer, of the ISTE WB Section. He is the current honorary Secretary of the Computer Society of India, Kolkata Chapter. He is also the Executive Committee Member of the IETE, Kolkata Centre. He has published over Sixty papers in various international journals, conference proceedings, and book chapters. He is the Editor-in-Chief of American Journal of Advanced Computing (AJAC), Smart Society, USA. He is the lead author of "A Text Book on Mastering Digital Electronics: Principle, Devices, and Applications" and co-editor of the six books. He has also co-authored another book and is currently processing four edited books in reputed international publishers like Springer, CRC Press, De Gruyter, etc. Presently he is also processing three more textbooks; those are now in press. His areas of research interests include Computational Intelligence, Cognitive Radio, Sensor Networks, AI/ML, Network Security, Different Computing Techniques, IoT, WBAN (e-healthcare), Expert Systems.

Dr. Sergey Gorbachev received a Ph.D. degree in National Research Tomsk State University, Russia, in 2003. He worked as a Senior Researcher at the International Laboratory Systems of technical vision, National Research Tomsk State University. He is currently a Professor with the School of Artificial Intelligence, Chongqing University of Education, China. He is an Academician of the Russian Academy of Engineering. He has published 8 monographs, 20 book chapters, 18 patents and certificates of computer programs, and more than 160 papers in reviewed journals, and proceedings of conferences. His research interests include neural-fuzzy networks, ensemble models, soft computing, deep learning, quantum-inspired computing, image processing, data mining, and neutrosophic cognitive maps.

Dr. Khan Muhammad received his PhD in Digital Contents from Sejong University, South Korea in February 2019. He was an Assistant Professor in the Department of Software, Sejong University from March 2019 to February 2022. He is currently the director of Visual Analytics for Knowledge Laboratory (VIS2KNOW Lab) and an Assistant Professor (Tenure-Track) in the Department of Applied AI, School of Convergence, College of Computing and Informatics, Sungkyunkwan University, Seoul, South Korea. His research interests include intelligent video surveillance, medical image analysis, information security, video summarization, multimedia data analysis, computer vision, and smart cities. He has registered 10 patents and contributed more than 220 papers in peer-reviewed journals and conference proceedings in his research areas. He is an Associate Editor/Editorial Board Member for more than 15 journals. He was among the most highly cited researchers in 2021 and 2022, according to the Web of Science (Clarivate).

Dr. Mario Köppen received his Masters degree in solid-state physics at Humboldt-University of Berlin in 1991. Afterward, he worked as a scientific assistant at the Central Institute for Cybernetics and Information Processing in Berlin. From 1992 to 2006, he worked with the Fraunhofer Institute for Production Systems and Design Technology and achieved a doctoral degree at the Technical University Berlin. He has published more than 150 peer-reviewed papers in conference proceedings, journals, and books and played an active role in various conferences, incl. the WSC online conference series on Soft Computing in Industrial Applications, and the HIS conference series on Hybrid Intelligent Systems. He is a founding member of the World Federation of Soft Computing and since 2016 Editor-in-Chief of Applied Soft Computing journal. In 2006, he became a JSPS fellow at the Kyushu Institute of Technology in Japan, a Professor at the Network Design and Research Center (NDRC) in 2008, and Professor at the Graduate School of Creative Informatics of the Kyushu Institute of Technology in 2013.

List of contributors

Aniruddha Nag
Air India, West Bengal, India

Arindam Mitra
Adamas University, West Bengal, India

Atishna Samantaray
Indian Institute of Engineering Science and Technology, Shibpur, West Bengal, India

Ankita Pramanik
Indian Institute of Engineering Science and Technology, Shibpur, West Bengal, India

Aarya Senan Surasenan
Bharathiar University, Tamil Nadu, India

Aparna Ramakrishnan
Bharathiar University, Tamil Nadu, India

Arindam Sadhu
Greater Kolkata College of Engineering and Management, West Bengal, India

Arnab Naha
Acharya Prafulla Chandra College, West Bengal, India

Aparajita Bhattacharya
Adamas University, West Bengal, India

Arpita Chakraborty
Bengal Institute of Technology, Kolkata, West Bengal, India

Binod Kumar Singh
University of Petroleum and Energy Studies, Dehradun, Uttarakhand, India

Bikramjit Sarkar
JIS College of Engineering, West Bengal, India

Eshani Sadhukhan
St. Xavier's University, West Bengal, India

Labhvam Kumar Sharma
Bengal Institute of Technology, Kolkata, West Bengal, India

Mehtab Alam
Jamia Hamdard, New Delhi, India

M. Afshar Alam
Jamia Hamdard, New Delhi, India

Madorina Paul Das
University of Calcutta, West Bengal, India

Parijat Roy
Adamas University, West Bengal, India

Prasun Ghosal
Indian Institute of Engineering Science and Technology, Shibpur, West Bengal, India

Prerona Saha
Bengal Institute of Technology, Kolkata, West Bengal, India

P.F. Steffi
Cauvery College for Women (Autonomous), Tamil Nadu, India

P.F. Mishel
Bharathidasan University, Tamil Nadu, India

Ravi Ranjan
Bengal Institute of Technology, Kolkata, West Bengal, India

Rahul Deb Das
IBM, Germany

Surajit Debnath
Women's Polytechnic, Tripura, India

Safdar Tanweer
Jamia Hamdard, New Delhi, India

Shishupal Kumar
Indian Institute of Information Technology, Nagpur, Maharashtra, India

https://doi.org/10.1515/9783110767681-205

Trung Hieu Nguyen
Banking University Ho Chi Minh City, Vietnam

Totakura Bangar Raju
University of Petroleum and Energy Studies, Dehradun, Uttarakhand, India

Van Chien Nguyen
Thu Dau Mot University, Vietnam

Yukthi R Aithal
Global Academy of Technology, Bangalore, Karnataka, India

Faisal Shah Khan
Dark Star Quantum Lab Inc., USA

Farheen Siddiqui
Jamia Hamdard, New Delhi, India

Harsha Haridasan
Bharathiar University, Tamil Nadu, India

Ihtiram Raza Khan
Jamia Hamdard, New Delhi, India

Jyoti Sekhar Banerjee
Bengal Institute of Technology, Kolkata, West Bengal, India

Johnson Retnaraj Samuel and Selvan Christyraj
Sathyabama Institute of Science and Technology (Deemed to be University), Tamil Nadu, India

Jackson Durairaj and Selvan Christyraj
Sathyabama Institute of Science and Technology (Deemed to be University), Tamil Nadu, India

Kamarajan Rajagopalan
Sathyabama Institute of Science and Technology (Deemed to be University), Tamil Nadu, India

Kumari Nidhi Lal
Visvesvaraya National Institute of Technology, Nagpur, India

Kunal Das
Acharya Prafulla Chandra College, West Bengal, India

Lam Oanh Ha
Thu Dau Mot University, Vietnam

Snigdha Sen
Global Academy of Technology, Bangalore, Karnataka, India

Sougata Mazumder
Indian Institute of Engineering Science and Technology, Shibpur, West Bengal, India

Snahasish Karmakar
Indian Institute of Engineering Science and Technology, Shibpur, West Bengal, India

Soham Guhathakurata
Bengal Institute of Technology, Kolkata, West Bengal, India

Sayak Saha
Bengal Institute of Technology, Kolkata, West Bengal, India

Soumyadip Daripa
Bengal Institute of Technology, Kolkata, West Bengal, India

Sagnick Biswas
Bengal Institute of Technology, Kolkata, West Bengal, India

Soumik Gangopadhyay
Institute of Engineering & Management, West Bengal, India

Sayanee Bandyopadhyay
Indian Institute of Engineering Science and Technology, Shibpur, West Bengal, India

Subhasree Bhattacharjee
Narula Institute of Technology, West Bengal, India

Sahil Zaman
Acharya Prafulla Chandra College, West Bengal, India

Suman Kumar Roy
National Institute of Technology, Surathkal, Karnataka, India

Thirumalaiyammal B
Cauvery College for Women (Autonomous), Tamil Nadu, India

Soumik Gangopadhyay, Aniruddha Nag*, and Eshani Sadhukhan

A retrospective journey of world in pandemic

Abstract: COVID-19 pandemic is one of the biggest catastrophes of this century. Since January 2020, global COVID-induced mortality attains new record every day and continues its hegemony even in 2022. Nations are fighting the waves after waves of the attacks of this pandemic. The humiliating devastation, nonguaranteed preventive option, and zero definite treatment have left humanbeings in extreme despair. Inestimable escalation in victimization has already created a mismatch between current rate of occupancy in clinical establishments, quarantine centers, and skilled care demand. Emergence of such pandemic is not new but uncommon. History has evidenced the outbreaks of major diseases like cholera, plague, swine flu, AIDS, SARS-Cov, and Mars-Cov. Each pandemic has challenged the very fundamental existence of mankind. The mutual relationship among cause and effect of infection is heterogeneous and complex. It has been observed that epidemics, endemics, and pandemics are caused by zoonotic pathogens, that is, bacteria, virus, or parasite, that are transmitted to humans through environment or direct contact, food, water, or animals. Irrespective of several speculative theories, exploring the right mechanism of transmission and establishing methods needs to control and prevent the incidences. Vaccination is the only path of salvation from such a pandemic. Rather, a fusion of treatment and prevention has the ability to escape such attack. During any pandemic, survival instinct has driven human community into a behavioral shift. But every pandemic leaves the same question, Are we ready to face the next one? This chapter has summarized and fundamentally addressed the historical emergence of different pandemic among human community of the world. Moreover, a brief outcome of management of COVID-19 pandemic has also been observed.

1 Introduction

Like human race, infectious diseases have spread across the world. Since prehistoric times, the continuous expansion of human populations has led to successive invasions of increasing numbers of different pathogens [20]. Communicable diseases represent ample threat to human survival across the nations but, at a variable degree. The

***Corresponding author: Aniruddha Nag**, Manager, Air India, Indai, e-mail: anirunag@gmail.com, ORCID ID: 0009-0008-1585-1437
Soumik Gangopadhyay, Department of Business Administration, Institute of Engineering and Management, Kolkata, West Bengal, India, e-mail: soumik74@gmail.com, soumik.gangopadhyay@iemcal.com, ORCID ID: 0000-0003-4115-472X
Eshani Sadhukhan, Research Scholar, St. Xavier's University, Kolkata, India

https://doi.org/10.1515/9783110767681-001

expanded human race as a result of extended trade, worldwide reach, and interaction between humans and animals are the reasons behind spread of infectious disease so fast. Optimum use of land induced by population explosion, climate change [10], international travel, and not obeying precautions further has aggravated the situation. Furthermore, exploitation of use of land and climatic condition play a vital role in the transmission of pathogens from animals to humans [22, 66]. The terms endemic, epidemic, and pandemic represent the deterioration of health status. The term basically differs due to its disparity of spread in geographic areas [28]. History has also evidenced the use of infectious agents (e.g., *Bacillus anthracis*, *Yersinia pestis*, and Variola virus) as biological weapons to destroy the financial and nonfinancial health of other nation. COVID-19 is the latest inclusion in the category of pandemic. Coronavirus has been suspected as such an initiative by few observation-based speculation. Few researches also hypothesized the spread of novel coronavirus as none other than a clandestine plan to destabilize the global economy par se health. Interestingly, in this twenty-first century, no pandemic has any resemblance with the magnitude of novel COVID-19 pandemic. As of now, definite treatment is yet to be invented which can successfully eradicate coronavirus. The fusion of scientific treatment and techniques of intervention may arrest or avoid such pandemic in future [80, 82]. Further, prevention is better than cure. In addition, to control these infections, clinical and nonclinical measures are essential to curb the intensity on human being. Emergence of many pandemic has challenged the very existence of mankind. Hence, global surveillance with clinical advancement to combat viruses is the need of the hour.

This chapter is a historical review of major epidemics, endemics, and pandemics that have troubled mankind such as plague, cholera, influenza, malaria, HIV, and different strains of coronavirus. The chapter is a compilation of pandemic and its versatile impact on mankind.

2 Historical panorama

Apart from COVID-19, the current century has evidenced at least five pandemics including H1N1 in 2009, polio in 2014, and Ebola pandemic (2014 and 2016 in West Africa and 2019 in Congo) [61] (see table 1, 2 & 3).

2.1 The antonine plague

The first known pandemic that attacked the human race was the Antonine plague (also known as Plague of Galen) in the year 165 and it continued up to AD 180. The name Galen came from the name of the physician. It affected the Roman Empire and

Table 1: Outbreak of different diseases.

Time period/ year of initiation	Disease outbreak	Geography	No. of victims	Impact
165–180	Antonine plague		5 million death	
735–737	Japanese smallpox		1 million death	
1,347–1,351	Bubonic plague pandemic (black death)	Afro-Eurasia, America	30–50% European mortality [17]	Humongous social and economic crisis [53]
1,520	Smallpox (first viral epidemic)	America	More than 50% mortality among few communities [36]	Destruction of indigenous population of North and South America [18]
1,629–1,631	Italian plague	Italy	1 million death	Disrupted labor supply and productivity
1,665	Great plague	London	100,000 death	
1881	Fifth cholera pandemic	Global	>1.5 million death (9.7/10,000) [11]	Victimization of Russian clinician [24]
1918	Spanish flu influenza pandemic	Global	Estimated 20–100 million mortality [37]	Huge GDP loss in Australia, Canada, the UK, and the USA [46]
1957	Asian flu influenza pandemic	Global	0.7–1.5 million death (2.4–5.1 death/10,000) [62]	Here also huge GDP loss in Canada, Japan, the UK, and in USA as a result economic disaster [46]
1968	Hong Kong flu influenza pandemic also known as 1968 flu pandemic	Global	Approximately 1 million mortality [47]	Loss of US $23–26 billion in the USA [38]
1981	HIV/AIDS pandemic	Global	>70 million infections, 36.7 million death (WHO)	Loss of approx. 2–4% growth in GDP in Africa [19]
2003	SARS pandemic	Four continents, 37 nations	8,098 possible cases, 744 deaths [63]	Loss in Hong Kong SAR US $4 billion, US $3–6 billion in Canada; and US $5 billion in Singapore [39]

Table 1 (continued)

Time period/ year of initiation	Disease outbreak	Geography	No. of victims	Impact
2009	Swine flu influenza pandemic	Global	1.51–5.75 lakh death (0.2–0.8/10,000) [16]	Loss of US $1 billion GDP in the Republic of [40]
2012	MERS epidemic	22 nations	1,879 cases, 659 deaths [5]	US $2 billion loss in the Republic of Korea, resulted cumulative loss of US $14 billion [33, 50]
2013	West Africa Ebola virus epidemic	10 nations	28,646 cases, 11,323 deaths [69]	Liberia, Guinea, Sierra Leone lost US $2 billion [35]
2015	Zika virus pandemic	76 nations	2,656 cases of microcephaly or malformation of central nervous system [70]	US $7 to US $18 billion in Latin America and the Caribbean experienced maximum loss [61]
2019	COVID-19 pandemic	Global	53.83 crore people affected, 63.20 lakh death till June 22, 2022	Global recession

Table 2: Few factors behind worldwide respiratory infections.

Factor	Variables
Virus	Fast transmission
	Survive outside the human body (in droplets, in stools, or any intermediate animal hosts)
	It transmits from an infected person
	Genetically stable, able to genetic recombine, gene exchanges, and gene adoptions
	Viral load determines the severity of disease, basically the formula is high viral means to high severity
Natural	Seasonal change, climatic change, weather, or temperature can affect the transmission and viability

Table 2 (continued)

Factor	Variables
Environment	Potentiality of the virus and human vulnerability
	Extreme harsh weather condition such as climate change
	Air pollution plays a vital role in the transmission and stability of the virus
Demographic/social variables	Demographic factors, e.g., population density, age, gender, and pattern of household
	Awareness of hygiene, practice, and social issues
	Construction of house, types of house, locality, free, and open space
	Social networks, mixing patterns with neighborhoods, working conditions and space, religious practices, and commuting medium
	Road infrastructure and socioeconomic conditions
	National and international travel plays an important role
	Crowded areas: e.g., schools, colleges, hospitals, cinemas, theaters, police barracks old age homes, religious places, and prisons
Human host	Susceptibility to the specific virus; passive immunity to children
	Animal-to-human and human-to-human transmission
	Ability of asymptomatic carriers to transmit the virus
	Short term postexposure immunity among infected
	Severity and lethality of the disease
	Disease pattern, spectrum varies with age and comorbidities and also related potential to spread

Table 3: Recent epidemic.

Emerging disease	Primary animal carrier	Escalating animal carrier	Major impact in countries/continents	Approximate years
HIV-AIDS	Primates		Global impact but worst sufferer Africa	1970 to till date
Ebola	Bats or nonhuman primates	Great apes and forest duikers	Entire Africa (East, Central, West)	Major epidemic in 2015 (variable effect)
Nipah	Pigs	Humans	Malaysia and Singapore	1999

Table 3 (continued)

Emerging disease	Primary animal carrier	Escalating animal carrier	Major impact in countries/continents	Approximate years
Severe acute respiratory syndrome (SARS)	Bats	Civet cats	Originated from China and spread to many other nations	2003
Middle East respiratory syndrome (MERS)	Bats	Camels	East Africa and Middle east	2008 onward
Avian flu (H5N1)	Wild aquatic birds	Poultry (ducks, geese, swans, gulls, and terns)	From Asia to rest of the countries	2005–2010
Swine flu (H1N1)	Pigs		Across the globe	2009
COVID-19	Bats	To be revealed	Originated in China to multiple	December 2019 to present
Monkeypox	Animals including human being	Squirrels, Gambian-pouched rats, dormice, nonhuman primates	Originated in 11 African countries	1970, 2017, 2018, 2019, 2021, 2022

transmitted through soldiers after returning from near east. Estimated 5 million people died due to the disease [6]. It was believed to have travelled via trade routes of Romans and spread to China. Rome observed an estimated death of more than 2,000 people died in each day [23].

2.2 Japanese smallpox epidemic

The first record is of this epidemic occurred in August AD 735 that affected Japan and claimed the life of one-third of the entire population [5]. In AD 737, another epidemic occurred affected all classes and became a cause of great mortality. This is said to have been the greatest epidemic known in Japan of the then era and was followed by another in the summer and autumn of the year [59]. This small pox epidemic was the first-recorded epidemics. In AD 790, another epidemic said to have affected persons of 30 years of age or older, but its authenticity has not been proved due to inadequate record [32].

2.3 Plague of Justinian

Between AD 541 and AD 549, this was originated from Egypt that spread across the Roman Empire to end the life of 100 million people. Most likely it was originated and carried from Africa to Constantinople through rats during shipment of grain from Egypt. This plague affected nearly half of the population of Europe and wreaked havoc [8].

2.4 Black death

The *Yersinia pestis* (*Y. pestis*) bacterium that spreads mostly by fleas on rodents and other animals is responsible for this devastating epidemic that struck Europe and Asia from AD 1346 and lasted to AD 1353. It was one of the most fatal pandemic recorded in human history. Almost 75–200 million victims died [7].

2.5 New world small pox

Smallpox is an acute contagious and deadly contagious disease. Variola virus spread through rodent to give birth of fresh victims. European travellers carried this virulent disease along with them to the new world that was unaware of this deadly disease. So, they fall prey to this deadly disease easily. Smallpox claimed the millions of life of inhabitants of Mexico and America. Moreover, it was imported to Australia that devastated the Aboriginal population [74].

2.6 Great plague of London

Started from 1665 to 1666, within a year of Great Plague of London, deadly epidemic of plague killed almost 100,000 residents of London and it was found that rats and fleas were the carrier of this devastated disease.

2.7 Italian plague

Another plague which is known as Italian plague also known as Great plague of Milan ravaged many regions of Italy and recorded approximately 200,000 deaths between 1629 and 1631. This was a type of Bubonic Plague. It has not only claimed life of people but also hit economy of Italy very hard [74].

2.8 Cholera pandemic

Between 1817 and 1923, the first six cholera pandemics hit the world occurred consecutively and continuously one after another over time and caused by the bacteria known as Vibrio Cholerae. It was believed that the pandemics originated from Indian subcontinent. India, Russia, England, entire Europe, and many other countries were badly affected. Proposed reason behind such outbreak were migration, pilgrimage, and other commercial activities. Since 1817, seven cholera pandemics hit the world. Few affected Europe and some reached to the United States. In the first three pandemics, an estimated death of around 15 million Indian were observed between 1817 and 1860. The third cholera pandemic also killed 1 million Russians. It spreaded like a wild fire everywhere and killed few lakhs people from Mecca to England.

2.9 Third plague

People know this as Black Death that wreaked havoc in Medieval Europe and killed about half of the population. Europe was also affected by the plague during the third plague pandemic. This originated in 1894 at Yunnan, China and has spread to Hong Kong and India and then to Europe. From remote Chinese province of Yunnan the plague reemerged in 1855 to spread further. It killed almost 12 million victims of India and China and claimed over 15 million from the rest of the world including Australia. Plague is classified into three types – bubonic, pneumonic, and septicemic based on their difference in signs, symptoms, and affected body parts.

2.10 Yellow fever

The Yellow fever virus evolved in Africa and was brought to America during the slave trade era. The virus spread by infected mosquitoes which is found commonly to areas of Africa and South America. Mosquito and monkeys are the carrier of this virus. Tropical South America and sub-Saharan Africa still dominate in rate of occurrence of this disease. Approximately, more than 1 lakh people lost their life due to this fever.

2.11 Russian flu

Russian flu was one of more pandemics of the nineteenth century that affected badly in Russia in the year 1889 and stayed upto 1891 [60]. This epidemic had broken out in St. Petersburg in November 1889. The deadly pandemic "Asiatic flu" (also termed as "Russian flu," Russian influenza, "the Russian epidemic") killed almost 1 million victims within a year. This was a respiratory viral pandemic, which has been referred as an earlier coronavirus pandemic [30].

2.12 Spanish flu

One of the deadliest pandemic in the human history is Spanish flu influenza epidemic or Spanish influenza pandemic of 1918–1919 that sacrificed an estimated 25 million life (alternative research claimed 40–50 million). Incidence of Spanish flu is a contribution of H1N1 influenza virus that transmits from one human individual to other through airborne respiratory secretions.

2.13 Asian flu

Asian flu is one of the deadliest global pandemic influenza in the human history occurred in the year 1957–1958 caused by a virus subtype H2N2. It was originated in Guizhou, southern China. This influenza also killed 1 million residents of the world.

2.14 Hongkong flu

The year 1968 has evidenced another influenza pandemic caused by H3N2 virus. Existence of two genes of avian influenza virus turns this virus unique. This epidemic initiated in Hong Kong and spread rapidly to India, northern Australia and sacrificed 1 million lives worldwide. More than 65 years older were dominating among them. Further it subsided into an endemic around the world as a seasonal influenza.

2.15 HIV/AIDS

HIV or human immunodeficiency virus causes AIDS and turns the victim nonimmune that leads to zero ability to fight infections. The virus can be transmitted through intravenous route, that is, contact with infected blood, semen, or vaginal fluids. According to UNAIDS, 36.3 million (alternatively estimated 27.2–47.8 million) lives have been lost due to AIDS-related illnesses since the emergence of this epidemic [83]. Our world is still not free from this virus.

2.16 Swine flu

The flu attacked first time in 2009. In resemblance with Spanish and Russian flu, this flu was also caused by the H1N1 influenza virus as a new strain of the virus. The US CDC (Centre for Disease and Control Prevention) estimated that 150,000–575,000 people died from this viral pandemic in the very first year of its outbreak.

2.17 SARS

In 2002–2004, worldwide around 8,000 people suffered by Severe Acute Respiratory Syndrome Coronavirus (SARS-CoV or SARS-CoV-1), out of which 770 people died. World Health Organization sent an alert to all nations on its first arrival in China [84, 85].

2.18 Ebola

Ebola virus disease, formerly known as Ebola hemorrhagic fever, is caused by a deadly virus. It is believed that those who handled infected chimpanzees, gorillas (dead/alive) in Congo and Gibon were the first victim of this virus. The symptoms are severe bleeding, organ failure that can lead to death. During 2014–2016, around 11,000 people died because of this virus in Africa.

2.19 MERS

Middle East respiratory syndrome (MERS), also known as Camel flu, is a viral respiratory disease caused by a novel coronavirus (Middle East Respiratory Syndrome Coronavirus, or MERS-CoV) that was first identified in Saudi Arabia in 2012. It is believed that from camel this flu has been spread. Till date around 800 people have died in this flu. Mostly, it has been found in the Middle East and far east Asian countries.

2.20 Monkeypox

After coronavirus world is reeling in fear of monkeypox, the latest lethal virus which has already killed around 100 people around the world. World Health Organization cautioned people after 724 confirmed cases of monkeypox have been reported from 13 non-EU/EEA countries and expressed their concern on this. Monkeypox is caused by the monkeypox virus, a member of the same family of viruses as smallpox, having symptoms very similar to smallpox though it is less severe. This virus belongs to the Orthopoxvirus genus of the Poxviridae family. According to researchers, there are two monophyletic groups of monkeypox virus, that is, the West African monophyletic group and the Congo Basin (Central African) monophyletic group. The name monkeypox coined from the initial discovery of the virus in monkeys in a Danish laboratory in 1958. Though monkeypox is not new, the first human case was found long back in a child in the Democratic Republic of the Congo in 1970. A recent hypothesis has observed that anyone who has had close contact with an infected individual can get monkeypox. The incubation period of monkeypox is usually from 6 to 13 days but can range from 5 to 21 days. Initially with symptoms like fever, rash, and swollen lymph nodes, it may create further complications that may lead to death.

Other than all the communicable diseases, world community is also in noncommunicable diseases endemic that needs change in subjective lifestyle to mitigate [27].

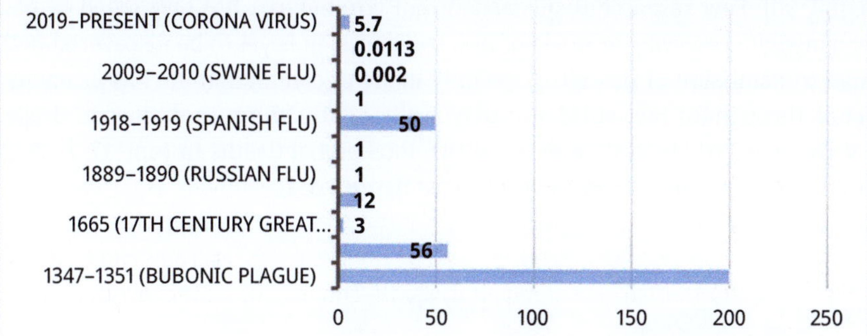

	1347–1351 (Bubonic Plague)	1520 (Smallpox)	1665 (17th Century Great Pleague)	1855 (The Third Plague)	1889–1890 (Russian Flu)	1899–1923 ((6th Cholera Outbreak)	1918–1919 (Spanish flu)	1968–1970 (Hongkong flu)	2009–2010 (swine Flu)	2014–2016 (Ebola)	2019–Present (Corona Virus)
Death in Million	200	56	3	12	1	1	50	1	0.002	0.0113	5.7

Figure 1: Death toll due to pandemics.

3 COVID-19 pandemic

COVID-19, SARS-CoV-2 is a communicable disease caused by the coronavirus. 'CO' "VI," "D," and 19 stands for "Corona," "virus," disease, and the year of its occurrence, respectively. Outbreak of COVID-19 pandemic initially came into limelight in a wholesale seafood market of Wuhan, Hubei province of China. Since then, the disease has swiftly travelled across the world, affecting every continent except Antarctica. COVID-19's emergence in China toward the end of 2019 triggered a global threat to human existence. It is a primary cause of hospitalization and mortality among the middle and elderly across all impacted countries. The virus is extremely contagious and can be spread via intimate contact or droplets [67]. Close contact with infected human subjects via sneezing, coughing, respiratory droplets, or aerosols spread the virus to transmit from person to person [12]. By inhaling through the nose or mouth, these aerosols can enter the human respiratory system [52, 54]. Individuals infected with COVID-19 experienced versatile symptoms including fever, cough, exhaustion, and breathing trouble as well as severe pneumonia with respiratory trouble followed by shock, which resemble to all other coronavirus illnesses [6]. There is a disparity in symptoms of COVID-19 disease among adults and children. COVID-19 is a pulmonary illness that damage lung tissues and also also other tissues and organs [68, 73]. Coronaviruses could be transmitted by the virus-infected blood products during transfusion. The WHO has classified it as a pandemic [86, 90]. Few researches speculated that coronavirus has originated in bat, but the intermediate reservoir or mode of first transmission is yet to be discovered [88]. Inter-human transmission of this virus, the only mode of contamination, has promoted the incidence throughout the world. Coronavirus is a 80–120 nm in diametric single-stranded RNA virus [31]. According to the WHO, total global deaths in June 17, 2022, is 6,314,972 (out of total victims 535,863,950) [89] (see figure 1 & 2).

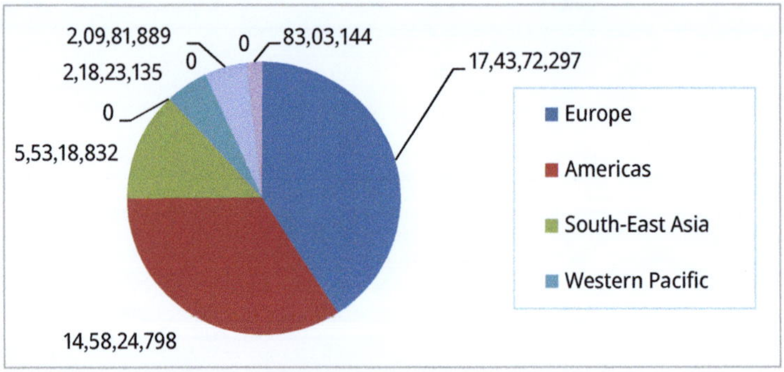

Figure 2: Global statistics of COVID-19 mortality.

This virus can spread from mouth or nose secretions of an infected person as droplets during cough, sneeze, speak, or spit. Unexpected emergence, unguaranteed treatment option, and inestimable mortality rate have compelled to impose "lock down" in every nation to break the contagious infection chain of COVID-19 [31, 65]. In search of sustenance and viability, viruses are always mutating to develop a new variant, or strain, of a virus to form which is quite evident for novel coronavirus too. A variant sometimes act in different ways. The following is the list of seven variants of coronavirus. The virus has fortified by multiplying its strains. Alpha, beta, gamma, and delta are the four main subgroupings of coronaviruses. Currently, omicron and XE are the "variant of concern" as it spreads faster than the existing viruses [90] (see table 4).

Table 4: Types of strains of coronavirus [91].

Types of coronavirus	Symptoms
SARS-CoV-2 (severe acute respiratory syndrome coronavirus 2) [91]	Severe acute respiratory syndrome, shortness of breath, weaken immunity system, fever, cough, and even death
SARS-CoV (severe acute respiratory syndrome)	Headache, muscle aches, dry cough, and difficulty in breathing and death
MERS-CoV (Middle East respiratory syndrome)	Cough, fever, and shortness of breath and pneumonia
Strains	Subclassification of coronavirus strain
HCoV-229E	Alpha
HCoV-NL63	Alpha
HCoV-OC43	Beta
HKU1	Beta
SARS-CoV	Beta
MERS-CoV	Beta
SARS-CoV-2	Alpha, beta, gamma, delta

Incidence and prevalence of COVID pandemic is not a mere healthcare problem. Interdisciplinary issues and complexity of environmental health issues are the part and parcel of this crisis. The studied transmission dynamics of COVID-19 have revealed a variety of environmental factors, that is, meteorological conditions, outdoor and interior air quality, relative humidity, fomites, water and waste water, solid waste, and soil that can influence COVID-19 transmission [49]. COVID-19 airborne transmissions are highly influenced by air quality index, NO_2, particulate matter, and temperature [21]. In fact, the transmission of coronavirus is a function of pollutant air to human transmission and human-to-human transference as the combination of low wind speed and high pollution levels encourages the spread of the virus [12, 13]. Exposure risk variables have strong association with demographic, socioeconomic, and environmental factors. COVID-19 spread may be hampered by the effects of poor air quality in unsustainable ecosystems [14].

3.1 Future threat and beyond omicron

With the evolution of omicron, XE (BA.1, BA.2) variants of COVID-19, the problem of pandemic compounded. Rate of infection and intensity of attack were observed to be very high, although morbidity rate has gone significantly decreased [76]. Newly developed vaccines, antiviral drugs are trying to arrest the transmission of the diseases and impact on host-cell replication along with nonclinical behavioral interventions such as wearing mask and social distancing to stop transmission of virus. But it doesn't mean complete eradication of COVID-19 from the world. On the contrary, according to the researchers and virologists, due to high tendency and capability of mutation, SARS-CoV-2 eradication needs a strategic action. Research on variants of interest and variants of concern will unfold the future of coronavirus and its impact on global residents [80].

3.2 Management of COVID-19

3.2.1 Treatment, mitigation, and prevention

Management of COVID victims includes isolation, treatment of asymptomatic individuals, supportive care, and measures. In absence of effective pharmaceutical interventions, social isolation, quarantine, adequate rest, and medication have been widely adopted all over the world to restrict COVID-19 incidence and save the structure of the human race.

3.2.2 Prevention

Several WHO approved COVID-19 vaccines have been administered among the world community via mass vaccination campaign across the globe [82]. Selective preventive measures for behavioral changes have also been implemented by administrative authorities of all the countries.

3.2.3 Vaccine

Only mass vaccination can design the path of salvation from COVID pandemic [43, 45]. Few vaccines have led to side effects such as fever, chills, fatigue, and headache [79]. There are ample cases of repeat victimization that have been witnessed among vaccinated adults (see table 5).

3.2.4 Medicinal approach

COVID-19 infection has spread around the globe, posing a clinical concern among public and healthcare workers. Being a brand-new virus, there isn't much information available about it. Further, no specific guaranteed antiviral therapies or vaccinations are available for COVID-19 illness at this time [44]. In absence of definite treatment,

Table 5: List of COVID-19 vaccines.

Vaccine brand	Types of component viral vaccines	Marketer
NUVAXOVID	Protein subunit	Novavax Inc. USA
COVOVAX (NOVAVAX)	Protein subunit	Serum Institute of India [75]
SPIKEVAX	RNA	Moderna
COMIRNATY	RNA	BioNTech/Pfizer
AD26.COV2.S	Nonreplicating viral vector	Janssen (Johnson & Johnson)
VAXZEVRIA	Nonreplicating viral vector	AstraZeneca/Oxford
COVISHIELD	Nonreplicating viral vector	Serum Institute of India (Oxford/AstraZeneca) [77]
COVAXIN	Inactivated	Bharat Biotech
SPUTNIK V	Adenoviral-based	The Gamaleya Research Institute
COVILO	Inactivated	Sinopharm (Beijing)
CORONAVAC	Inactivated	Sinovac

unexpected growth of virus has been combatted through the symptomatic primary treatment. Antiviral medicines such as Hydroxychloroquine and Azithromycin were found relatively effective in treating COVID-19 [34, 55]. Remdesivir, Favipiravir, Tocilizumab, Itolizumab, Ivermectin, Casirivimab-imdevimab, and Baricitinib were also found significantly effective in treating critical patients of COVID-19 [63–65]. Telemedicine has shown a new path of expanding the scale of treatment of victims as it can easily reach to remote geography. Several other RPA and AI-based devices or gadgets have been discovered for detection, mitigation, and treatment of COVID victims.

3.2.5 Social distancing

Several behavioral preventive measures such as social or physical distancing, use of face coverings or masks, quarantine of the victims, ventilation of indoor spaces, covering faces against coughs and sneezes, frequently washing hands, avoiding frequent touch of mouth by unwashed hands, and keeping hands away from the face in public were identified to clear out infectious aerosol (as it can circulate due to inadequate ventilation within enclosed space) have been suggested to minimize the risk of transmissions to decrease the probability of spread of infection, virologists, and doctors. WHO and the US CDC have also published guidelines for individuals to keep risk of transmission at bay. Further, WHO has also recommended the use of personal protective equipment PPE) in health care service functioning, domestic care operations, during serving travelers and handling of cargo as a mandatory practice all over the world. Further, in adherence with such guidelines doctors, chemists, health workers, and nurses are using PPE kit at the work place mandatorily for all their encounters with the patients to escape the risk of transmission [15]. Many countries have used social distance as their major tactics to stop the incidence of COVID-19 since early March 2020. Closure of offline educational institution, working from home, embargo on public meetings, and restrictions on free movement of subjects outside their residence are some techniques of social distancing tactics adopted around the world to decrease viral spread via asymptomatic carriers of SARS-CoV-2. With such safeguards in place, infection rates, death rates, and the number of patients requiring intensive care are predicted to decrease [40, 41, 57]. Social distancing, a time-tested method adopted following the end of World War I during an influenza pandemic a century ago, is now being used again during COVID-19 pandemic [29].

3.2.6 Personal protective equipment

SARS-CoV-2 has infected both care givers and patients in hospitals all around the globe due to the rapid dissemination of the virus by symptomatic or asymptomatic carriers. With current research pointing to human-to-human transmission of the virus via respiratory droplets, close contact and a number of precautions have been practiced to arrest the spread of infections. As health care personnel are becoming more exposed to the virus, they must properly adhere with the clinical protocols and wear PPE [71].

Maintaining a safe distance (minimum 1 m) from others, not touching mouth, nose, or eyes, washing hands often or using an alcohol-based liquid to clean hands, and use of mask to cover one's nose and mouth when coughing or sneezing or are all examples of personal hygiene precautions. Despite the fact that the US Centers for Disease Control and Prevention has advised the public to use nonmedical masks to escape transmission of infection which was declared ineffective by the WHO on April 6, 2020, and declared [72].

3.2.7 Testing and contact tracing

As SARS-CoV-2 spreads by respiratory droplets and close contact, many countries have used "contact tracing" in conjunction with testing to combat the disease's spread. The WHO has released laboratory testing recommendations for SARS-CoV-2, which includes instructions on how to collect, package, and ship specimens effectively. It also includes instructions for performing real-time reverse transcriptase polymerase chain reaction testing of the collected samples. This test can trace unique virus RNA sequences. The ELISA (enzyme-linked immunosorbent assay) is another non WHO recommended test

[1]. South Korea adopted innovative techniques of testing at drive-through stations for instant tracing and tracking and to break the chain of contamination [42, 56]. Israel has developed a device to be used all the time up to 15 days after his/her arrival from an international tour. Individuals who may have been exposed are tested and encouraged to self-isolate for 14 days (later 7 days) if tested positive. The goal of this technique was to stop the virus from spreading by isolating those who are asymptomatic.

4 Outcome of COVID pandemic

COVID-19 has given birth of many discoveries. Several robots and AI-supported diseases tracing device, sanitizing tunnels came into practice (see figure 3). AditShortage in skilled clinical and paramedical staff has potentiated the crisis of COVID pandemic [25]. But the pandemic-induced crises are not only confined in medical or paramedical field. Pandemic have potentiality to create devastating socioeconomic and economic crises in the affected nations. COVID-19, the global epidemic, has resulted in changing structure of morbidity and mortalities among the global residents as well as financial loss of values [2]. COVID-19 has blocked the social progress by many ways.

The effect is mostly visible in different segment such as

A) Healthcare [48]
  - Improper diagnosis, quarantine, and treatment of affected or suspected individuals
  - Disruption in delivery supply chain of healthcare service of patients with or without health problems other than COVID-19
  - Unexpected overload on clinicians
  - Huge health risk of physician and para-medical professionals [26]
  - Overload on drug manufacturing and chemist shops
  - Necessity of health safety and security

B) Economic [4]
  - Intermittent production of essential goods
  - Disruption of supply chain of FMCG & FMCD goods
  - Slowing down commercial activity
  - Poor market transaction
  - Steep fall in commercial activity that leads to loss of revenue

C) Social [58]
  - Improper or no functioning of different service sector.
  - Cancellation or postponement of tournaments and events
  - Embargo on flexible movement of common people
  - Disruption in religious and cultural celebration
  - Inestimable fear psychosis common people
  - Social distancing between family members and peers

- Prohibition on free movement of people
- Closure of entertainment options such as movie, sports clubs, gymnasiums, and swimming pools.
- Shift of offline education to online mode.

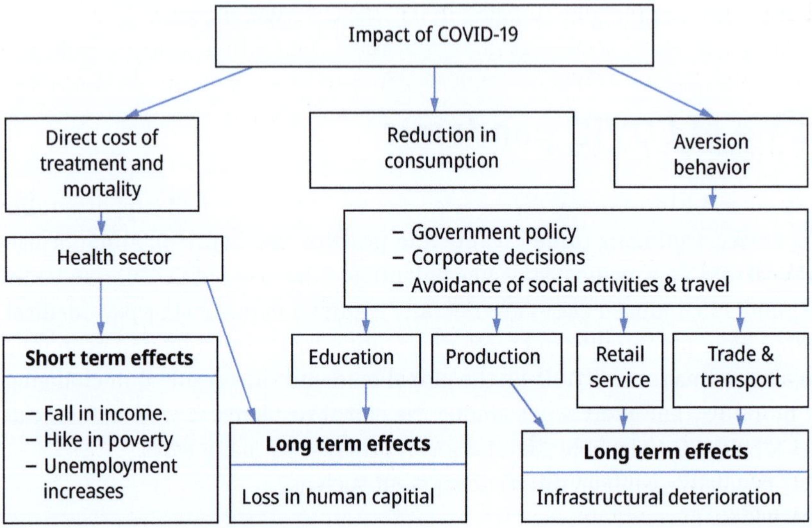

Figure 3: Outcome of COVID-19.

4.1 Health in all policy

Corona has pushed human being in dire straits. Objective and subjective intervention strategies are very much dependent on severity of a pandemic [9]. With the advent of COVID, pulse oximeter, oxygen cylinder, sanitizer, and thermometer were purchased at random out of panic. Naturally, there was a surge in consumption of immune boosters to fight novel coronavirus for building immunity. The concept of "immune boosting" is often used to market nonscientific, partially proven, questionable products, and therapies and thus misled common people. "Immune boosting," buzzword of the world, has turned into a trending topic during the pandemic. Since the outbreak, pharmaceutical corporates are promoting several vitamins and minerals as savior through social media hype to fulfill their commercial interests. This relevance of opting immune-boosting among common people and the mediating role of COVID-19 in influencing such behavior were found to be a by-product of "infodemic." The surge in inorganic growth of sales in immune boosters is the outcome of such behavior to escape COVID-19 infection. Organic immune boosters are going to get better preference for such purchase even in future.

4.2 Physical to digital

Due to escalated probability of infection and perceived threat of physical existence, virtual working pattern became priority. A complete shift of consumer preference from offline to online may not be feasible option across every sphere of our life. A new digital era is converging which is objectively focused. But, online is going to be a parallel alternative in many sectors such as education, purchase of daily convenience goods, and banking. During COVID-19 pandemic-induced lockdown, pupils developed post-traumatic stress disorder [3]. Telemedicine has expanded the inorganic reach of treatment to remote residents [22]

5 Conclusion

Pandemic creates a volatile, uncertain, complex, and ambiguous situation. The most important question is how to prevent pandemic? We found that initially, bacteria were the dominating root cause of most of the pandemics. But, since the incidence of Avian flu pandemic, it is quite evident that different virus has started ruling and its attack is unpredictable. The virus is almost invincible as it can unexpectedly change its genetic structure and mutate very fast that turns it. We have zero guaranteed option of prevention or treatment option for onslaught of virus [51].

During COVID pandemic, perceived value of individuals has shifted from growth mindset to the principles of self-existence or sustenance. An orbit shift in every sphere of life has been observed due to compulsion. COVID-19 pandemic is bound to generate several changes in perceived value of utility. This is going to influence purchase attitude of consumers. The prime objective was survival rather than growth as an immediate impact of emergence of this viral outbreak. Will it leave a lasting impression among common people ? Long-term existence of such attitude will be a function of subjective degree of fear mongering. Health or healthy lifestyle will be considered as a principle theme in purchasing any utility product by millennial and z generation. Due to fear mongering health is a new term of purchase. Medicine and treatment will subjectively get first preference than any other option. Our society, economy, behavior, and lifestyle all have been changed in this "Hybrid New Normal." From marketing point of view, brand narrations to advertising content will show a new pattern. Pharmaceutical industry will comparatively prosper among all industries. Even a complete shift of manpower to machine power to cope up with the changing situation is signaling the emergence of a new paradigm. AI-supported advanced technologies and more effective ways or smart techniques are needed to combat future pandemics. History has taught us about the attack of diseases oriented dire consequences. But preparation to combat COVID pandemic leaves a food for thought for all of us, that is, are we ready to face the next one?

References

[1] Abbasi, J. The promise and peril of antibody testing for COVID-19. JAMA, 2020, 323(19), 2020. https://doi.org/10.1001/jama.2020.6170.
[2] Allocati, N., Petrucci, A., Di,, Giovanni, P., et al. Bat–man disease transmission: Zoonotic pathogens from wildlife reservoirs to human populations. Cell Death Discovery, 2016, 2, 16048. https://doi.org/10.1038/cddiscovery.2016.48.
[3] Alkhamees, A. A., Aljohani, S. M. The psychological impact of COVID-19 pandemic on the students of Saudi Arabia. The Open Public Health Journal, 2021, 14, 12–23. https://doi.org/10.2174/1874944502114010012.
[4] Alon, I., Li, S. COVID-19 response: Democracies v authoritarians. The American Spectator, 27 March, 2020. https://spectator.org/covid-19-response-democracies-v-authoritarians/.
[5] Arabi, Y. M., Balkhy, H. H., Hayden, F. G., Bouchama, A., Luke, T., et al. Middle east respiratory syndrome. New England Journal of Medicine, 2017, 376(6), 584–594.
[6] Backer, J. A., Klinkenberg, D., Wallinga, J. Incubation period of 2019 novel Coronavirus (2019-nCoV) infections among travelers from Wuhan, China. Euro Surveillance, 2020, 25(5), 1–6.
[7] Bean, J. M. W. The black death: The crisis and its social and economic consequences. In: Williman, D. (eds.) The Black Death: The Impact of the Fourteenth-century Plague; Papers of the Eleventh Annual Conference of the Center for Medieval & Early Renaissance Studies. Binghamton, NY: Center for Medieval & Early Renaissance Studies, 1982, 23–38.
[8] Bollet, A. J. Plagues and Poxes. New York: Demos, 1987.
[9] Brauer, F. The final size of a serious epidemic. Bulletin of Mathematical Biology, 2019, 81(3), 869–877.
[10] Brooke, J. A., Global Antiquity, 500 BC–AD 542. In: In climate change and the course of global history: A rough journey (Studies in Environment and History). Cambridge: Cambridge University Press, 2014, 317–349. https://doi.org/10.1017/CBO9781139050814.011.
[11] Chisholm, H. Cholera. Encyclopedia Britannica, 1911, 11(6), 265–266.
[12] Coccia, M. How do low wind speeds and high levels of air pollution support the spread of COVID-19? Atmospheric Pollution Research, 2021, 12(1), 437–445.
[13] Coccia, M. An index to quantify environmental risk of exposure to future epidemics of the COVID-19 and similar viral agents: Theory and practice. Environmental Research, 2020, 191, 110155. https://doi.org/10.1016/j.envres.2020.110155.
[14] Coccia, M. How (un) sustainable environments are related to the diffusion of covid-19: The relation between Coronavirus disease 2019, air pollution, wind resource and energy. Sustainability, 2020, 12 (22), 9709.
[15] Das, D., et al. Personal protective equipment for COVID-19: A comprehensive review. In: Garg, L., Chakraborty, C., Mahmoudi, S., Sohmen, V. S. (eds.) Healthcare Informatics for Fighting COVID-19 and Future Epidemics. Cham: EAI/Springer Innovations in Communication and Computing. Springer, 2022. https://doi.org/10.1007/978-3-030-72752-9_7.
[16] Dawood, F. S., Iuliano, A. D., Reed, C., Meltzer, M. I., Shay, D. K., et al. Estimated global mortality associated with the first 12 months of 2009 pandemic influenza a h1n1 virus circulation: A modelling study. The Lancet Infectious Diseases, 2012. 12(9), 687–695.
[17] DeWitte, S. N. Mortality risk and survival in the aftermath of the medieval black death. PLoS ONE, 2014. 9(5), e96513. https://doi.org/10.1371/journal.pone.0096513.
[18] Diamond, J. Guns, Germs, and Steel: The Fates of Human Societies. New York: Norton, 2009.
[19] Dixon, S., McDonald, S., Roberts, J. AIDS and economic growth in Africa: A panel data analysis. Journal of International Development, 2001, 13(4), 411–426.

[20] Dobson, A. P., Carper, E. R. Infectious diseases and human population history: Throughout history the establishment of disease has been a side effect of the growth of civilization. Bioscience, 1996, 46, 115–126.
[21] Domingo, J. L., Marquès, M., Rovira, J. Influence of airborne transmission of SARS-CoV-2 on COVID-19 pandemic: A review. Environmental Research, 2020, 188, 109861.
[22] El-Sayed, A., Kamel, M. Climatic changes and their role in emergence and re-emergence of diseases. Journal Environmental Sciences and Pollution Research, 2020, 27, 22336–22352. https://doi.org/10.1007/s11356-020-08896-w.
[23] Fears, J. R. The plague under marcus aurelius and the decline and fall of the roman empire. Infectious Disease Clinics of North America, 2004, 20, 65–77.
[24] Frieden, N. M. The russian cholera epidemic, 1892–93, and medical professionalization. Journal of Social History, 1977, 10(4), 538.
[25] Gangopadhyay, S., Ukil, A. Being resilient to deal with attrition of nurses in private COVID-19 hospitals: critical analysis with respect to the crisis in Kolkata, India. In: Garg, L., Chakraborty, C., Mahmoudi, S., Sohmen, V. S. (eds) Healthcare Informatics for Fighting COVID-19 and Future Epidemics. Cham: EAI/Springer Innovations in Communication and Computing. Springer, 2022, 353–363. https://doi.org/10.1007/978-3-030-72752-9_18.
[26] Gangopadhyay, S., Ukil, A., Chatterjee, S. Emerging paradigm of smart healthcare in the management of COVID-19 pandemic and future health crisis". In: Chakraborty, C., Khosravi, M. R. (eds.) Intelligent Healthcare. Singapore: Springer, 2022, 455–478. https://doi.org/10.1007/978-981-16-8150-9_20.
[27] Gangopadhyay, S., Chakraborty, S. A model of strategic communication for clinical premises based on perceived risk of NCDs: A study of Kolkata, India. International Journal of Business Innovation and Research 25(3), 353–364, 2022.
[28] Grennan, D. What is a pandemic? JAMA, 2019, 321, 910.
[29] Hatchett, R. J., Mecher, C. E., Lipsitch, M. Public health interventions and epidemic intensity during the 1918 influenza pandemic. Proceedings of the National Academy of Sciences of the United States of America, 2007, 104(18), 7582–7587.
[30] He, D., Dushoff, J., Day, T., Ma, J., Earn, D. J. Mechanistic modelling of the three waves of the 1918 influenza pandemic. Theoretical Ecology, 2011, 4(2), 283–288.
[31] Huang, C., Wang, Y., Li, X., Ren, L., Zhao, J., Hu, Y. Clinical features of patients infected with 2019 novel Coronavirus in Wuhan, China. Lancet, 2020 395, 497–506.
[32] Irwin, F., Smallpox in Japan. Public Health Reports, 1910, XXV(35), 1205–1208.
[33] Jain, S., Kamimoto, L., Bramley, A. M., Schmitz, A. M., Benoit, S. R., et al. Hospitalized patients with 2009 H1N1 influenza in the United States, April–June 2015. New England Journal of Medicine, 1935–44, 361(20), 2009.
[34] Jin, Y. H., Cai, L., Cheng, Z. S., et al. A rapid advice guideline for the diagnosis and treatment of 2019 novel Coronavirus (2019-nCoV) infected pneumonia (standard version)". Military Medical Research, 2020, 7(1), 4.
[35] Jonas, O. B. Pandemic risk. In: Background Paper for World Development Report 2014: Risk and Opportunity. Washington, DC: Managing Risk for Development, World Bank, 2013.
[36] Jones, D. S. The persistence of american indian health disparities. American Journal of Public Health, 2006, 96(12), 2122–2134.
[37] Johnson, N. P., Mueller, A. S. J. Updating the accounts: Global mortality of the 1918–1920 'Spanish' influenza pandemic. Bulletin of the History of Medicine, 2002, 76(1), 105–115.
[38] Kavet, J. A perspective on the significance of pandemic influenza. American Journal of Public Health, 1977, 67(11), 1063–1070.
[39] Keogh-Brown, M. R., Smith, R. D. The economic impact of SARS: How does the reality match the predictions? Health Policy, 2008, 88(1), 110–120.

[40] Kim, Y. W., Yoon, S. J., Oh, I. H. The economic burden of the 2009 pandemic H1N1 influenza in Korea. Scandinavian Journal of Infectious Diseases, 2013, 45(5), 390–396.
[41] Koo, J. R., Cook, A. R., Park, M., et al. Interventions to mitigate early spread of SARS-CoV-2 in Singapore: A modelling study. Lancet Infectious Diseases, 2020, 20(6), 678–688.
[42] Kucharski, A. J., Russell, T. W., Diamond, C., et al. Early dynamics of transmission and control of COVID-19: A mathematical modelling study. Lancet Infectious Diseases, 2020, 20(5), 553–558.
[43] Lee, V. J., Chiew, C. J., Khong, W. X. Interrupting transmission of COVID-19: Lessons from containment efforts in Singapore. Journal of Travel Medicine, 2020, 27(3), taaa039.
[44] Liu, W., Morse, J. S., Lalonde, T., Xu, S. Learning from the past: Possible urgent prevention and treatment options for severe acute respiratory infections caused by 2019-nCoV. Chemistry and Biochemistry, 2020.
[45] Lu, H. Drug treatment options for the 2019-new Coronavirus (2019-nCoV). Biosci Trends. (2020). https://doi.org/10.5582/bst.2020.01020.
[46] McKibbin, W. J., Sidorenko, A. A. Global Macroeconomic Consequences of Pandemic Influenza. Sydney, Australia: Analysis, Lowy Institute for International Policy, 2006.
[47] Mathews, J. D., Chesson, J. M., McCaw, J. M., McVernon, J. Understanding influenza transmission, immunity, and pandemic threats. Influenza and Other Respiratory Viruses, 2009, 3(4), 143–149.
[48] Neogi, S. B., Preetha, S. G. Assessing health systems' responsiveness in tackling COVID-19 pandemic. Indian Journal of Public Health, 2020, 64(6), 211–216.
[49] Núñez-Delgado, A. SARS-CoV-2 in soils. Environmental Research, 2020, 190, 110045.
[50] Park, J., Kim, J. Hong Kong sets 'Serious' response to South Korea's MERS outbreak. Reuters, 2015.
[51] Patel, V., Chisholm, D., Dua, T., Laxminarayan, R., Medina-Mora, M. E. (eds): Mental, neurological, and substance use disorders. In: Disease Control Priorities. 3rd edition. Vol. 4, Washington, DC: World Bank, 2015. https://doi.org/10.1596/978-1-4648-0426-7.
[52] Phan, L. T., Nguyen, T. V., Luong, Q. C., Nguyen, T. V., Nguyen, H. T., Le, H. Q. Importation and human-to-human transmission of a novel Coronavirus in Vietnam. The New England Journal of Medicine, 2020, 382(9), 872–874. https://doi.org/10.1056/NEJMc2001272.
[53] Platt, C. King Death: The Black Death and Its Aftermath in Late-Medieval England. Oxon U.K: Routledge, 2014.
[54] Riou, J., Althaus, C. L. Pattern of early human-to-human transmission of Wuhan 2019 novel Coronavirus (2019-nCoV), December 2019 to January 2020. Euro Surveillance: Bulletin Europeensur Les Maladies Transmissibles = European Communicable Disease Bulletin, 2020, 25(4), 2000058. https://doi.org/10.2807/1560-7917.ES.2020.25.4.2000058.
[55] Rolain, J. M., Colson, P., Raoult, D. Recycling of chloroquine and its hydroxyl analogue to face bacterial, fungal and viral infections in the 21st century. The International Journal of Antimicrobial Agents, 2007, 30, 297–308, 2007. https://doi.org/10.1016/j.ijantimicag.2007.05.015.
[56] Salathe, M., Althaus, C. L., Neher, R., et al. COVID-19 epidemic in Switzerland: On the importance of testing, contact tracing and isolation. The Swiss Medical Weekly, 2020, 150, w20225. 2020.
[57] Shim, E., Tariq, A., Choi, W., et al. Transmission potential and severity of COVID-19 in South Korea. International Journal of Infectious Diseases, 2020, 93, 339–344.
[58] Singh, M. K., Neog, Y. Contagion effect of COVID-19 outbreak: Another recipe for disaster on Indian economy. Journal of Public Affairs, 2020, 20, e2171. https://doi.org/10.1002/pa.2171.
[59] Smith, B. F. Smallpox in Japan. Public Health Reports (1896–1970), 1995, 25(35), 1205–1208.
[60] Smith, B. F. The Russian influenza in the United Kingdom. Social History of Medicine, 1995, 8(1), 55–73. https://doi.org/10.1093/shm/8.1.55.
[61] UNDP (United Nations Development Programme): A Socio-Economic Impact Assessment of the Zika Virus in Latin America and the Caribbean: With a Focus on Brazil, Colombia, and Suriname. Synthesis report, UNDP, New York. 2017.

[62] Viboud, C., Simonsen, L., Fuentes, R., Flores, J., Miller, M. A., et al. Global mortality impact of the 1957–1959 influenza pandemic. Journal of Infectious Diseases, 2016, 212(11), 738–745.
[63] Wang, M. D., Jolly, A. M. Changing virulence of the sars virus: The epidemiological evidence. Bulletin of the World Health Organization, 2004, 82(7), 547–548.
[64] Wang, C., Horby, P. W., Hayden, F. G., Gao, G. F. A novel Coronavirus outbreak of global health concern. Lancet, 2020.
[65] Wang, M., Cao, R., Zhang, L., Yang, X., Liu, J., Xu, M. Remdesivir and chloroquine effectively inhibit the recently emerged novel Coronavirus (2019-nCoV) in vitro. Cell Research, 2020, 30(3), 269–271. https://doi.org/10.1038/s41422-020-0282-0.
[66] White, R. J., Razgour, O. Emerging zoonotic diseases originating in mammals: A systematic review of effects of anthropogenic land-use change. Mammal Review, 2020, 12201. https://doi.org/10.1111/mam.12201.
[67] Wölfel, R., Corman, V. M., Guggemos, W., Seilmaier, M., Zange, S., Müller, M. A., Niemeyer, D., Jones, T. C., Vollmar, P., Rothe, C., Hoelscher, M. Virological assessment of hospitalized patients with COVID-2019. Nature, 2020.
[68] Zou, L., Ruan, F., Huang, M., Liang, L., Huang, H., Hong, Z., Guo, Q. SARSCoV-2 viral load in upper respiratory specimens of infected patients. New England Journal of Medicine, 2020, 382(12), 1177–1179.
[69] WHO. Ebola situation report. Weekly data report, April 15. 2016.
[70] WHO. Situation report: Zika virus, microcephaly, guillain-barré syndrome. Weekly data report, February 2. 2017.
[71] WHO. Rational use of personal protective equipment for Coronavirus disease (COVID-19) and considerations during severe shortages, 2020. https://apps.who.int/iris/bitstream/handle/10665/331695/WHO-2019-nCov-IPC_PPE_use-2020.3-eng.pdf.
[72] WHO. Advice on the use of masks in the context of COVID-19, 2020. www.who.int/publications-detail/advice-on-the-use-of-masks-in-the-community-during-home-care-and-in-healthcare-settings-in-the-context-of-the-novel-Coronavirus-(2019-ncov)-utbreak\.
[73] World Health Organization. Clinical Management of Severe Acute Respiratory Infection When Novel Coronavirus (2019-nCoV) Infection Is Suspected: Interim Guidance. 2020.
[74] www.weforum.org/agenda/2020/03/a-visual-history-of-pandemics.
[75] www.Coronavirus.gov.hk/eng/index.html.
[76] www.euro.who.int/en/media-centre/sections/statements/2022/statement-risk-remainshigh-in-eastern-europe-and-central-asia-with-arrival-of-covid-19-omicron-variant.
[77] www.moh.gov.sg/covid-19.
[78] www.ncbi.nlm.nih.gov/books/NBK525302/table/pt5.ch17.sec3.table1/.
[79] https://covid19.trackvaccines.org/types-of-vaccines/.
[80] www.euro.who.int/en/media-centre/sections/statements/2022/statement-risk-remains-high-in-eastern-europe-and-central-asia-with-arrival-of-covid-19-omicron-variant.
[81] www.who.int/teams/health-product-policy-and-standards/assistive-and-medical-technology/medical-devices/ppe/ppe-covid.
[82] https://covid19.who.int/.
[83] www.gov.uk/government/publications/long-term-evolution-of-sars-cov-2-26-july-2021/long-term-evolution-of-sars-cov-2-26-july–2021.
[84] www.healio.com/news/infectious-disease/20210219/qa-after-covid19-what-is-the-next-threat.
[85] www.unaids.org/en/resources/fact-sheet.
[86] World Health Organization Best Practices for the Naming of New Human Infectious Diseases (PDF) (Report). World Health Organization (WHO). May 2015. hdl:10665/163636.
[87] Scientific brief: SARS-CoV-2 and potential airborne transmission. COVID-19 Published Science and Research.U.S. Centers for Disease Control and Prevention (CDC). 11 February 2020.

[88] Centers for Disease Control and Prevention. 5 April 2020. What to do if you are sick. U.S. Centers for Disease Control and Prevention (CDC).Archived from the original on 14 February 2020.

[89] Coronavirus Disease 2019 (COVID-19) – prevention & treatment. U.S. Centers for Disease Control and Prevention (CDC). 10 March 2020. Archived from the original on 11 March (2020).

[90] WHO-China Joint Mission, Report of the WHO-China Joint Mission on Coronavirus Disease 2019 (COVID-19), 2020. https://www.who.int/docs/default-source/coronaviruse/who-china-joint-mission-on-covid-19-final-report.pdf.

[91] World Health Organization, Coronavirus disease 2019 (COVID-19) Situation Report – 47, 2020. https://www.who.int/docs/default-source/coronaviruse/situation-reports/20200307-sitrep-47-covid-19.pdf?sfvrsn=27c364a4_2.

Parijat Roy, Arindam Mitra*

A review on AI-based medical image analysis for reliable and rapid diagnosis of SARS-CoV-2

Abstract: AI, or artificial intelligence, is precise simulation of human intelligence by machines. AI and computer-aided diagnosis are routinely used in medical imaging. In the context of the COVID-19 pandemic, early and accurate diagnosis of COVID-19 cases reduce the spread and mortality caused by SARS-CoV-2, the causative agent of COVID-19. AI has been used to improve the precise detection of COVID-19 cases. The gold standard for the detection of SARS-CoV-2 is by reverse transcription polymerase chain reaction (RT-PCR). However, RT-PCR is a time-consuming process that can give false-negative results and requires skillful laboratory technicians, which may not be possible in some resource-constrained regions. Contrastingly, AI-based screening and detection of specific changes in X-ray and CT scan images of suspected COVID-19 patients can offer a cost-effective, speedy, and accurate diagnosis of clinical cases. Convolutional neural network (CNN), a deep learning algorithm, can improve the accuracy and reliability of diagnosis of COVID-19 from chest X-rays. An enormous amount of training data is required to make accurate predictions of clinical cases via CNN. Several pretrained models such as GoogLeNet, AlexNet, VGG, and open databases such as GitHub can help the training of deep learning networks. This chapter will provide an overview of AI, machine learning, and deep learning-based strategies to improve the specificity, sensitivity, and accuracy for diagnosing SARS-CoV-2.

1 Introduction

The worldwide crisis caused by SARS-CoV-2 has resulted in more than 5.5 million deaths and infected around 355 million individuals as of January 24, 2022. Sometimes the daily affected count rose to 300,000 at some places. These threatening numbers demand prompt medical assistance and infrastructure. Improving early screening and diagnosis of the disease are critical steps in assisting professionals related to the healthcare department to save lives during this pandemic. These data might not be

Acknowledgment: PR would like to thank his parents for their unwavering support.

***Corresponding author: Arindam Mitra,** Department of Biological Sciences, School of Life Science and Biotechnology, Adamas University, Kolkata, West Bengal, India,
e-mail: arindam.mitra@adamasuniversity.ac.in, ORCID ID – 0000-0002-1591-6164
Parijat Roy, Department of Biological Sciences, School of Life Science and Biotechnology, Adamas University, Kolkata, West Bengal, India

https://doi.org/10.1515/9783110767681-002

accurate as many cases remain unreported with more death tolls. The healthcare professional should be given the adequate infrastructure to detect the presence of the virus rapidly. The gold standard to detect the presence of SARS-CoV-2 uses the reverse transcription polymerase chain reaction (RT-PCR) of swab samples from patients. However, a limitation of this method is frequent false-negative cases when the virus concentration is not high enough in some individuals. One approach involves the use of artificial intelligence (AI) in the interpretation of chest X-rays and CT scans of patients to improve the accuracy of diagnosis in a time-efficient manner. A critical aspect of imaging techniques involves the processing of data. AI techniques that employ various deep learning methods have proved to be remarkably successful in medical imaging as deep learning has the capability of advanced feature extraction. Advanced neural networks classify individuals based on their respiratory patterns [1]. AI enables machines to become efficient, understand queries, process, link large data sets, and draw meaningful conclusions. Automated diagnostic approaches are being developed based on these applications, enhancing the accuracy and speed of diagnosis. It will assist in early notification of diagnosis to the frontline healthcare workers, and they can determine the severity of the condition in the patients and initiate appropriate treatments.

2 Review of literature

From the detailed research going on COVID-19 and ways to detect, tackle, and stop the spread of virus, it is evident that AI plays a very important role. Scientists worldwide have acknowledged this method and has presented their findings in different journals. Some recent findings in this field are (I) Qi et al. [3] proposed a machine learning-based CT radiomics model to predict the time required for a patient to stay in hospital with pneumonia associated with SARS-CoV-2 infections; (II) Gozes et al. [4] developed a U-Net model for detecting anomalies in lung CT images; (III) Jin et al. [5] created an AI method to diagnose COVID-19 more quickly. This approach uses a two-step process to screen COVID-19 patients based on CT image segmentation of lung lesions [5]. Arun et al. [6] proposed a new type of COVID-19 lung infection segmentation deep network named Inf-Net. It can automatically identify the infected area from chest CT [6]. Ma et al. [7] implemented a model for COVID-19 detection that detects and determines its severity. The model is popularly known as the random forest model [7]. Wang et al. [8] using a two-step transfer learning strategy designed a fully automatic deep learning system using raw CT images for COVID-19 diagnostic and prognostic analysis. Li et al. [9] proposed a 3D DL system for diagnosing COVID-19 named COV-Net based on lung CT scans using ResNet50. Ghosal and Tucker [10] developed a DL approach based on Bayesian convolutional neural networks (BCNN) to assess the uncertainty in DL solutions in order to enhance the COVID-19 diagnosis from the chest X-ray database. Gaal et al. [64] proposed a model for the segmentation of the lung images which will extract features related to pneumonia. The model was known as Attention-U-Net. He et al. [70] proposed a framework for joint assessment of severity of the infection and also segment the lung lobes. Ni et al. [65] proposed a deep learning model, convolutional MVPNet, and 3D U-Net for the detection of infection from CT scans. The results were sensitivity: for detecting patient sensitivity: 100%; for per-lung lobe lesion: 0.96%; AUC was around 87% and 88%. Panwar et al. [66] used VGG-16 as a DL model and designed a framework for faster detection of infection. He achieved a sensitivity of 97.62%, specificity of 78.57%, and an accuracy of 88.10%. Based on XGBoost classifier, Burdick et al. [67] proposed a model for the prediction of requirement of ventilator in COVID-19-affected patients [68]. Toraman et al. [82] used an ML model, CapsNet to identify COVID-19 infections from chest X-ray. He achieved an accuracy of 89%, sensitivity of 84%, and specificity of 92%. For screening of COVID-19 pneumonia from other types of pneumonia, Murphy et al. [71] designed a model, CAD4COVIDX-RAY, and achieved an AUC score of 0.81 and specificity of about 85%. Song et al. used a model BigBGAN for differential diagnosis of COVID-19 pneumonia from other types of pneumonia from chest CT images. After external validation 0.85 AUC was achieved. Shuai et al. used inception transfer learning model to predict COVID-19 cases from chest CT images. They managed to get an accuracy of 89% and a specificity of 88% [72]. Deshpande et al. [73] gave a research overview for screening, diagnosing, monitoring, and spreading the awareness about the pandemic by the use of human radio signals with the help of AI. Fong et al. [74] used polynomial neural network with corrective feedback to forecast the spreading of the pandemic with a very low error rate.

Combining chest imaging and AI will facilitate fast and accurate disease diagnosis and identify patients with various other complications with severe outcomes. However, there are limitations to using these techniques including the expensive use of CT scans and the immobility of these machines, significantly restricting it to some clinical and diagnostic settings. Apart from some hardware and economic limitations, there are many software limitations. Many ML models used for study may not be ready for clinical use [11]. The lack of data in some studies is another bottleneck to rely on these systems entirely. In a nutshell, we can say that AI is beneficial if correct data, good infrastructure, and skilled professionals are available.

3 Deep learning approaches for COVID-19 detection

We have seen how much AI is helpful in the detection of COVID-19. But there are some challenges to the ways by which it is used. Patients with COVID-19 often show some irregularities in their chest X-ray or their CT scans, and many lung diseases show identical results as COVID-19. For this reason, and faster and more accurate results, some new approaches have been devised that work on deep learning and machine learning [12]. The most common DL algorithms used for COVID-19 detection are convolutional neural network (CNN), deep neural network (DNN), recurrent neural network (RNN), graph neural network (GNN), and vision transformers. A DL mechanism used for classifying COVID-19 patients is DenseNET201 [13]. DL is the current flag-bearing program of AI. However, this DL requires many datasets and accurate and fast computing sources. There is always a scarcity of reliable datasets as the pandemic is ongoing, and the data may change as the virus mutates and gives new symptoms. Deep transfer learning (DTL) can be employed in this situation as it learns from one task and can implement and work on another job [14].

3.1 Convolutional neural network

A CNN is a DL algorithm that takes the input of images, processes it, finds learnable features, and differentiates one image from the other [15]. A CNN has many levels like convolutionary, nonlinear, pooling, and completely linked levels. CNNs are regularized versions of completely connected networks, where all the neurons in one layer are connected to the other in the next layer. They are named because they use a mathematical operation "convolution" in place of general matrix multiplication in at least one of its layers [16] (see figure 1).

Convolutional layers, the building blocks of CNN, combine the inputs received and process the inputs received and processed them to form a new input and then pass the result to the subsequent layers. Each convolutional neuron processes information just for its receptive field. Convolutional networks sometimes include "local pooling" or "global pooling" simultaneously with the traditional pooling layers. Pooling layers are used to lessen data sizes by combining all the received outputs at one layer into a single neuron in the next upcoming layer. There are two types of pooling that are generally used: max and average. Max pooling is used by the maximum value of each local cluster in a feature map, and average pooling uses the average value in the feature map [17, 18].

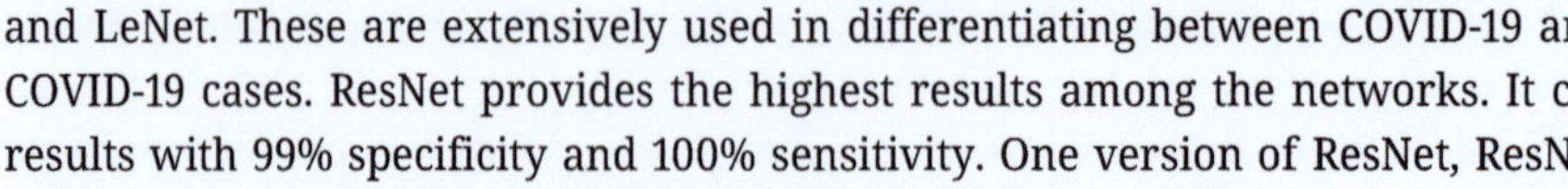

Figure 1: Basic work structure of convolutional neural network.

There are various architectures of CNN available, namely AlexNet, GooGleNet, ResNet, and LeNet. These are extensively used in differentiating between COVID-19 and non-COVID-19 cases. ResNet provides the highest results among the networks. It can give results with 99% specificity and 100% sensitivity. One version of ResNet, ResNet101 is being confirmed and concluded by the radiologist that it can be used as an instrument in radiology departments as a high sensitivity model for the detection of COVID-19 in patients. A group of scientists aiming to segment the anomalies in COVID-19 chest CT images proposed anamorphic depth embedding-based lightweight CNN, called Anam-Net [19]. The results from the chest CT scans showed that the model could give good Dice similarity scores for abnormal and normal regions in the lung. This model was also deployed on embedded systems to determine how suitable the method is for point of care platforms. For classification, deep feature extraction is done, for that pretrained deep CNN models are used like ResNet50, ResNet101, and VGG19. The accuracy of the ResNet50 came around 92.6% [20].

An automated system for disease identification has been developed to assist various health professionals and physicians diagnose COVID-19, which also showed a decrease in mortality risks. They automatically put LSTM and CNN models to diagnose COVID-19 from the chest X-ray images. CNN and LSTM both had a huge work, CNN extracted deep functions, and LSTM was employed in identifying extracted elements. The proposed method was successful as the results showed very high accuracy, specificity, and sensitivity. It also showed 98.9% F1 score [21].

3.2 Deep neural network

An artificial neural network is an algorithm designed to emulate the learning approach used by professionals to gain certain types of knowledge. The advanced version of the conventional artificial neural network is the deep neural network.

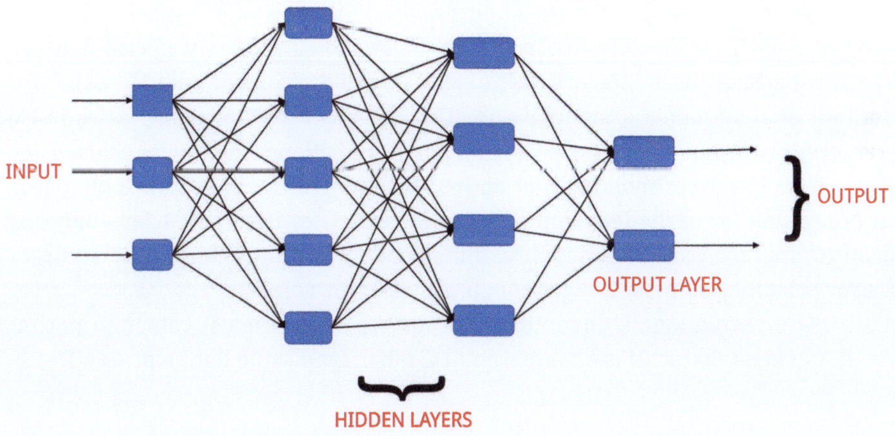

Figure 2: Typical architecture of deep neural network.

Wherever an item is expressed as a layered collection of primitives, DNN architectures build integrated models [22]. The extra levels alter the makeup of options from the lower layers [23].

DNNs are a type of feedforward network in which data travels from the input to the output layer without being processed again (see figure 2). The DNN starts by creating a map of virtual neurons and assigning random integer values, or "weights," to the connections between them. If the network fails to recognize a certain pattern accurately, the weights associated with the inputs grow and result in an output between zero and one. The weights would be changed by the Associate in Nursing algorithmic program [24]. That is, the algorithmic software will check for new factors until it identifies the appropriate mathematical transformation to process the data.

The scale (number of layers and range of units per layer), learning rate, and initial weights should all be considered when training DNNs. Because of the cost in time and machine resources, sweeping through the parameter area for optimal parameters may not be possible. Many techniques, such as batching (directly computing the gradient on a large number of coaching samples rather than individual examples) [25], can help speed up calculation. Because of the suitability of such process designs for matrix and vector computations, large process capabilities of many-core architectures (such as GPUs or the Intel Xeon Phi) have resulted in significant training speedups [26].

3.3 Recurrent neural network

A recurrent neural network (RNN) is a type of artificial neural network which is used for solving ordinal or temporal problems like language translation and speech recognition. They are distinguished from other neural networks as they use the previous inputs to influence the current inputs [27–30]. There are four types of RNN generally used: (a) one to one; (b) one to many; (c) many to one; and (d) many to many. Apart from these three types of RNN architecture are in use: (a) bidirectional recurrent neural network (BRNN); (b) long-short-term memory (LSTM); and (c) gated recurrent units (GRUs).

Indrajit et al. designed a model named COVID-Deep Predictor, which uses LSTM as a recurrent neural network for performing the predictions. The model achieves an accuracy of 99.51% [68]. Abdelfatah et al. [69] highlighted the importance of speech signal processing for early detection of the infection. They used LSTM for analyzing the acoustic characteristic of cough, breathing, and voice. They achieved an accuracy of 98% for breathing sounds, 97% for cough, and 88% for voice.

LSTMs are revolutionary invention and very specific when it comes to performance. It is evident that RNN is an important DL pillar against the fight with COVID-19.

3.4 Graph neural networks

This is an ongoing hot topic among various researchers and academicians. These are used as an inference tools for determining connections between graphs. In computer science, a graph is a data structure containing two components: nodes and edges. They capture the dependence of graph via messages passing through some specific

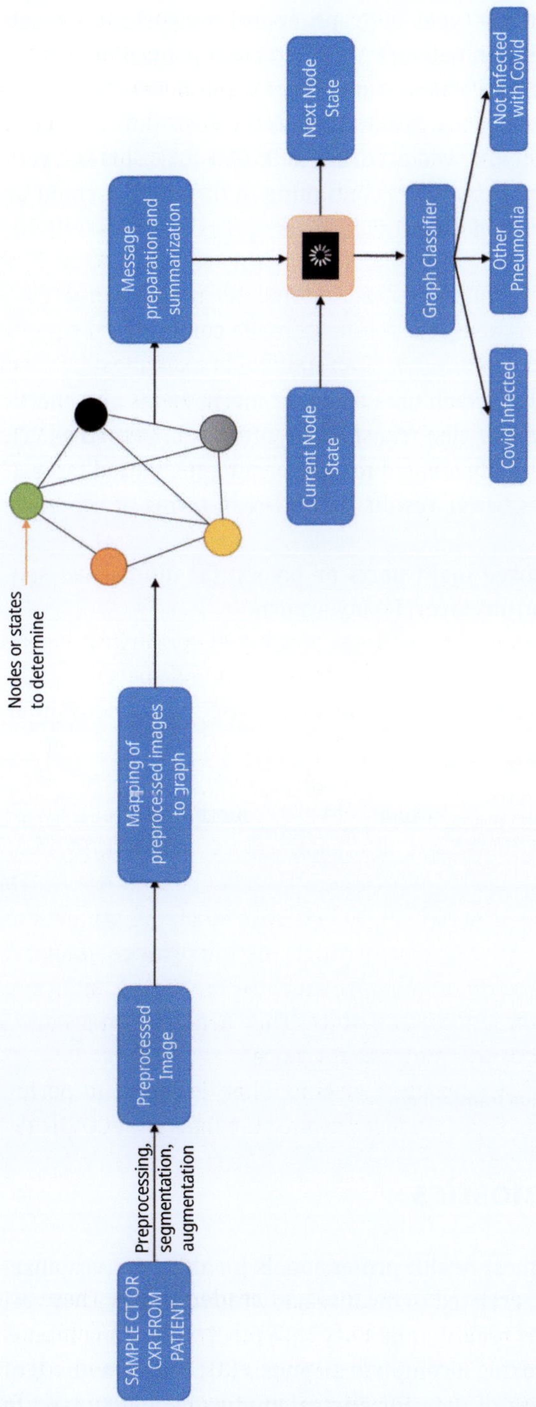

Figure 3: Basic workflow of GNN.

nodes [62] (see figure 3). There are three types of graph neural networks: (a) graph convolutional network; (b) graph attention network; (c) gated graph neural network.

Some GNN models that are used by various researchers include GraphCovidNet and ResGNetC. They achieve remarkably good results such as for ResGNetC, the sensitivity comes at 92.23%, specificity at 99.15%, and accuracy at 95.91% [63]. This is a very promising way to detect COVID-19 and research is continuing in this field. It could be one of the most important replacements of CNN.

3.5 Vision transformers

A transformer is a deep learning model which uses different mechanisms and checks each significant part of the input data. A vision transformer, often abbreviated as ViT, is a model based on transformer originally created for performing text-based tasks. If trained with enough data often gives better results than CNN in terms of accuracy, sensitivity, and specificity.

The transformer encoder has three main parts or layers: (a) multi-head self-attention layer; (b) multilayer perceptrons layer; (c) layer norm.

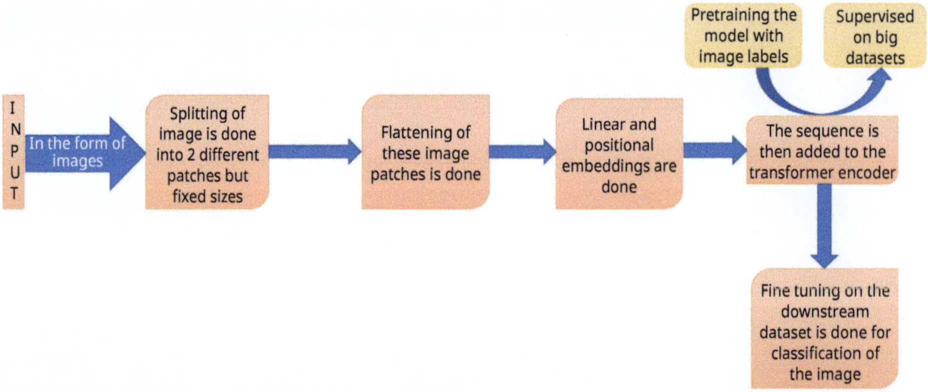

Figure 4: Basic process of detection using vision transformers.

4 AI for COVID-19 diagnostics

The first step of treatment used by most health professionals includes the visualization and study of different parameters related to the disease, which helps in early and easy diagnosis of the disease. I, in this regard, might say that medical imaging is used as the primary data source before making a complete diagnosis [31]. One drawback of the medical imaging is the processing of data for clinical studies. AI has proved to give accurate results in identifying imaging abnormalities.

AI is a technology that involves the use of different algorithms to understand complicated data. Clinical examinations using computer-aided diagnostics have shown great accuracy and sensitivity for the detection of radiographic abnormalities, which when applied in public health sectors prove to improve the disease understanding, course of the disease, and its effects, so in a nutshell we can say that it is a great tool in improving public health standards. The use of AI in medical imaging diagnostics is currently under extensive tests and trials. This also helps to enhance tissue-based detection and classification.

It was the year 2019, the world faced the onset of COVID-19. Soon it was declared a pandemic by the WHO, and unexpectedly the cases kept on rising. The health officials constantly recommended to "break the chain" and to stop the spread, almost every country imposed lockdowns. However, the situation continued to worsen, more and more people got infected and, many cases go unreported. In India, there were consecutive three waves of COVID-19, the second one being the most dangerous, as the death toll was the record high. Based on serosurveys, household data, and official data, it was estimated that almost 4 million people have died in India at the end of the second wave

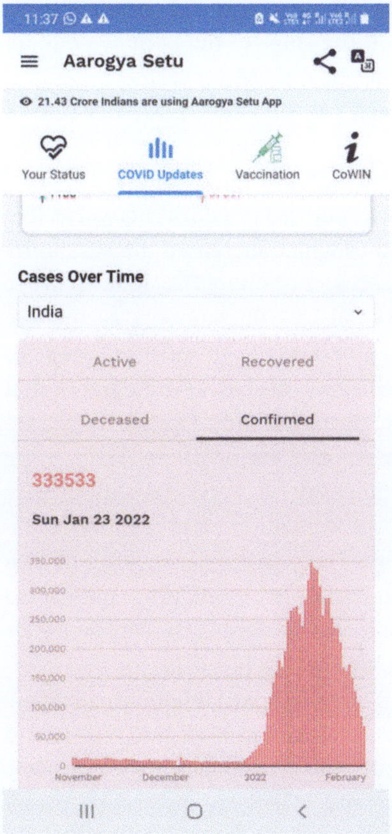

Figure 5: The number of COVID-19 cases per day in India. The number reaches more than 300,000 cases per day where the role of AI along with the medical imaging modalities is justified.

(see figure 5). This extreme data urges the medical health practitioners to outperform. However, they were also helpless because of the shortage of perfect health infrastructure, facilities, and medicines. The disease understanding was also not there as epidemiological data were insufficient, which is very commonplace in an ongoing pandemic. Early detection is essential to treat and stop the spread of diseases like COVID-19. The conventional methods of RT-PCR fail to address the situation. Even though it is economical, but when the number of cases that can be handled exceed the threshold limit these slow procedures does not work. The RT-PCR takes almost 5–6 h for a single sample to be tested. Researchers working on various models for the detection of COVID-19 have presented the use of AI in their literature. They have shown how AI is used to process the data obtained from different radiological tests, specially from chest X-ray and CT scans.

4.1 AI in diagnosis of COVID-19 using chest X-ray

CXR is the most common type of diagnostic imaging method. It may be used in determining the order of treatment for COVID-19. It can be considered an effective, rapid, and low-cost tool used in detecting COVID-19. It can help in identifying different signs of pneumonia. Its sensitivity is highly dependent on the stage of the patient's pulmonary infection, the technical quality of the study, and the disease's severity.

This technique's major problem is the low specificity rate and sensitivity rate of CXR. To address this problem scientists worldwide worked and thought of using AI for easy and risk-free detection of COVID-19. On this account they employed several techniques under AI, they are automated ML algorithms, use of neural networks like CNN and DNN, and deep transfer learning approaches which increased the sensitivity to 97–100%, specificity from 30–40% to 95–98%, precision of up to 97%, and accuracy to 83–97% [32–36]. Accuracy can be further improved by using support vector machines, which works on the principle of dividing the datasets in different steps of training and test subsets. One hundred percent accuracy is also achievable but in that case transfer learning must be used twice [37, 38]. Output neuron keeping is yet another method which is used to increase training speeds and performance [39].

The images obtained from CXR for COVID-19 can easily be correlated with disease severity; thus AI can be used for monitoring the disease evolution and identifying patients with need of critical or intensive care units. The criteria of working of CXR using AI is based on the degree of opacity found in the lungs and its geographical extent over there which gave the severity scores, and the patients risk can be determined on a 4-point scale – normal, mild, moderate, and severe [40, 41].

One of the ways opted for diagnosis of COVID-19 using CXR was lesion visualization. They performed object detection, where the object was a lesion caused by COVID-19 and displayed the affected area of the lung. To easily detect the ground glass opacity region, attention and heat maps were employed in the processing [42]. Some researchers prefer to do the step of segmentation so as to remove the unwanted regions on the image of the lungs. This is done as it increases the efficiency in disease detection. On this account a way of segmentation is using Watershed algorithm, which provides a complete segregation of the essential features or feature regions for diagnosis [43].

With the help of AI, CXR images can also be used as a tool in the differential diagnosis of COVID-19 pneumonia from other types of pneumonia. A group of scientists proposed a model which does the work in three steps, and it was seen that the process helped to reduce the training time and the size of the training sets. They used a feature extractor, feature selector, and an SVM classifier. Using these steps an overall accuracy was found to be coming at about 98% [44]. To achieve the best accuracy the AI models should be perfectly trained; CXR images must be obtained in different body positions, like postero-anterior and latero-lateral, and the processing of these must be differentiated. The AI model must be trained separately for children, adults, and elderly groups and also the CXR processing would have to be done separately.

CXR is the most widespread imaging technique used for diagnosis; however, if the reading of the images from the X-ray is being done by non-certified or a less expert person, chances of getting error increase multiple folds. Even its sensitivity is lower than CT scans. This can lead to false negatives as the images might appear normal in the early phase of the disease when the virus has just entered the body and infection has not started. Many DL methods are used to improve the prediction accuracy. The degree of confidence is a very important factor in a diagnosis, and it is very much essential for the trust of the health professionals. Researchers addressing to this problem proposed a DL model, BCNN (Bayesian convolutional neural network). It works by combining what is known about the response to determine the uncertainty in the diagnosis for the prediction of COVID-19. Bayesian model increased the accuracy of the normal model from 85% to 92% [45].

4.2 AI in diagnosis of COVID-19 using CT scans

The use of AI for diagnosis or for the prognostic study of the infection of COVID-19 on CT images was investigated. Machine learning approaches or models and also DL models, algorithms when applied to CT images, improved the accuracy of diagnosis and predicted the outcomes of the infection. COVID-19 cases can be detected early and managed in a well-classified framework with the help of numerous AI algorithms.

Researchers working worldwide on various algorithms, models, all wanted a faster and accurate diagnosis of COVID-19. Some worked upon sources limited to health professionals and some worked on open-source platforms. One group of scientists worked upon a DenseNet algorithm model for the detection of COVID-19 on high-resolution computed tomography. They confirmed that the model can perform a human level performance and one can get the results of the test within 30 s [46]. Another group of scientists created a cloud-based AI platform which was made in an open access tool. This used a UNet++ model for the detection of COVID-19 [47].

To make COVID-19 evaluation easier, a standardized score called CO-RADS was created. It grades the level of risk of infection or suspicion value in a 5-point scale where 1 means very low and 5 means the patient is at very high risk [48]. A group continued this work and came up with CO-RADS AI which was made for automated assessment of suspicion score. This approach has three steps: first, U-Net is used to segment lesions, then CT severity score is predicted based on the percentage of afflicted tissue per lobe, and finally, the CO-RADS value is assessed. This high-throughput model gave a high-diagnostic performance in detection of COVID-19 [49]. Another researcher developed a method for the diagnosis of COVID-19 and developed a CNN-tailored DNN. This CNN-tailored DNN gave higher AUC of 0.9808 as compared to normal DNN [50]. This has a very important role in the triaging, which help in rapid isolation of infected people and avoiding delayed treatment which would otherwise be of great concern (Table 1).

To avoid subjective, time-consuming, and complex evaluations, multiple AI models are being designed to divide or classify the patients into various severity stages. This also helps in improving the clinical decision process. A group of researchers devised an algorithm to divide patients into three categories: moderate, severe, and extreme. The COVID-19 CHDSET dataset [51] was used to train this method. These models were enough to classify the patient's severity, suppose a patient with a high severity score was admitted to the ICU first. But, if two or more patients have same severity scores and infrastructure is not up to the mark then which patient should get more weightage. To address this a DL-based prognostic model was developed by a group of scientists which predicted the probability of patient's death within 14 days. They designed an advanced CNN model, which they called 3D-CNN De-COVID19-Net, and this gave higher AUC of 0.943 in the identification of severe patient's as compared to normal CNN models. They used this to identify high risk patients that may die within two weeks and hence they can assign ICUs to them before hand as an attempt to save the lives [52].

The differentiation of COVID-19 from other types of pneumonia is critical and very important for early diagnosis and pandemic control. A Chinese study developed a model known as COVNet which is a three-dimensional DL model used for the detection of COVID-19 and to differentiate it from other types of community acquired pneumonia. There was an automatically generated heatmap in the model known as Grad-CAM, which helped in the interpretation of the results. A red color is shown in the suspected regions [53].

These were some areas which is covered in this chapter, apart from these there were numerous other models, hypothesis, algorithms designed by various scientists worldwide. The two imaging modalities X-ray and CT scans are extensively used in the detection, diagnosis, assessment of severity, and in differentiating with other types of pneumonia. However, imaging provides a partial information, and AI does the actual work of combining the data and various clinical manifestations, laboratory results, and data from other learning tools to give the final verdict. AI has proved to be the best helping hand of the physicians, radiologists, and researchers.

Table 1: Different models used for the prediction of COVID-19.

Modality	Model	Accuracy and sensitivity, area under curve (AUC)	References
CXR	CNN-LSTM	Accuracy: 98.5% Sensitivity: 99%	Islam et al. [21]
CXR	CVDNet	Accuracy: 97% Sensitivity: 100%	Ouchicha et al. [36]
CXR	BCNN	Accuracy: 92%	Ghosal and Tucker [10]
CT	DenseNet201	AUC: 0.79–0.97	Chatzitofis et al. [51]
CT	ResNet50	Accuracy: 95%	Gozes et al. [4]
CT	U-Net++	Precision: 95% Sensitivity: 100%	Chen et al. [47]
CT	ML	Accuracy: 87.9% Sensitivity: 90.7%	Shi et al. (2020) [75]
CT	Random Forest	Accuracy: 87.5%	Tang et al. (2020) [76]
CT	CNN	Accuracy: 89.5%	Wang et al. [8]
CT	COVNet	Accuracy: 96% Sensitivity: 90%	Li et al. [9]
CXR and CT	CNN configured DNN	Accuracy: 96.29%	Mukherjee et al. (2020) [81]
CXR	ResNet	AUC: 0.952 Sensitivity: 96%	Zhang et al. (2020) [80]
CXR	CNN	Accuracy: 98.3% Sensitivity: 96.7%	Chowdhury et al. [34]
CXR	ResNet50	Accuracy: 94.4%	Hall et al. (2020) [77]
CXR	EfficientNet	Accuracy: 91.4% Sensitivity: 90%	Luz et al. (2020) [78]
CXR	CNN	Accuracy: 97.97%	Jain et al. (2020) [79]

5 AI-based SARS-CoV-2 detection protocol or working system

This portion of the chapter deals with the processes or the workflow of the models used for the detection of COVID-19 strains. This includes in detail discussion of steps required for a successful detection.

[72] Wang, Shuai, Bo Kang, Jinlu Ma, Xianjun Zeng, Mingming Xiao, Jia Guo, Mengjiao Cai et al. "A deep learning algorithm using CT images to screen for Corona Virus Disease (COVID-19)." European radiology 31 (2021): 6096–6104.

[73] Deshpande, G.; Batliner, A.; Schuller, B.W. AI-Based human audio processing for COVID-19: A comprehensive overview. Pattern Recognit. 2021, 122, 108289.

[74] Fong, Simon James, Gloria Li, Nilanjan Dey, Rubén González Crespo, and Enrique Herrera-Viedma. "Finding an accurate early forecasting model from small dataset: A case of 2019-ncov novel coronavirus outbreak." arXiv preprint arXiv:2003.10776 (2020).

[75] Shi, Feng, Jun Wang, Jun Shi, Ziyan Wu, Qian Wang, Zhenyu Tang, Kelei He, Yinghuan Shi, and Dinggang Shen. "Review of artificial intelligence techniques in imaging data acquisition, segmentation, and diagnosis for COVID-19." IEEE reviews in biomedical engineering 14 (2020): 4–15.

[76] Shi, Feng, Jun Wang, Jun Shi, Ziyan Wu, Qian Wang, Zhenyu Tang, Kelei He, Yinghuan Shi, and Dinggang Shen. "Review of artificial intelligence techniques in imaging data acquisition, segmentation, and diagnosis for COVID-19." IEEE reviews in biomedical engineering 14 (2020): 4–15.

[77] Hall, Lawrence O., Rahul Paul, Dmitry B. Goldgof, and Gregory M. Goldgof. "Finding covid-19 from chest x-rays using deep learning on a small dataset." arXiv preprint arXiv:2004.02060 (2020).

[78] Luz, Eduardo, Pedro Lopes Silva, Rodrigo Silva, and Gladston Moreira. "Towards an efficient deep learning model for covid-19 patterns detection in x-ray images." arXiv preprint arXiv:2004.05717 710 (2020).

[79] Jain, Rachna, Meenu Gupta, Soham Taneja, and D. Jude Hemanth. "Deep learning based detection and analysis of COVID-19 on chest X-ray images." Applied Intelligence 51 (2021): 1690–1700.

[80] Zhang, Jianpeng, Yutong Xie, Yi Li, Chunhua Shen, and Yong Xia. "Covid-19 screening on chest x-ray images using deep learning based anomaly detection." arXiv preprint arXiv:2003.12338 27 (2020): 141.

[81] Mukherjee, Himadri, Subhankar Ghosh, Ankita Dhar, Sk Md Obaidullah, K. C. Santosh, and Kaushik Roy. "Deep neural network to detect COVID-19: one architecture for both CT Scans and Chest X-rays." Applied Intelligence 51 (2021): 2777–2789.

[82] Toraman S, Alakus TB, Turkoglu I. Convolutional capsnet: a novel artificial neural network approach to detect COVID-19 disease from X-ray images using capsule networks. Chaos, Solitons Fractals. 2020;140:110122

Binod Kumar Singh*, Totakura Bangar Raju

Measuring association between COVID-19 with DASS-21 variables: a pilot study

Abstract: Depression, stress, and anxiety are major issues affecting the society among many age groups of humans over a period of time. Off late, COVID-19 pandemic has brought a jump in a phenomenal increase in the cases among younger age group population. This research work attempts to explore various DASS-21 variables among millenials and Gen-Z adults due to COVID-19. A strong association among DASS-21 variables and COVID-19 was established among the Gen-Z and millenials. Based on the survey, various factors were ranked to understand the COVID-19 affect on DASS-21 variables. It is found that gender and educational qualifications played no role in affect of COVID-19 on the Gen-z and millenials. Uncertainty in jobs and business emerges out to be a major cause of depression, anxiety, and stress. The results obtained could help psychologists and government bodies to take appropriate steps to improve the mental health conditions of the Gen-z and millenials in the society.

1 Introduction

In December 2019, pneumonia of unknown etiology reported in Wuhan, a city in China. On February 11, 2020, the International Committee on Taxonomy of Viruses (ICTV) named the virus the Severe Acute Respiratory Syndrome Coronavirus 2 (SARS-CoV-2), and World Health Organization (WHO) announced the disease caused by the virus is called coronavirus disease 2019 (COVID-19) [1]. Due to its highly transmissive nature, the COVID-19 spread to other regions [2]. On March 11, 2019, WHO (World Health Organization) had declared the COVID-19 a pandemic [3]. In India, on March 4, 2020, the country has reported five confirmed cases of COVID-19. As per the ministry of health in India, since the last week of March 2021, COVID-19 patients are increased by 1.5 times [4]. In India, the first time new 103,558 COVID cases reported on April 4, 2021, which is the highest number of new COVID cases in India since March 4, 2020.

The speedy diffusion of the virus and increasing inflow of diseased cases and deaths create panic, depression, stress, and anxiety in public. According to a Chinese survey, more over half of respondents assessed the epidemic's psychological impact as serious or severe [5]. In Austria, 37.7% population has reported a powerful psychological impact,

***Corresponding author: Binod Kumar Singh,** School of Business, University of Petroleum and Energy Studies, Dehradun, Uttarakhand, India
Totakura Bangar Raju, School of Business, University of Petroleum and Energy, Studies, Dehradun, Uttarakhand, India

https://doi.org/10.1515/9783110767681-003

and one out of ten is suffering from DASS-21 variables [6]; 64.7% of 442 respondents in Istanbul had depression symptoms; 51.6% had anxiety; and 41.2% had stress [7]. COVID-19 has a moderate-to-severe influence on 50.43% of respondents in Spain, according to a survey of 2,530 people [8]. COVID-19 impacts health workers and general people leading to anxiety, stress, and depression [9, 10].

In Australia and New Zealand, 21.6% of people experience moderate-to-severe depression, 28.6% have moderate-to-severe anxiety, and 28.6% have mild to extremely severe stress [11]. *The British Journal of Psychiatry* study during lockdown stress level in the younger population had increased from 13% to 24%. Also, there has been an increase in stress by 34% and also 40% of people have insomnia.

Due to COVID-19, many people have lost their family members or someone in the family ill. Many people deprive of job for a more extended period and the younger generation also deprived of the quality of education. All these problems increased depression, stress, and anxiety [12–14]. Many colleges, as well as universities, have moved from offline education to virtual education. Such situations create an unhealthy environment and impact the psychological health of the population [13–15]. Due to the global economic recession, many qualified professionals passed out from good universities/institutions waiting a more extended period for getting a job [16].

The younger population across the globe is facing a high level of depression, stress, and anxiety during the COVID-19. The younger generation is worried about career growth, primary and higher education, and future uncertainties due to COVID-19. The younger generation suffers from mental and psychological stress, leading to depression, anxiety, stupor, and numerous physiological stress [10].

Some researches were also carried out to assess the psychological effects of the COVID-19 pandemics on healthcare workers [17–20].

India is the second-largest country in terms of population. India's population is the youngest in the aging world. Also, in India median age will be 28 years by 2022 [21]. In India younger generation have more depression levels, stress levels, and anxiety. As per APA's 2020 survey, Gen-Z adults (having ages between 18 and 23 years) and millennials (having periods between 24 and 41 years) have the highest stress level compared to other generations. They have the highest level of symptoms of depression [22]. An online survey shows that 40.5% of people informed of stress or depression, and 74.1% have reported a middle level of stress. A study conducted by the Indian Psychiatry Society, due to COVID-19 in India, has increased mental illness from 15% to 20% [23]. The leading cause(s) of such depression, stress, and anxiety during COVID-19 are loneness due to lockdown, illness, death of a family member(s), social distancing, and uncertainty related to job and business. Due to these, there has been an increase in depression level, stress level, and anxiety [23].

The literature review is in Section 2, the methodology is in Section 3, the data analysis is in Section 4, and the results and comments are shown in Section 5. The study concludes with implications in Section 6, and the final section discusses the study's future scope.

There is a need to study DASS-21 variables of the age group between 15 and 29 due to suicidal attempts and death worldwide. So, in this paper, an attempt is made to measure the association between COVID-19 with DASS-21 variables viz. depression, stress, and anxiety among Gen Z-adults and millennials.

2 Literature review

Lenzo et al. [24] investigated DASS-21 between healthcare workers. In this study, DASS-21 is used to measure depression, anxiety, and stress, and Flexible Regulation of Emotional Expression scale is used to measure emotional expression. In this study researchers have also used context sensitivity index for measuring relative nods and also determined nods nonappearance.

Marijanović et al. [25] used DASS-21 to examine depression, anxiety, and stress levels in healthcare and administrative staff in five Oncology Institutions in Bosnia and Herzegovina during COVID-19 pandemic and observed that COVID-19 has significant impact on DASS-21 variables in oncology Institutions in Bosnia and Herzegovina. In this study cross-sectional data has been taken from healthcare and administrative staffs during COVID-19 pandemic using questionnaire.

Vaughan et al. [26] used DASS-21 variables to investigate mental health measurement in a post-COVID-19 world among athletes and non-athletes, finding that sport-specific measures of mental health, such as tiredness, mental strain, anxiety, and depression, improve its efficacy in the sport setting. During COVID-19, researchers used particular sport-related tools to measure mental health, such as the Sport Anxiety Scale, Athlete Burnout Questionnaire, and Athlete Psychological Strain Questionnaire. The DASS-21's internal consistency, factor structure, invariance, and convergent validity were all examined.

Regarding the COVID-19 pandemic Vahedian-Azimi et al. [27] examined the level of psychological suffering across four segments of an Iranian population. Here researchers have collected cross-sectional data from four different groups which include community population, COVID patients, medical staff, and medical students and used ANOVA to compare the severity of stress, anxiety, and depression between these groups. The study implies that COVID-19 patients and medical students have a higher risk of mental illness since they have less experience than professional medical workers and the general public.

Wang et al. [5] investigated the impact of COVID-19 on Asians' physical and mental health using data from seven Asian middle-income countries and observed that protective factors were observed to include gender, group retention, occupation, trust in doctors, high likelihood of survival, and less time spent on health information.

McKinsey [28] has studied on coronavirus and its effect on global economic sentiment. As per report the overall economic optimism continues to decline due to COVID-19. The geopolitical instability is the most critical factor and the geopolitical conflicts as a risk to near-term growth in their own economies.

A study on the economic impact of COVID-19 on core industries and the Hispanic workforce was produced by Klein and Smith [29]. According to the research, the financial vulnerability to the pandemic, as well as the recession's racially unequal effects across six select metropolitan zones, necessitated centralized federal coverage to deal with the areas and populations most hit by the COVID-19 recession.

Nicola et al. [30] studied on the COVID-19's socioeconomic effects. COVID-19 has socioeconomic effects on various parts of the global economy according to this study. In all areas of the economy, social distance, self-isolation, and travel limitations have resulted in a reduction in the workforce and the loss of employment.

The health, emotional, and economic effects of the COVID-19 pandemic on people with chronic diseases in India were researched by Singh et al. [31]. According to their research, people with chronic diseases, particularly those in impoverished, rural, and downgraded communities, have had difficulty accessing healthcare and have been badly socially and financially impacted by the COVID-19 pandemic.

3 Methods

The survey was utilized largely to collect data and 1,302 respondents were chosen through sampling in this study. The majority of the data for this analytical study came from primary sources, but secondary sources were also used on occasion. A direct interview and a questionnaire were employed as data collecting methods to get the relevant information from the primary sources. The target population is from India's largest cities, with one individual serving as a sampling unit.

A layout of methodology is as given below:

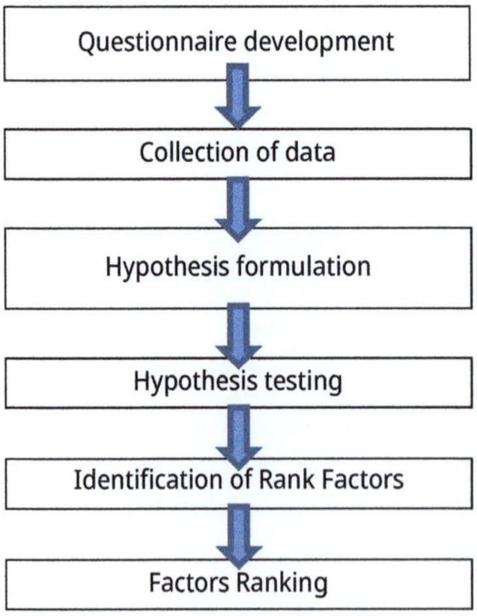

The three essential variables of DASS-21 are depression, anxiety, and stress [32]. These variables are measured based on seven proclamations. Here, a five-point scale is used from 1 to 5 (1 – normal, 2 – mild, 3 – moderate, 4 – severe, and 5 – extremely severe) for measuring the level of mental health of Gen Z-adults and millennials during COVID-19. Further, three important demographic factors like age, gender, and educational qualification are used for hypothesis formulation.

The following hypotheses formulated for measuring the association between DASS-21 variables with demographic components of Gen-Z adults and millennials.

Ho: There is no association between age and the DASS-21 variables.

Ho: There is no association between gender and the DASS-21 variables.

Ho: There is no linkage between educational qualification and the DASS-21 variables.

For studying association between qualitative or categorical variable Chi-square test for testing hypotheses has been used [33]:

$$\chi^2 = \sum_{i=1}^{n} \frac{(O_i - E_i)^2}{E_i} \quad \text{where} \sum_{i=1}^{n} E_i = \sum_{i=1}^{n} O_i$$

A contingency table is prepared in this study, and the degree of freedom is based on $(r-1)(s-1)$. Here r and s represent row and column, respectively [33].

Also, in this study, responses are collected related to five critical factors of depression, stress, and anxiety during COVID-19 among Gen Z-adults and millennials viz., loneness due to lockdown, social distancing, uncertainty related to job and business, death of the family member(s), and illness of family member(s) from respondents.

Rank is assigned to five factors viz., loneness due to lockdown, social distancing, and uncertainty related to job and business, death of the family member and illness of family member and requested respondents to rank them according to their preference and assigned a rank from 1 to 5. Here rank 1 having weight 5, rank 2 having weight 4, rank 3 having weight 3, rank 2 having weight 2, and rank 1 having weight 1.

4 Data analysis

The study aims at assessing the impact of COVID-19 on Gen Z-adults and millennials. The research shows that out of 1,302 respondents, 67.97% are male, and the rest are female (Figure 1). Out of 1,302 respondents, 55.53% of respondents are having age 24 and above. Out of 1,302 respondents, 30.87% are undergraduates, 39.48% are postgraduates, and the rest pursue higher education (Figure 2).

Also, the association between demographic factors (age, gender, and educational qualification) with DASS-21 variables (depression, stress, and anxiety) established. Here chi-square test is used to measure such associations. The chi-square test is applied for each DASS-21 variables with age, gender, and education (Tables 2–4).

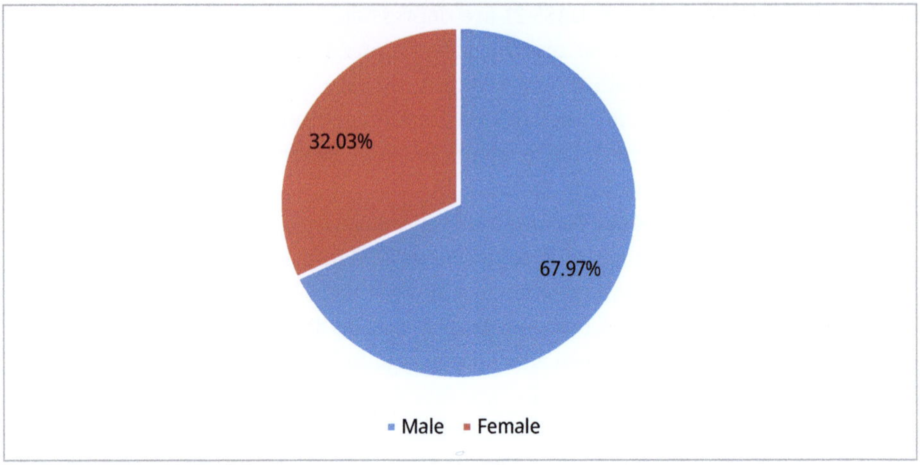

Figure 1: Demographic distribution of the respondents.

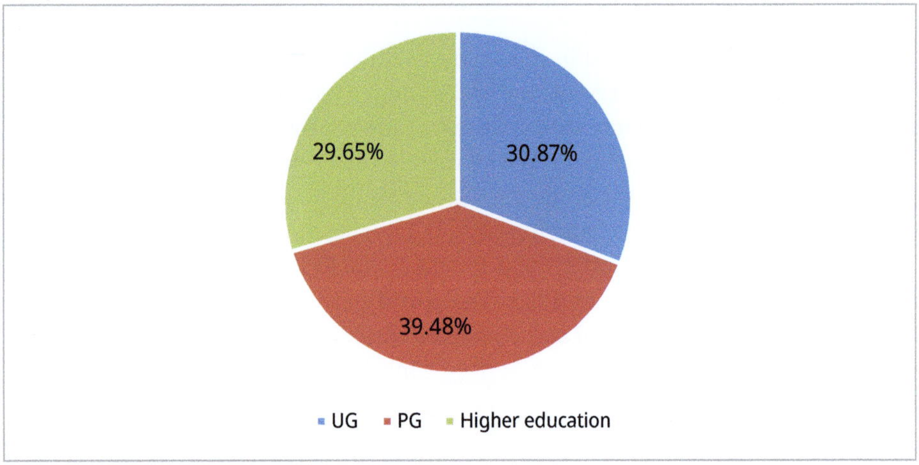

Figure 2: Distribution of educational qualification of respondents.

Table 1: Percentage of Gen Z-adults and millennials with DASS-21 variables.

	Normal	Mild	Moderate	Severe	Extremely
Depression	6.25%	7.4%	38.66%	26.38%	21.29%
Stress	9.42%	7.81%	45.065	28.73%	8.96%
Anxiety	21.37%	5.51%	17.47%	8.73%	46.89%

Table 2: Association between age with depression, stress, and anxiety.

Depression level						
Age	**Normal**	**Mild**	**Moderate**	**Severe**	**Extremely severe**	**Significant***
18–20	2.84%	3.19%	40.07%	33.69%	20.21%	Yes
21–23	4.04%	4.38%	38.72%	34.01%	18.85%	
24–26	7.29%	6.70%	39.07%	28.57%	18.37%	
Above 26	3.95%	5.52%	43.42%	28.16%	18.95%	
Stress level						
Age	**Normal**	**Mild**	**Moderate**	**Severe**	**Extremely severe**	**Significant***
18–20	4.61%	6.38%	50%	23.40%	15.60%	Yes
21–23	6.42%	7.77%	41.55%	26.35%	18.24%	
24–26	8.75%	11.08%	37.90%	23.91%	18.37%	
Above 26	6.32%	8.68%	43.95%	22.37%	18.68%	
Anxiety level						
Age	**Normal**	**Mild**	**Moderate**	**Severe**	**Extremely severe**	**Significant***
18–20	18.44%	16.31%	21.99%	21.99%	21.28%	Yes
21–23	14.48%	13.13%	19.87%	27.95%	24.58%	
24–26	12.83%	12.83%	23.03%	27.99%	23.32%	
Above 26	10.79%	15.79%	17.89%	28.68%	26.84%	

*It is based on experimental and tabulated value with 10% significance level.

Table 3: Association between gender with depression, stress, and anxiety.

Depression level						
Gender	**Normal**	**Mild**	**Moderate**	**Severe**	**Extremely severe**	**Significant***
Male	14.92%	19.10%	21.81%	22.82%	21.36%	No
Female	16.07%	21.10%	24.22%	19.66%	18.94%	
Stress level						
Gender	**Normal**	**Mild**	**Moderate**	**Severe**	**Extremely severe**	**Significant***
Male	14.01%	18.53%	22.37%	23.50%	21.58%	No
Female	15.11%	21.82%	24.70%	18.71%	19.66%	
Anxiety level						
Gender	**Normal**	**Mild**	**Moderate**	**Severe**	**Extremely severe**	**Significant***
Male	13.79%	18.08%	16.95%	25.88%	25.31%	No
Female	17.03%	15.35%	13.91%	26.38%	27.34%	

*It is based on experimental and tabulated value with 10% significance level.

Table 4: Association between educational qualification with depression, stress and anxiety.

Depression level						
Education qualification	**Normal**	**Mild**	**Moderate**	**Severe**	**Extremely severe**	**Significant***
UG	12.19%	18.41%	34.33%	20.90%	14.18%	No
PG	14.40%	18.48%	31.13%	18.68%	17.32%	
Higher education	10.62%	13.99%	31.87%	24.35%	19.17%	
Stress level						
Education qualification	**Normal**	**Mild**	**Moderate**	**Severe**	**Extremely severe**	**Significant***
UG	11.69%	17.91%	36.82%	20.40%	13.18%	Yes
PG	14.20%	17.51%	33.27%	18.29%	16.73%	
Higher education	10.10%	13.47%	34.46%	23.83%	18.13%	
Anxiety level						
Education qualification	**Normal**	**Mild**	**Moderate**	**Severe**	**Extremely severe**	**Significant***
UG	15.42%	17.16%	17.91%	27.36%	22.14%	No
PG	16.93%	17.12%	18.48%	23.93%	23.54%	
Higher education	13.21%	15.28%	14.25%	30.57%	26.68%	

*It is based on experimental and tabulated value with 10% significance level.

Ranking based on weighted scores was used to investigate the numerous elements that contribute to depression, stress, and anxiety during COVID-19 (Tables 5 and 6).

Table 5: Various factors responsible for depression, stress, and anxiety.

	No. of respondents				
Rank factors	1	2	3	4	5
Loneness due to lockdown	10.83%	14.52%	13.98%	28.34%	32.33%
Social distancing	7.53%	12.83%	20.74%	27.57%	31.34%
Uncertainty related to job and business	56.14%	23.35%	6.91%	8.83%	4.76%
Death of a family member(s)	8.76%	28.57%	31.18%	18.36%	13.13%
Illness of family member(s)	16.74%	20.74%	27.19%	16.90%	18.43%

Table 6: Ranking of various factors.

Factors	**Weighted score**	**Percentage**	**Rank**
Loneness due to lockdown	3,166	16.21	4
Social distancing	3,094	15.84	5
Uncertainty related to job and business	5,433	27.82	1
Death of a family member(s)	3,925	20.09	2
Illness of family member(s)	3,912	20.03	3

5 Results and discussion

The study shows that out of 1,302 respondents, 33.17% are depressed, 33.41% are stressed, and the rest have anxiety. Out of 432 respondents, 38.65%, 26.38%, and 21.29% had moderate, severe, and extremely severe depression. Out of 435 respondents, 46.89% respondents have extremely severe anxiety. Also, 45.05% of respondents have a moderate stress level, and 28.73% have extreme stress (Table 1).

Table 2 explains the linkage between age with depression, stress, and anxiety level. It indicates a significant relationship between age with depression, stress, and anxiety level among Gen-Z adults and millennials. About 40.07% of respondents having an age group (18–20), 38.72% respondents having an age group (21–23), 39.07% respondents have an age group (24–26), and 43.42% respondents have a moderate depression level. There is the highest level of depression in the age 26 and above against the others. About 50% of respondents having an age group (18–20), 41.55% respondents having an age group (21–23), 37.90% respondents have an age group (24–26), and 43.95% of respondents have a moderate stress level. There is the highest level of stress in the age 26 and above against the others. Also, about 21.99% of respondents having an age group (18–20), 27.95% of respondents having an age group (21–23), 27.99% of respondents have an age group (24–26), and 28.68% respondents have a severe anxiety level. There is the highest level of stress in the age 26 and above against the others.

As per Table 3, there is no association between gender with depression, stress, and anxiety among Gen-Z adults and millennials. About 21.81% of male respondents and 24.22% female respondents have a moderate depression level. There is a higher level of depression in males as compared to females. About 22.37% of male respondents and 24.70% female respondents have a moderate stress level. There is a higher level of stress in males as compared to females. Also, about 25.88% of male respondents and 26.38% of female respondents have a severe anxiety level. There is a higher level of anxiety in males as compared to females.

Table 4 explains the association between education qualification with depression, stress, and anxiety level. It is observed there is no linkage between educational qualification with depression and anxiety among Gen-Z adults and millennials. But, there is a significant relationship between education qualification with stress among Gen-Z adults and millennials. About 34.33% of undergraduate respondents, 31.13% post-graduate respondents, and 31.87% of respondents pursuing higher education have a moderate depression level. There is the highest level of depression in post-graduate respondents. About 36.82% of undergraduate respondents, 33.27% of post-graduate respondents, and 34.46% of respondents pursuing higher education have a moderate stress level. There is the highest level of depression in respondents having post-graduate qualifications against the others. Also, about 27.36% of undergraduate respondents, 23.93% post-graduate respondents, and 30.57% of respondents pursuing higher education have a severe anxiety level. There is the highest level of anxiety in respondents having post-graduate qualifications against the others.

Table 5 summarizes the various factors responsible for depression, stress, and anxiety.

Table 6 summarizes the ranking of various factors. It is clear from the table that the most critical aspects of depression, stress, and anxiety among Gen-Z adults and millennials are uncertainly related to job and business during COVID-19. The second significant factor in the study is in line with the previous research conducted by the Indian psychiatric society that shows that during the pandemic, the death of a family member is the leading cause of depression, stress, and anxiety.

From Table 2, one interesting finding is that the normal-to-moderate levels of depression are high in the age group of 24–26. However, moderate-to-extremely severe levels of depression recorded for the people in the age group above 26. From Table 2, the results confirm higher stress levels in the higher age groups. Similar observations can also be in accord for anxiety and age groups shown in Table 2. These attributes could be due to unemployment or the threat of unemployment in the COVID scenario. The age groups of 24–26 or above 26 are the segments that generally go for employment after completing graduation or post-graduation in the Indian scenario. The same derived from Table 4. Indian social structure is also with male domination, and he is the primary bread earner in the family. Thereby, a strong association of depression, anxiety, and stress can be seen in males than in females from Table 3.

Based on the above study, psychologist and the government agencies need to understand that the gender and educational qualification have no role to play while treating mental health issues due to DASS-21 variables.

6 Conclusion

This study indicates that age is a significant factor in measuring DASS-21 variables during COVID-19. This study also shows that Gen-X adults and millennials are affected mainly by COVID-19. There is the highest level of depression, stress, and anxiety among Gen-X adults and millennials. As far as the significant factor for depression, stress, and anxiety during COVID-19 is concerned, uncertainty related to job and business perceived to be the most important factor by the respondents, followed by the death of a family member(s), illness of family member(s), loneness due to lockdown, and social distancing. Due to COVID-19, it is challenging to cope with uncertainty among Gen-Z adults and millennials. So, Gen-X adults and millennials need psychological support. In this challenging situation, mental wellness is the key factor to protect Gen-X adults and millennials. Gen-Z adults and millennials must start mindfulness and emotional release techniques for mental peace.

They must focus on the right food, sleep well, believe in others, daily yoga, listen to music, maintain a balance between workplace and home, and be focussed on work.

7 Future research direction

Researchers could formulate a new framework which could help in improving mental health of Gen-X adults and millennials in other countries.

References

[1] WHO. A report on Naming the coronavirus disease (COVID-19) and the virus that causes it, n.d. https://www.who.int/emergencies/diseases/novel-coronavirus-2019/technical-guidance/naming-the-coronavirus-disease-(COVID-2019)-and-the-virus-that-causes-it (accessed Jan 25, 2021).

[2] Bukhari, Q., Jameel, Y. Will coronavirus pandemic diminish by summer?. SSRN Electronic Journal, 2020. https://doi.org/10.2139/ssrn.3556998.

[3] Puliatti, S., Eissa, A., Eissa, R., Amato, M., Mazzone, E., Dell'Oglio, P., Rocco, B. COVID-19 and urology: A comprehensive review of the literature. BJU International, 2020, 125(6), E7–E14. https://doi.org/10.1111/bju.15071.

[4] Ministry of Health and Family Welfare, 2021. mohfw.gov.in. (accessed April 4, 2021).

[5] Wang, C., Tee, M., Roy, A. E., Fardin, M. A., Srichokchatchawan, W., Habib, H. A., et al. The impact of COVID-19 pandemic on physical and mental health of Asians: A study of seven middle-income countries in Asia. PLoS ONE, 2021, 16(2), e0246824. https://doi.org/10.1371/journal.pone.0246824.

[6] Traunmüller, C., Stefitz, R., Gaisbachgrabner, K., Schwerdtfeger, A. Psychological correlates of COVID-19 pandemic in the Austrian population. BMC Public Health, 2020, 20, 1395, 1–16. https://doi.org/10.1186/s12889-020-09489-5.

[7] Elbay, R. Y., Kurtulmuş, A., Arpacıoğlu, S., Karadere, E. Depression, anxiety, stress levels of physicians and associated factors in Covid 19 pandemics. Psychiatry Research, 2020, 290, 1–5. https://doi.org/10.1016/j.psychres.2020.113130.

[8] Gonzáleza, P. O., Gómezb, Á. P., Irurtiaa, M. J., Garcíab, R. D. L. Psychological effects of the COVID-19 outbreak and lockdown among students and workers of a Spanish university. Psychiatry Research, 2020, 290, 113108. 10.1016/j.psychres.2020.113108.

[9] Kang, L., Li, Y., Hu, S., Chen, M., Yang, C., Yang, B. X., Wang, Y., Hu, J., Lai, J., Ma, X., Chen, J., Guan, L., Wang, G., Ma, H., Liu, Z. The mental health of medical workers in Wuhan, China dealing with the 2019 novel coronavirus. Lancet Psychiatry, 2020, 7(3), e14. https://doi.org/10.1016/S2215-0366(20)30047-X.

[10] Wang, C., Pan, R., Wan, X., Tan, Y., Xu, L., Ho, C. S., et al. Immediate psychological responses and associated factors during the initial stage of the 2019 coronavirus disease (COVID-19) epidemic among the general population in China. International Journal of Environmental Research and Public Health, 2020, 17(5), 1729. https://doi.org/10.3390/ijerph17051729.

[11] Hammond, N. E., Crowe, L., Abbenbroek, B., Elliott, R., Tian, D. H., Donaldson, L. H., Fitzgerald, E., Flower, O., Grattan, S., Harris, R., Sayers, L., Delaney, A. Impact of the coronavirus disease 2019 pandemic on critical care healthcare workers' depression, anxiety, and stress levels. Australian Critical Care: Official Journal of the Confederation of Australian Critical Care Nurses, 2021, 34(2), 146–154. https://doi.org/10.1016/j.aucc.2020.12.004.

[12] Major, L. E., Eyles, A., Machin, S. Generation COVID: Emerging work and education inequalities, Centre for Economic Performance. The London School of Economics and Political Science, 1–14, 2020. https://cep.lse.ac.uk/pubs/download/cepcovid-19-011.pdf.
[13] Al-Rabiaah, A., Temsah, M. H., Al-Eyadhy, A. A., Hasan, G. M., Al-Zamil, F., Al-Subaie, S., Alsohime, F., Jamal, A., Alhaboob, A., Al-Saadi, B., Somily, A. M. Middle east respiratory syndrome-Corona Virus (MERS-CoV) associated stress among medical students at a university teaching hospital in Saudi Arabia. Journal of Infection and Public Health, 2020, 13. https://doi.org/10.1016/j.jiph.2020.01.005.
[14] Kafka, A. C. Shock, Fear, and Fatalism: As Coronavirus Prompts Colleges to Close Students Grapple With Uncertainty, The Chronical of Higher Education, 2020. https://www.chronicle.com/article/shock-fear-and-fatalism-as-coronavirus-prompts-colleges-to-close-students-grapple-with-uncertainty/ (accessed April 1, 2021).
[15] Razai, M. S., Doerholt, K., Ladhani, S., Oakeshott, P. Coronavirus disease 2019 (covid-19): A guide for UK GPs. BMJ, 2020, 368:m800. https://doi.org/10.1136/bmj.m800.
[16] Sahu, P. Closure of Universities Due to Coronavirus Disease 2019 (COVID-19): impact on education and mental health of students and academic staff. Cureus, 2020, 12(4), e7541. https://doi.org/10.7759/cureus.7541.
[17] Cao, W., Fang, Z., Hou, G., Han, M., Xu, X., Dong, J., Zheng, J. The psychological impact of the COVID-19 epidemic on college students in China. Psychiatry Research, 2020, 287, 112934. https://doi.org/10.1016/j.psychres.2020.112934.
[18] Gupta, A. K., Mehra, A., Niraula, A., Kafle, K., Deo, P. S., Singh, B., Sahoo, S., Grover, S. Prevalence of anxiety and depression among the healthcare workers in Nepal during the COVID-19 pandemic. Asian Journal of Psychiatry, 2020, 54, 1–3. 10.1016/j.psychres.2020.113108.
[19] Liao, Q., Cowling, B. J., Lam, W. W. T., Ng, D. M. W., Fielding, R. Anxiety, worry and cognitive risk estimate in relation to protective behaviors during the 2009 influenza A/H1N1 pandemic in Hong Kong: Ten cross-sectional surveys. BMC Infectious Diseases, 2014, 14, 1–11. https://doi.org/10.1186/1471-2334-14-169.
[20] Qiu, J., Shen, B., Zhao, M., Wang, Z., Xie, B., Xu, Y. A nationwide survey of psychological distress among Chinese people in the COVID-19 epidemic: Implications and policy recommendations. General Psychiatry, 2020, 33(2), e100213. https://doi.org/10.1136/gpsych-2020-100213.
[21] Ghosh, M. D. Youth can be a clear advantage for India. The Hindu, 2020. https://www.thehindu.com/opinion/lead/youth-can-be-a-clear-advantage-for-india/article30897179.ece (accessed March 1, 2021).
[22] Stieg, C. More than 7 in 10 Gen-Zers report symptoms of depression during pandemic, survey finds, 2020. https://www.cnbc.com/2020/10/21/survey-more-than-7-in-10-gen-zers-report-depression-during-pandemic.html (accessed March 1, 2021).
[23] India Today. Report on 20% increase in patients with mental illness since coronavirus outbreak: Survey, 2020. https://www.indiatoday.in/india/story/20-per-cent-increase-in-patients-with-mental-illness-since-coronavirus-outbreak-survey-1661584-2020-03-31 (accessed April 4, 2021).
[24] Lenzo, V., Quattropani, M. C., Sardella, A., Martino, G., Bonanno, G. A. Depression, anxiety, and stress among healthcare workers during the COVID-19 outbreak and relationships with expressive flexibility and context sensitivity. Frontiers in Psychology, 2021, 12, 623033. doi: 10.3389/fpsyg.2021.623033.
[25] Marijanović, I., Kraljević, M., Buhovac, T., Cerić, T., Mekić Abazović, A., Alidžanović, J., Gojković, Z., Sokolović, E. Use of the depression, anxiety and stress scale (DASS-21) Questionnaire to assess levels of depression, anxiety, and stress in healthcare and administrative staff in 5 oncology institutions in bosnia and herzegovina during the 2020 COVID-19 Pandemic. Medical Science Monitor: International Medical Journal of Experimental and Clinical Research, 2021, 27, e930812. https://doi.org/10.12659/MSM.930812.

[26] Vaughan, R. S., Edwards, E. J., MacIntyre, T. E. Mental health measurement in a Post Covid-19 world: Psychometric properties and invariance of the DASS-21 in athletes and non-athletes. Frontiers in Psychology, 2020, 11, 590559. doi: 10.3389/fpsyg.2020.590559.
[27] Vahedian-Azimi, A., Moayed, M. S., Rahimibashar, F., Shojaei, S., Ashtari, S., Pourhoseingholi, M. A. Comparison of the severity of psychological distress among four groups of an Iranian population regarding COVID-19 pandemic. BMC Psychiatry, 2020, 20, 402.
[28] McKinsey. A report on The coronavirus effect on global economic sentiment, 2022. https://www.mckinsey.com/business-functions/strategy-and-corporate-finance/our-insights/the-coronavirus-effect-on-global-economic-sentiment (accessed April 26, 2022).
[29] Klein, A., Smith, E. Report on Explaining the economic impact of COVID-19: Core industries and the Hispanic workforce. Brookings Mountain West, February 5, 2021. https://www.brookings.edu/research/explaining-the-economic-impact-of-covid-19-core-industries-and-the-hispanic-workforce/ (accessed March 1, 2022).
[30] Nicola, M., Alsafi, Z., Sohrabi, C., Kerwan, A., Al-Jabir, A., Iosifidis, C., Agha, M., Agha, R. The socio-economic implications of the coronavirus pandemic (COVID-19): A review. International Journal of Surgery (London, England), 2020, 78, 185–193. https://doi.org/10.1016/j.ijsu.2020.04.018.
[31] Singh, K., Kondal, D., Mohan, S., et al. Health, psychosocial, and economic impacts of the COVID-19 pandemic on people with chronic conditions in India: A mixed methods study. BMC Public Health, 2021, 21(685). https://doi.org/10.1186/s12889-021-10708-w.
[32] Lovibond, S. H., Lovibond, P. F. DASS-21, in: Manual for the Depression Anxiety & Stress Scales, Psychology Foundation, Sydney, 1995.
[33] Singh, B. K. A study on investors` attitude towards mutual funds as an investment option. Journal of Asian Business Strategy, 2011, 1(2), 8–15. https://search.proquest.com/docview/1417594348?pq-origsite=gscholar&fromopenview=true.

Atishna Samantaray, Sayanee Bandyopadhyay, Ankita Pramanik*

Novel algorithm for COVID-19 variant detection from chest X-rays

Abstract: COVID-19 has cost 5 million lives worldwide and destabilized the economic and healthcare systems in just two years. An important strategy to combat COVID-19 is to propose a fast and accurate method of screening infected persons. One such efficient technique of screening is doing radiology examinations using chest X-rays. It was found in earlier studies that people affected with COVID-19 display abnormalities in chest radiography images. A large number of works detecting COVID-19 are presently available; however, the works do not give a high accuracy of detection. Motivated by this drawback, a deep network-based solution to determine COVID-19 from X-rays of the chest has been proposed here. With the advent of the different variants of the COVID-19 virus determining whether a patient is affected by COVID-19 is not enough. The variant of the COVID-19 also needs to be determined. The proposed work also provides an efficient algorithm for variant detection, that is, delta, omicron, or alpha variant. The proposed algorithm is split into two stages: detection of COVID-19 is undertaken in the first stage and in the next stage, the variant detection of COVID-19 is done for patients whose test results are COVID-19 positive. The proposed CNN model is inspired by the residual network model ResNet50. The suggested convolutional neural network model is inspired by the residual network model ResNet50. The model proposed is efficient and produces a high accuracy of 99.47% for stage 1 of the algorithm, that is, COVID-19 detection and an accuracy of 98.46% for stage 2, that is, COVID-19 variant detection on the used dataset obtained from images of patients of eastern India.

1 Introduction

In the past 2 years, mankind has witnessed one of the biggest disasters of the century – the COVID-19 pandemic. Within a span of 2 years, a staggering number of about 387 million have been affected by the virus. This virus has caused over 5 million deaths [1] and has caused the global economic and healthcare systems to collapse. The symptoms of COVID-19 often range from fever, headache, cough, fatigue, pneumonia, shortness of breath (dyspnea), and loss of smell and taste.

The degree of severity and virulence of COVID-19 varies from variant to variant. Some COVID-19 variants require hospitalization and for some recovery at home

*Corresponding author: **Ankita Pramanik**, Department of Electronics and Telecommunication Engineering, IIEST, Shibpur, West Bengal, India
Atishna Samantaray, Sayanee Bandyopadhyay, Department of Electronics and Telecommunication Engineering, IIEST, Shibpur, West Bengal, India

https://doi.org/10.1515/9783110767681-004

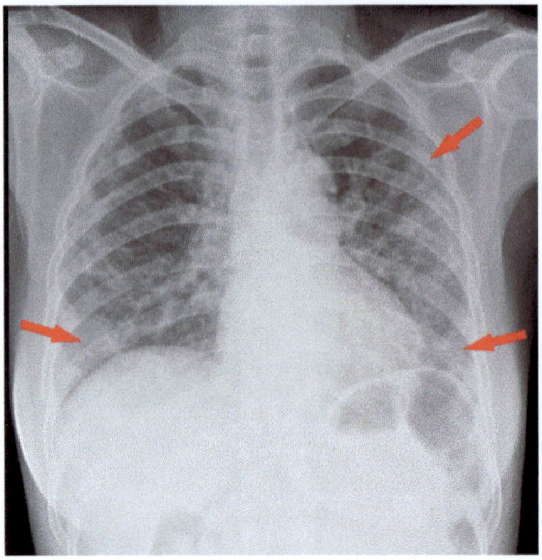

Figure 1: Ground glass opacity in a patient affected by COVID-19.

suffice. To make matters worse, these variants are present in the same geographical location at the same time. So, determining the COVID-19 variant is essential to determine the course of treatment for the affected people.

RT-PCR is the accepted norm for detecting COVID-19 infection. However, this test takes time and is limited by the availability of the testing reagents. It has been seen that it is possible to detect if a person has been affected by COVID-19 by a careful study of chest X-rays or chest CT scans. Ground glass opacity (GGO) is manifested in chest X-rays of an affected patient. GGO in such patients is most often bilateral, peripheral, and lower zone predominant. Figure 1 presents the chest image of a COVID-19-positive patient. In the X-ray, the following abnormalities are observed:

COVID-19 variant detection

- rounded airspace opacities mainly in the lower and peripheral lobe and
- multifocal rounded opacities and nodules.

The abnormalities caused by COVID-19 are pointed by red arrows in Figure 1. In the past 2 years, several classification models such as DenseNet201 [2], VGG-16/19, and Inceptionv3 [3] have been proposed for detecting COVID-19 through X-rays or CT scans of the chest. However, the existing works did not offer satisfactory accuracy. Moreover, an efficient algorithm for variant detection is presently not available. The need of the hour is to design more accurate and fast models to not only detect COVID-19 but also ascertain its variant. CT scan images consist of images from multiple angles and so COVID-19 detection algorithms give more accurate results on CT scan images as compared to X-ray images. However, a CT scan is expensive compared to an X-ray and is not always available in rural hospitals. This work uses X-rays of the chest for detecting COVID-19 and its variant.

To address the above issues, the authors have presented a deep network-based solution inspired by a convolutional neural network (CNN) and the residual network model ResNet50. The proposed model works in two stages. In the first phase, the algorithm aims to detect if a person is a COVID-19 positive. If the patient is detected as COVID-19 positive, then the second stage of the algorithm is executed. In the second stage of the model, the SARS COV2 variants, that is, omicron (B.1.1.529) or delta (B.1.617.2) or alpha (B.1.1.7) of concern, are detected from the COVID-19-positive scans.

The main contributions of this work can be summarized as follows:

- To illustrate the concepts of deep learning (DL) to perform image processing and classification
- To present a new deep CNN-rooted model which has the capability of extracting relevant features from COVID-19-positive chest X-rays
- To use those features for performing binary classification, that is, the model can distinguish between COVID-19-positive and COVID-19-negative chest X-rays
- To detect COVID-19 variants of concern such as alpha, delta, and omicron variants using relevant extracted features from COVID-19-positive images

The effectiveness of the proposed algorithm has been established by presenting a performance comparison of the new model with various state-of-art models. The remaining part of this chapter is organized as follows: Section 2 presents a summary of the current works on detecting COVID-19 using DL. The present work uses artificial neural network (ANN) to detect COVID-19 and also classify its variant. A brief description of ANN is given in Section 3. A brief introduction to the various computational tools and techniques applied here is compiled in Section 4. The algorithm proposed in this work is given in Section 5. Section 6 presents the model architecture. The data preparation and partitioning techniques used in this work are discussed in Section 7. The training, testing, obtained results, and the associated discussions are given in Section 8. The work is finally concluded in Section 9. The scope for future works is also discussed in the last section.

2 Literature review

With the advent of COVID-19, the world has seen a scramble for publishing COVID-related research. The very first paper on detecting COVID-19 automatically was published within 40 days of the advent of COVID-19 [4]. The work proposed three multivariate logistic regression models that worked on clinical features and semantics of radiological images and by distributing the patients into two groups consisting of 70 cases of COVID-19 and 66 cases of non-COVID-19 pneumonia, respectively, into validation ($n = 38$) cohorts and primary ($n = 98$), and then executing a series of tests like Kruskal–Wallis H, chi-square test, and Student's t-test. The authors compared 67 features and 1,745 lesions in the two sections.

Numerous research works in automatic COVID-19 detection have been undertaken since 2019 [4]. In [5], a DL-based classification model, that is a blend of support vector machine (SVM) and Resnet50 for detecting COVID-19 (excluding MERS, SARS, and ARDS) was given. It achieved an accuracy of 95.38%. The work in [6] used a ResNet-101-based CNN architecture which was pre-trained to identify objects from datasets in the range of millions. They then retrained the model to determine anomalies in chest X-ray images and achieved 82% of accuracy.

Hemdan et al. [7] developed a model named COVIDXNet, which is an amalgamation of seven different deep CNN architectures, namely, the second version of Google MobileNet and modified VGG19. The authors claimed that the performance of each model in analyzing the normalized values of intensities of input X-rays was acceptable and thereafter generated comparable performances between DenseNet and VGG19 with F_1-scores of 0.89 and 0.91 for negative and positive cases, respectively. The InceptionV3 produced the worst classification performance with an F_1-score of 0.00 for COVID-19 and normal cases had a value of 0.67.

Ahsan et al. [8] have attempted to detect symptoms of COVID-19 using eight types of DL models namely VGG16, VGG19, ResNet50, ResNet15V2, InceptionResNetV2, DenseNet201, MobilenetV2, and NasNetMobile. Two datasets having 400 CT scans and 400 chest X-ray images each and LIME that stand for local interpretable model-agnostic explanation were used. They concluded that the performance of NasNetMobile was the finest among all models in the category of X-ray images by achieving an accuracy of 93.94% with X-rays and 82.94% in CT scans, whereas MobileNetV2 achieved an accuracy of 95% on CT scans (best among all others) and something in between 81.5 and 95.2% on X-rays.

Mahmud et al. [9] have given a CNN architecture named CovXNet that utilizes convolution in a depthwise fashion and changing rates of dilation to extract features efficiently. They have also used a stacking algorithm and for COVID/normal cases gave an accuracy of 97.4%. Wang et al. [10] have created a DL-based CNN called COVIDNet. Adam optimizer was used to pre-train the model with ImageNet43 and COVIDx to produce performance accuracies of 98.4%, 98.8%, and 98.9% on VGG-19, ResNet-50, and COVID-Net, respectively. Hussain et al. [11] have developed a 22-layer CNN model, built on simple convolutional and max pool layers named CoroDet. It produces diagnostics on detecting COVID-19 automatically into two, three, and four classes from X-rays as well as images from CT scans. The authors have achieved accuracies of 99.1% for two-class classification. The authors have created one of the largest COVID-19 datasets available using the repositories [12–19].

The authors in [20] have put forward a CNN model, named DeTrac, an acronym for Decompose, Transfer, and Compose which presents a transfer learning model for detecting and classifying COVID-19 from radiological chest X-rays. The authors made use of a combination of two datasets where one contained X-ray photos of COVID-19 and SARS and the other had X-ray images of normal people collected from various hospitals. They have achieved an accuracy of 97.35%, specificity of 96.34%, a sensitivity of 98.23% with VGG19, thus attesting its efficiency on actual chest X-ray photographs. The authors have achieved 93.1% accuracy on DeTraC. In [21], the authors have proposed an AI-based deep Bayes-SqueezeNet framework capable of decision-making for diagnosing COVID-19. They have improved upon the traditional SqueezeNet architecture by making use of the Bayes optimization algorithm. Albahli et al. [22] have proposed three different pre-trained BiT models named DenseNet, InceptionV3, and Inception-ResNetV4 to identify COVID-19. Those three models provide uncertainty matrices and receiver-operating characteristic analysis. The authors have proposed the addition of an extra dense layer with 512 perceptrons for performance improvement of the existing pretrained model DenseNet and produce a classification efficiency of 92%. Ozturk et al. [23] proposed a CNN model constructed of 17 layers to produce accurate diagnostics on the binary classification of COVID-19 and normal. It used the DarkNet model. Based on the Xception architecture and ImageNet dataset, the work in [24] presented CoroNet. The work had an accuracy of 89.6% and 95% for four-class and three-class classification, respectively. Khasawneh et al. [25] have used CNN-based customized pre-trained DL models for diagnosing pneumonia induced by complications after COVID-19 from chest X-rays. The authors tested their model over various combinations of public and local datasets and have an accuracy of 98.7% on the combination of the dataset. Tuncer et al. [26] have proposed an automated chest X-ray image classification model to differentiate between pneumonia and COVID-19 using classification procedures like fuzzy tree creation, INCA-based feature selection, and multi-kernel local binary pattern (MKLBP)-based feature extraction. Using the fuzzy tree, they have created an F-transformation such that each X-ray image produces 15 variable images. The MKLBP then gives rise to features that are further worked upon by the exemplars. The authors have achieved 97.01% classification accuracy on cubic SVM. Chandra et al. [27] have produced an automatic COVID screening (ACoS) and obtained accuracy of 98.062% and 91.329% for phases 1 and 2, respectively. Shankar et al. [28] have used a barnacle mating optimization (BMO) and cascaded recurrent neural network (CRNN) to form the BMOCRNN model to determine the presence of COVID-19. They used the CRNN model for feature extraction, tuned its hyperparameter via the BMO algorithm, and obtained an average accuracy of 97.31%. The CNN model in [29] trained the model on a total of five variants of ResNet and inception and their combination [30] using the five-fold cross-validation method. The work inferred that the ResNet50 model has the best performance for detecting COVID-19. The ResNet101 and ResNet50 yielded the highest overall performance of 96.1%. Jamil and Rahman [31] have proposed a DL framework for detecting COVID-19 and classifying its variants into alpha, beta, gamma, and delta. They have used both CT scans and chest X-ray images as input data. In the first step of detection, a 2D wavelet transform was performed to get the spectrogram of images and the obtained spectrum is passed through a CNN, after which features are extracted and combined to build a vocabulary of features which is fed to an SVM classifier to detect the variant. Thus it can be seen that a large number of works on COVID-19 detection have been done. However, no significant work on variant detection has been done. The present work proposes not only a COVID-19 detection algorithm but also an algorithm to detect the variant of COVID-19. The proposed work gives better results than the existing works. The efficacy of the proposed algorithm for COVID-19 detection over the existing works has been presented in Section 8.

3 Artificial neural networks

The ANN (Figure 8), commonly referred to as neural networks, was first brought into light by a young mathematician named Walter Pitts and a neurophysiologist named Warren McCulloch in the year 1943. The structure of a neural network is identical to that of a human brain, consisting of a large number of neurons. An example of ANN is shown in Figure 6 and ANN after dropout is shown in Figure 7.

For handling images ANN treats pixel brightness as a distinct feature and feeds it to the neural network as input. However, to make this process a success, the neural network will have to consist of millions of neurons. Scaling down the images will help but at the cost of losing valuable information. So, to deal with images efficiently, a method was needed that would use as much data as possible, with a minimal number of calculations and parameter requirements. Hence, CNN came into play. CNN is a form of ANN that can detect meaningful patterns in data and this pattern detection specialization makes them useful for image analysis.

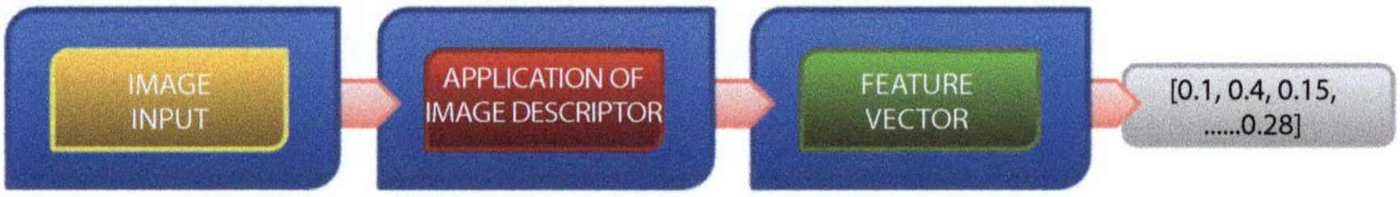
IMAGE INPUT
APPLICATION OF IMAGE DESCRIPTOR
FEATURE VECTOR
[0.1, 0.4, 0.15, ...0.28]

Figure 2: Demonstration of the feature extraction process.

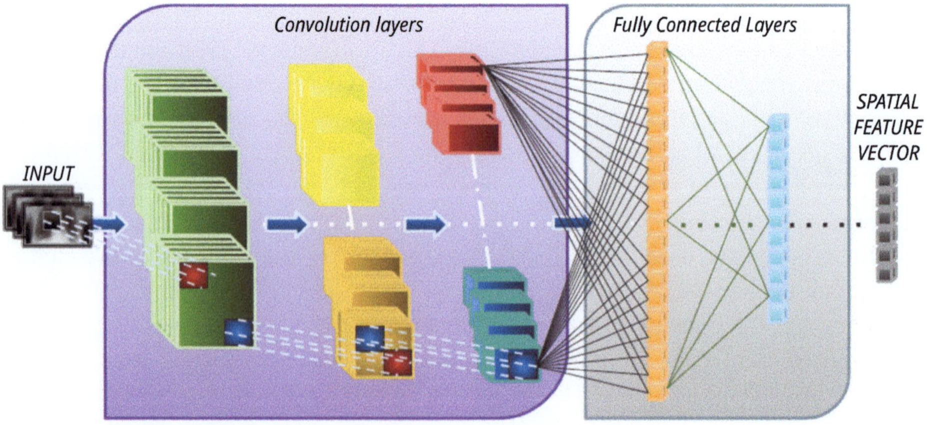

Figure 3: Spatial feature extraction.

The success of a CNN algorithm depends on two important processes: feature extraction and feature selection. The procedure of feature extraction, shown in Figure 2, plays a critical role in reducing data redundancy by dimensionality reduction without losing important information. It helps decrease the number of resources required for processing and also speeds up the machine learning process. Feature extraction is widely used in autoencoders, image processing, and bag-of-words (a technique for natural language processing).

Feature selection helps in determining the most appropriate features for the phenomena under consideration. Feature selection can be supervised or unsupervised.

3.1 Feature extraction using CNNs

CNN mainly consists of three layers: a convolutional layer, a pooling layer, and a fully connected (FC) layer. *The first few layers of a CNN extract low-level details or features namely colors and edges. With each passing layer, the complexity of the CNN increases exponentially. The layers toward the end are responsible for extracting higher-level features, gradually resulting in the identification of greater parts of the input image until the final intended output is achieved. Figure 3 demonstrates the spatial feature extraction using CNN.*

The convolutional layers are fed with elements like a set of digital filters and feature maps that perform the convolution operation on the input data. These filters are first randomly initialized and then later updated through back-propagation.

The pooling layer integrates the maps produced by the previous convolutional layer and downsizes its dimensions, acting as an "output dimensionality reduction layer" and deciding the threshold. It also reduces several parameters yielding two benefits: first, it compensates for the computation time during training and second, it helps combat the challenge of overfitting. The various kinds of pooling layers are max pooling, min pooling, average pooling, etc. The convolutional and pooling layers together form the feature extraction network, and the resultant extracted features from this network are further forwarded to a classifier network.

At the end comes the FC layer, also known as the dense layer. Here each input has a connection with every other neuron. The last FC layer is called the output layer, and for classification applications, it denotes the class scores. The output of the final convolutional layer or pooling layer is first flattened and then fed as an input to the FC layer.

To increase the accuracy of a DL model and dodge overfitting, a set of techniques called regularization is performed. Thus, regularization controls the complexity of the model by reducing the burden on the weights. So, post regularization the weights end up having a lesser impact on the loss function which displays the error between the actual and predicted label.

For regularization, CNNs provide an option to add dropout layers that either drop or make certain neurons in the network inactive resulting in the reduction of overfitting and causing quicker convergence. Other regularization techniques are L1 regularization and L2 regularization.

For feature detection, kernel convolution is an important step. Here, a kernel or filter, that is, a small-sized 2-D array is passed over the input image and further calculations are made. The values of the feature map are computed according to the given formula:

$$G[u,v] = (I * w)[u,v] = \sum_y \sum_x w[y,x] I[u-y, v-x]$$

where I is the input image, w is the kernel, and the row and column indices of the resultant matrix are given by u and v, respectively. Figure 4 shows the convolution operation on a micro-scale. It can be seen that when a 6×6 image undergoes convolution with a 3×3 kernel, a 4×4 feature map is obtained. There as on behind this is the availability of just 16 unique locations where the filter can be placed inside the image.

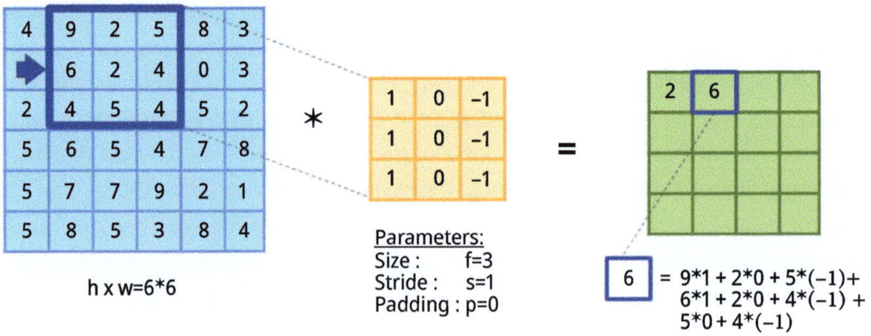

Figure 4: Convolution example.

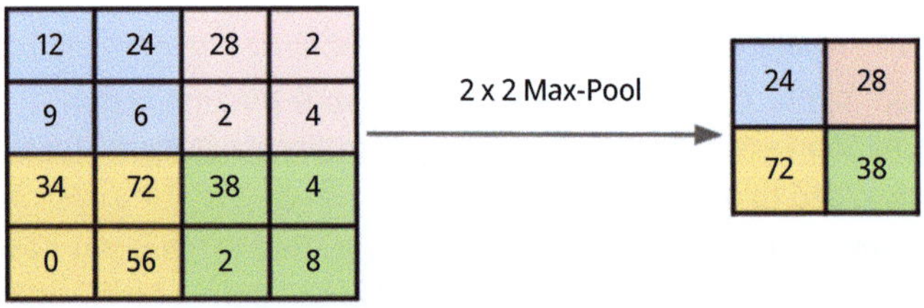

Figure 5: Depiction of max-pooling operation.

In CNN pooling layers are used for speeding up calculations and reducing the tensor size. In the max pool layer, the largest value in each region is chosen to replace the value in that location in the output. Max pooling operation is shown in Figure 5.

4 Computational tools and techniques

The various computational tools and techniques and the parameters to estimate the performance of the proposed model are discussed briefly here.

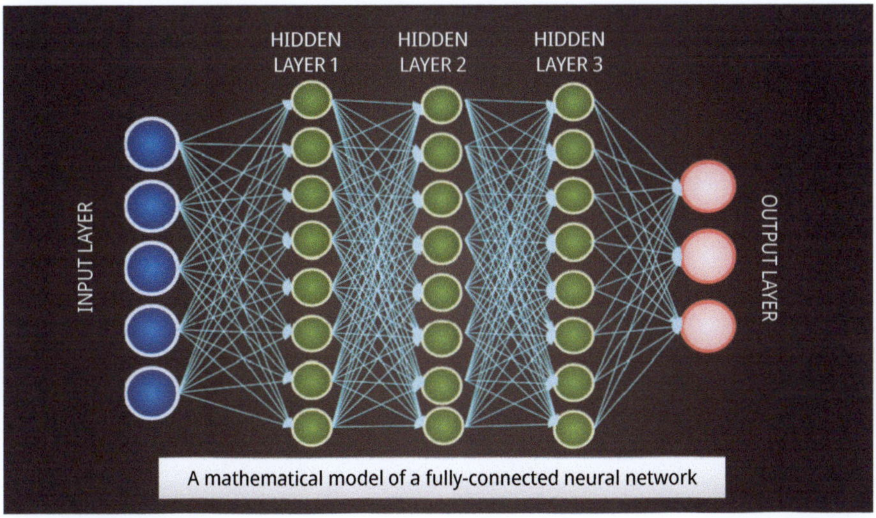

Figure 6: Neural networks.

4.1 Image classification

Image classification sequentially performs the tasks of image pre-processing (normalization), image segmentation, extraction of important features, and identification of the class to identify and classify the target object/image. CNN has revolutionized the field of image classification by being able to learn the basic geometry in the initial layers and developing to learn and extract key features in the deeper layers, resulting in more accurate classification of images.

4.2 Histogram of oriented gradient, local binary pattern, oriented FAST and rotated BRIEF, and support vector machine

Features can be extended by various techniques, namely histogram of oriented gradients (HoG), oriented FAST and rotated BRIEF (ORB), and local binary pattern (LBP). The feature descriptor tool HoG is very popular for extracting features from images. HOG calculates the instances of gradient orientation in local parts of an image. LBP [32] is a computationally simple and efficient texture descriptor used to define the local texture patterns of an image by thresholding the neighbors of each pixel and considering the result as a binary numeral. Harmonization of the modified version of the visual descriptor binary robust-independent elementary features (BRIEF) and the features from the accelerated segment test (FAST) keypoint detector is called the ORB. The features extracted by HOG, LBP, and ORB feature extractors from a COVID-19-positive delta variant diagnosed chest X-ray are shown in Figure 9.

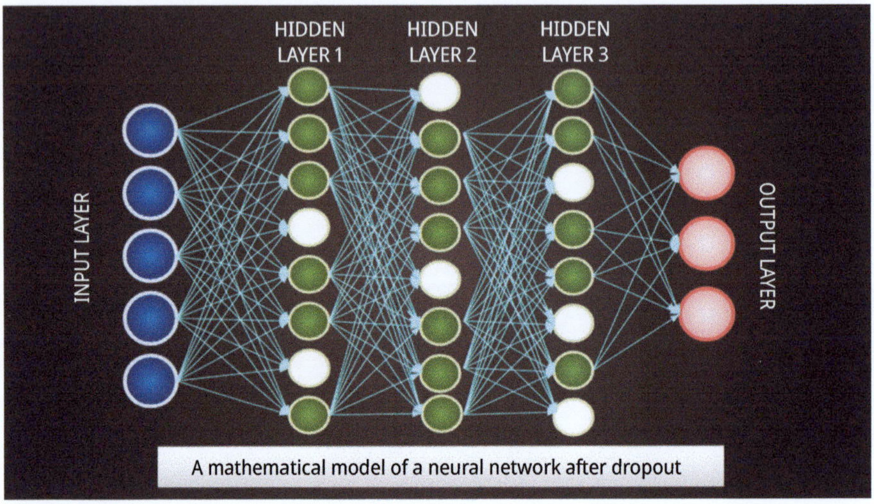

Figure 7: Neural networks after dropout.

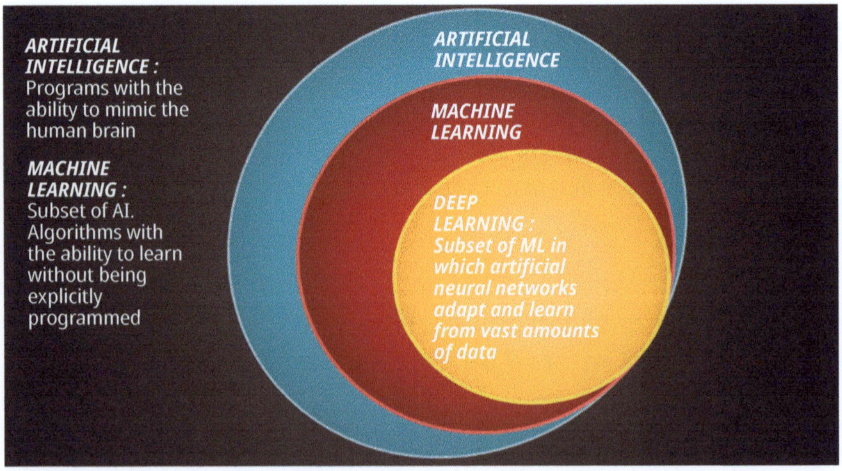

Figure 8: Relationship between artificial intelligence, machine learning, and deep learning.

A SVM is a supervised machine learning algorithm. It finds widespread applications in tasks of classification and regression. SVM can perform both linear and nonlinear classification. The kernel function is used to perform nonlinear classification. SVM performs well when kernels and the parameters of the kernels are selected properly.

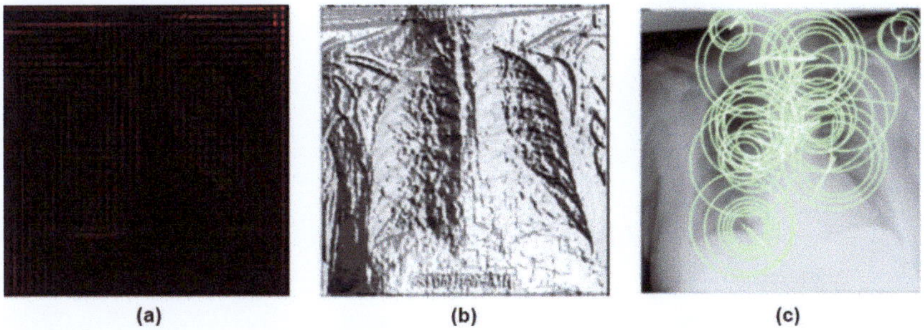

Figure 9: Illustration of features extracted by (a) HOG, (b) LBP, and (c) ORB feature extractors from a delta variant chest X-ray.

4.3 Performance metrics of a classification model

Different performance metrics are used to evaluate different algorithms. In the classification task, metrics like categorical-cross-entropy-loss, precision, F_1-score, and accuracy can be used. The following parameters are essential for defining the various performance metrics.

- **True positive:** In this case, both the actual and predicted classes of the data are true, that is, 1. It is a case of true positive (TP) when the person is truly COVID-19 positive and the model classifies his/her case as COVID-19 positive.
- **True negative:** In this case, both the actual and predicted classes of the data are false, that is, 0. It is a case of true negative (TN) when the person is COVID-19 negative and the model classifies his/her case as COVID-19 negative.
- **False positive:** In this case, the actual class of the data is false but the predicted class of the data is true (1). It is known as false-positive (FP) as the model has predicted incorrectly the case to be a positive one. Here when a COVID-19-negative person is predicted by the model as COVID-19 positive then it's an FP case.
- **False negative:** In this case, the actual class of the data is true (1) but the predicted class of the data is false (0). It is known as false-negative (FN) as the model has predicted incorrectly the case to be a negative one. Here when a COVID-19-positive person is predicted by the model as COVID-19 negative then it is an FN case.

In an ideal scenario the model should give zero FP and zero FN. The metrics used in the proposed work are:

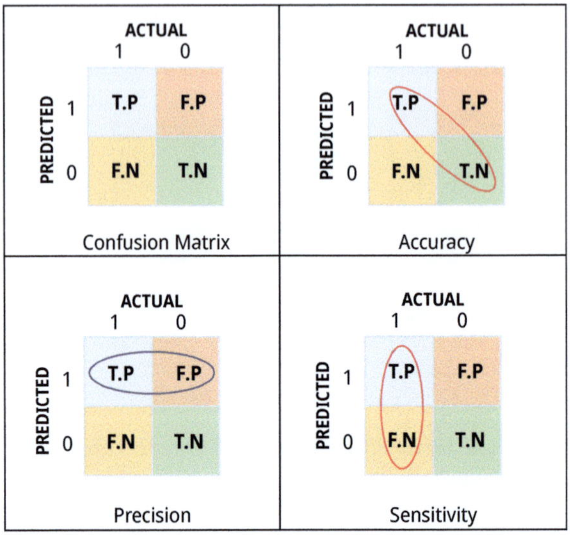

Figure 10: Confusion matrix, accuracy, precision, and sensitivity.

1. Confusion matrix

Labeling the target variables: COVID-19 positive as 1 and COVID-19 negative as 0. The confusion matrix as shown in Figure 10 is a two-dimensional table that allows one to visualize the performance of a model.

2. Accuracy

In any classification problem, accuracy, as shown in Figure 10, determines the number of accurate predictions produced by the model. It is calculated as follows:

$$\text{Accuracy} = \frac{\text{TN} + \text{TP}}{\text{FN} + \text{FP} + \text{TN} + \text{TP}} \tag{1}$$

When the data is balanced as in the proposed case, accuracy is a good measure.

3. Precision

Precision is a quantity that represents the degree of excellence of a positive prediction, that is, in this case it gives the proportion of patients detected with COVID-19 actually being COVID-19 positive. As can be seen from Figure 10, precision can be defined as follows:

$$\text{Precision} = \frac{\text{TP}}{\text{FP} + \text{TP}} \tag{2}$$

4. Recall or sensitivity

Recall tells what proportion of the X-rays that actually were COVID-19 positive was diagnosed by the model as COVID-19 positive. As can be seen from Figure 10, recall can be calculated as follows:

$$\text{Recall} = \frac{\text{TP}}{\text{FN} + \text{TP}} \tag{3}$$

5. F_1-score

F_1-score is a measure that incorporates both precision and accuracy. It is calculated as follows:

$$F_1\text{-score} = \frac{2 \times \text{Precision} \times \text{Recall}}{\text{Precision} + \text{Recall}} = \frac{\text{TP}}{\text{TP} + \frac{\text{FN}}{2} + \frac{\text{FP}}{2}} \tag{4}$$

5 Proposed algorithm

A smarter, high-accuracy COVID-19 detection algorithm is required to cater to the increased demand for faster and more accurate testing. Moreover, as several variants of COVID-19 have surfaced all over the world variant detection has become increasingly important for proper diagnosis. The proposed algorithm provides a solution for these two problems. The algorithm is outlined in two stages. In the first stage, COVID-19 detection is done. If a patient is COVID-19 positive, the algorithm moves to the second stage, where the variant of COVID-19 is detected. The presented algorithm is encapsulated in Algorithm 1.

Algorithm 1 Proposed algorithm

1: **Input**: Chest X-ray Image
2: **Stage 1**: Check if the image is COVID positive
3: **if** COVID positive **then**
4: Display message: **"Covid Positive"**
5: Go to **Stage 2**
6: **Stage 2**: Check for COVID variant
7: Display message: **"Covid variant is XY"** d XY may be Omicron or Delta or Alpha
8: **else**
9: COVID Negative
10: Display message: **"Covid Negative"**
11: **end if** 12: Input next chest X-ray image

To make the process faster, the proposed algorithm does not create very deep neural networks as they have the inherent issue of vanishing gradients while training. The first stage of the proposed model has been designed inspired by the ResNet50 which is neither too shallow nor too deep. In the second stage, variant detection is done by extracting spatial and handcrafted features from the COVID-19-positive images and forming a vocabulary of features vector from the features that have been extracted. The spatial features are being extracted using the first-stage image classifier and the handcrafted features are extracted using HoG, ORB, and LBP feature extractors. The vocabulary of features vector is used by a classifier to make the final decision of the variant type, that is, omicron, delta, or alpha.

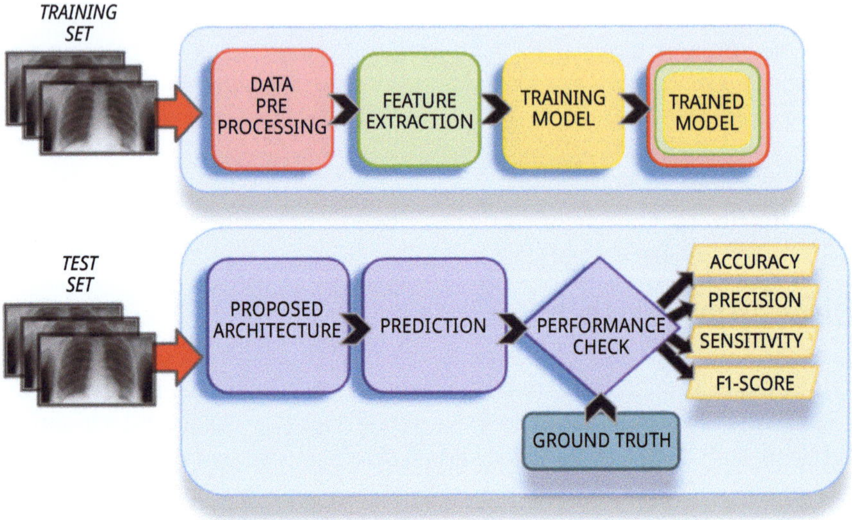

Figure 11: Block diagram of the proposed model, stage 1.

6 Model architecture

To develop an algorithm for the detection of COVID-19, various state-of-art classification models like VGG-16 [33], MobileNets [34], and InceptionV3 [3], were implemented on the dataset created. The performance obtained by those models is presented in Table 1. From Table 1 it can be inferred that ResNet50 [35] model gave the best precision of 97.8%. To further improve the performance, the authors then developed a 16-layer CNN model for classification. The layers of the proposed model are given in Table 2. Finally, the best out of the commonly used classification model, that is, ResNet50 and the 16-layer CNN model were combined to get the desired model.

Stages 1 and 2 of the suggested algorithm are demonstrated in Figures 12 and 13, respectively. Stage 1 is the classification model and it works in two phases, that is, training and testing. The block diagram of stage 1 is shown in Figure 11. The model in the first step is trained using a large number of images. After the training stage, testing is done and their performances are calculated by comparing with ground truth.

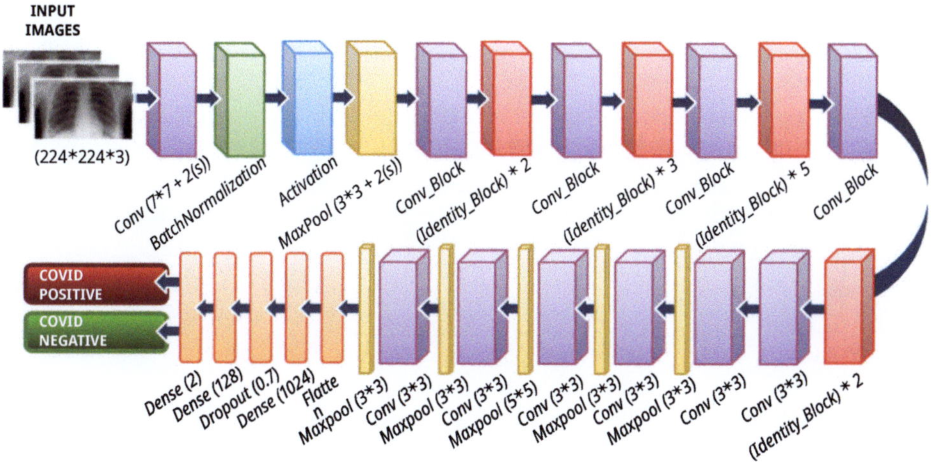

Figure 12: Proposed model: stage 1, that is, COVID detection stage.

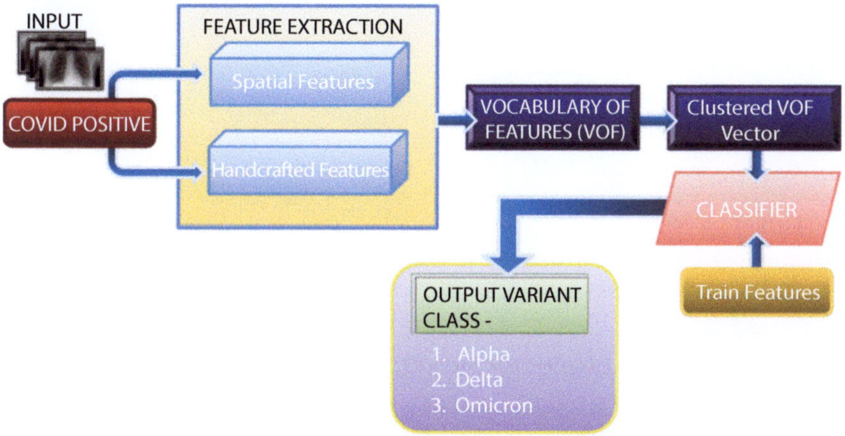

Figure 13: Convolutional and identity block.

It can be seen from Figure 11 that before implementation of the actual algorithm, preprocessing of the images is done. In this step, all the input gray-scale images which are usually of different sizes are resized into 224 × 224 pixels and then replicated in red, green, and blue planes to form an RGB-scale image of size 224 × 224 × 3. Then the images are passed to the first stage of the proposed model whose initial layers resemble the ResNet50 model. Skip connections as shown in Figure 14 are used in this model to overcome the gradients back-propagation while training, that is, the diminishing gradient issue. There are two shortcut modules in implementation, that is, an identity block and the convolution block. In the case of the identity block, the input has an identical dimension to the output. In the convolution block, which has a

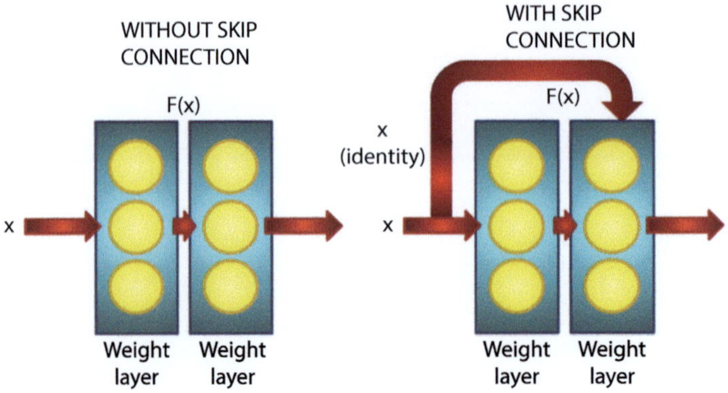

Figure 14: Skip connection illustration.

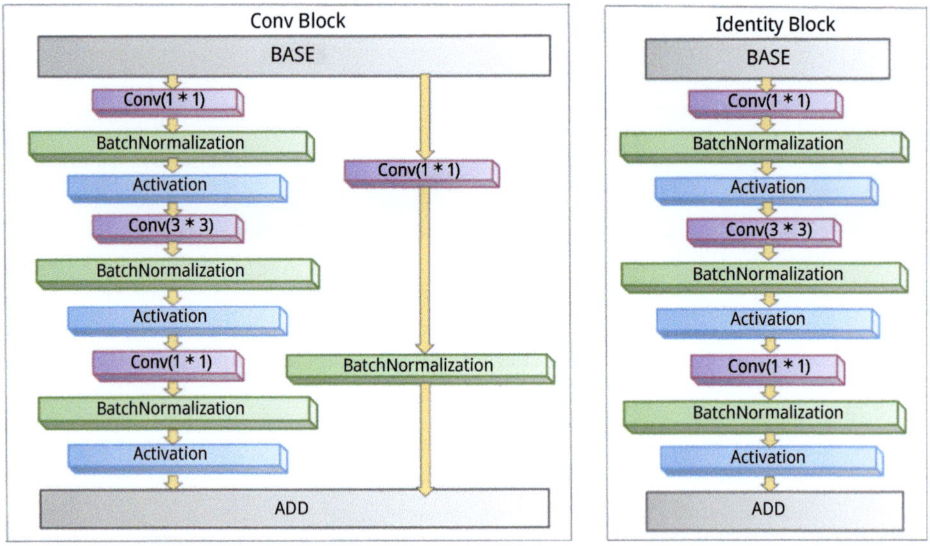

Figure 15: Convolutional and identity block.

Table 1: Performance comparison.

Model	Patient status	F_1-score	Recall	Precision
VGG-16	Positive	0.92	0.98	0.86
	Negative	0.94	0.96	0.93
InceptionV3	Positive	0.31	0.3	0.32
	Negative	0.52	0.5	0.55
MobileNetV2	Positive	0.68	0.88	0.56
	Negative	0.41	0.26	0.92

Table 1 (continued)

Model	Patient status	F_1-score	Recall	Precision
Densenet201	Positive	0.87	0.9	0.86
	Negative	0.95	0.92	0.98
Xception	Positive	0.69	0.62	0.78
	Negative	0.87	0.93	0.81
Ours	Positive	0.99	0.99	0.99
	Negative	0.99	0.99	1.00

convolution layer, the input dimensions are lesser than the output dimensions. Convolution layers of size 1 × 1 are added to both the blocks at the beginning and end of the network to implement the bottleneck design approach. The identity and convolution blocks are demonstrated in Figure 15.

Table 2: Layers of the first stage of the proposed algorithm.

Layer (type)	Param #	Connected to
input_1 (InputLayer)	–	–
Resnet 50 (50 layers)	23587712	input_1[0][0]
Conv_2d (Conv2D)	589856	conv5_block3_out[0][0]
Conv_2d_1 (Conv2D)	9248	Conv_2d[0][0]
max_pooling_2d (MaxPooling2D)	0	Conv_2d_1[0][0]
Conv_2d_2 (Conv2D)	18496	max_pooling_2d[0][0]
max_pooling_2d_1 (MaxPooling2D)	0	Conv_2d_2[0][0]
Conv_2d_3 (Conv2D)	73856	max_pooling_2d_1[0][0]
max_pooling_2d_2 (MaxPooling2D)	0	Conv_2d_3[0][0]
Conv_2d_4 (Conv2D)	73792	max_pooling_2d_2[0][0]
max_pooling_2d_3 (MaxPooling2D)	0	Conv_2d_4[0][0]
Conv_2d_5 (Conv2D)	18464	max_pooling_2d_3[0][0]
max_pooling_2d_4 (MaxPooling2D)	0	Conv_2d_5[0][0]
flatten (Flatten)	0	max_pooling_2d_4[0][0]
dense (Dense)	33792	flatten[0][0]
dropout (Dropout)	0	dense[0][0]
dense_1 (Dense)	131200	dropout[0][0]
dense_2 (Dense)	258	dense_1[0][0]

The proposed network does not follow the traditional approach of neural networks, that is, does not directly feed one layer to the next layer. The various layers of the presented architecture are shown in Table 2. If neural networks were actually universal function approximates, then they will have the ability to learn any simple or complex function which is not the case. So, in the proposed network extra layers have been skipped and the accuracy of the shallow sub-networks has been matched.

Pre-activation and batch normalization have been used as they give the best results. The batch normalization speeds up the training process and reduces the dependency on good weight initialization. Most of the convolution layers used in this work have a 3×3 filter size. Using larger kernels can turn out to be more expensive both in terms of computation and parameters. The first 50 layers resemble those of ResNet 50 with trainable parameters. The output of the 50th layer, that is, the identity block is fed to the simple CNN-based 16 layers. The hyper-parameters of the final 16 layers have been tuned to give optimal performance.

For the last 16 layers comprising the convolutional and max-pooling layers, the number of filters has been increased while decreasing the spatial feature map size at the same time so that too much information is not lost at a time. Finally, the outputs of the previous layer are flattened and fed to a dense layer consisting of 1,024 neurons and 70% of the input units have been randomly set to 0 at each step during training time to prevent overfitting. Then it is fed into a dense layer consisting of 128 neurons and ReLu activation (5) has been used for those neurons:

$$\begin{aligned} \text{ReLu}(x) &= x \text{ if } x \geq 0 \\ \text{otherwise ReLu}(x) &= 0 \end{aligned} \tag{5}$$

Finally the outputs of the previous dense layer are passed on to the final dense layer consisting of two neurons with softmax activation given as follows:

$$\sigma(\underline{x})_a = \frac{\exp x_a}{\sum_{b=1}^{k} \exp x_b} \tag{6}$$

where σ is the soft-max activation, $(\underline{x})_a$ is the input vector, exp x_a is the exponential function for $(\underline{x})_a$, K the number of classifier classes, and exp x_a is the exponential of the output vector. For the present case, the classifier is binary so $K = 2$. For the given class of the X-ray images, the softmax layer gives output 1 if COVID-19 positive gives 0. On classification of the X-ray image into COVID-19 positive, the image moves as an input to the next stage of the algorithm, that is, the stage that classifies it as omicron or delta or alpha variant.

The second stage of the presented model extracts features from the COVID-19 positive chest X-rays using HoG, LBP, and ORB. The spatial features are extracted using the proposed CNN-based model as described. Then a feature vector is formed using the normalized extracted features as a combination of handcrafted features extracted using the HoG, ORB, and LBP feature extractors in addition to spatial features. Then this feature vector is applied to an SVM classifier to get the final prediction, that is, whether the COVID-19-positive image is that of delta (B.1.617.2) or omicron (B.1.1.529) or alpha (B.1.1.7) variant.

7 Data preparation and partitioning

For developing and demonstrating the effectiveness of the DL algorithm, the images have to be partitioned into train and test sets. The partition is done randomly and in the ratio of 7:3, as is the norm to negate any possible sampling bias. The dataset was created by collecting images from various sources including [36–38] IEEE8023 [39, 40]. The test dataset consists of 948 COVID-19-negative chest radiograph images and 550 COVID-19-positive chest radiograph images out of which 455, 89, and 6 chest radiograph images are of alpha, delta, and omicron variants, respectively. As the dataset size is small, image augmentation has been done by flipping the chest X-rays. The first stage was trained over 75 epochs and the loss of the model over the epochs is demonstrated in Figure 16.

The COVID-19-positive images were passed on to the second stage and features were extracted using HoG, ORB, and LBP descriptors along with the spatial features extracted through the model proposed in atage 1. The test train split was used and the X-ray images of the chest consisting of alpha, delta, and omicron variants were again randomly split in the ratio of 7:3.

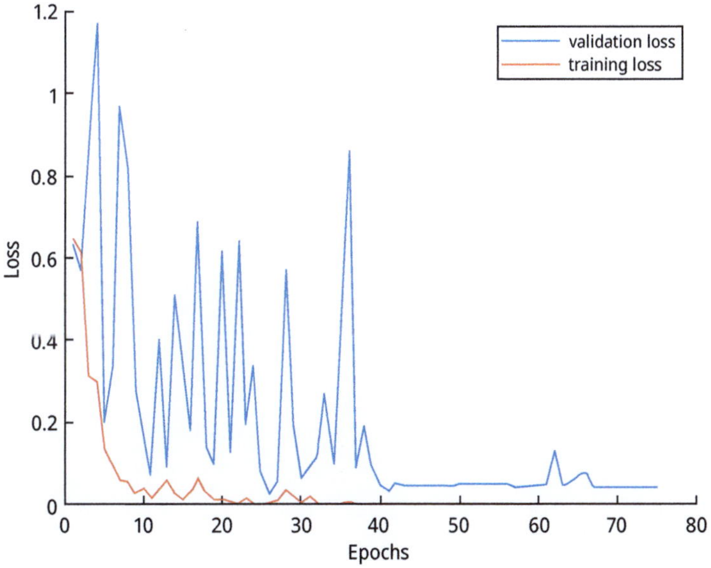

Figure 16: Training and validation loss of stage 1.

8 Results and discussions

The model was simulated in Jupyter Notebook on Lenovo Ideapad 330 with Intel(R) having Core(TM) i5-8250U CPU with a 1.60 GHz clock frequency having a 1.80 GHz processor and an 8 GB RAM. Stochastic-gradient descent is used as an optimizer and the code has been trained over 75 epochs with a batch size of 32 as trainable hyper-parameters.

The obtained training and validation accuracy for the proposed model are shown in Figure 22 and the comparison with various state of art models are shown in Figure 17 and Figure 18. The comparison in terms of training loss (Figure 19), and validation loss (Figure 20) for the COVID-19 detection stage are also presented.

The performance metrics which were calculated for the first stage had considered COVID-19 positive as class 1 and COVID-19 negative or normal chest X-ray as class 0. The model gives a training accuracy of 100% and a validation accuracy of 99.47% on our dataset which has been constructed from the patients of eastern India. The confusion matrix (discussed in 4.3) for the proposed first stage is shown in Figure 21a. It may be inferred from the given confusion matrix in Figure 21a that 1 FP and 0 FN cases have been obtained.

Figure 16 shows the validation and training accuracy of the first stage. In the proposed model, the stage has been trained over 75 epochs considering no over-fitting in the range. The proposed first stage of the model gives an accuracy of 0.9947 for the classification task.

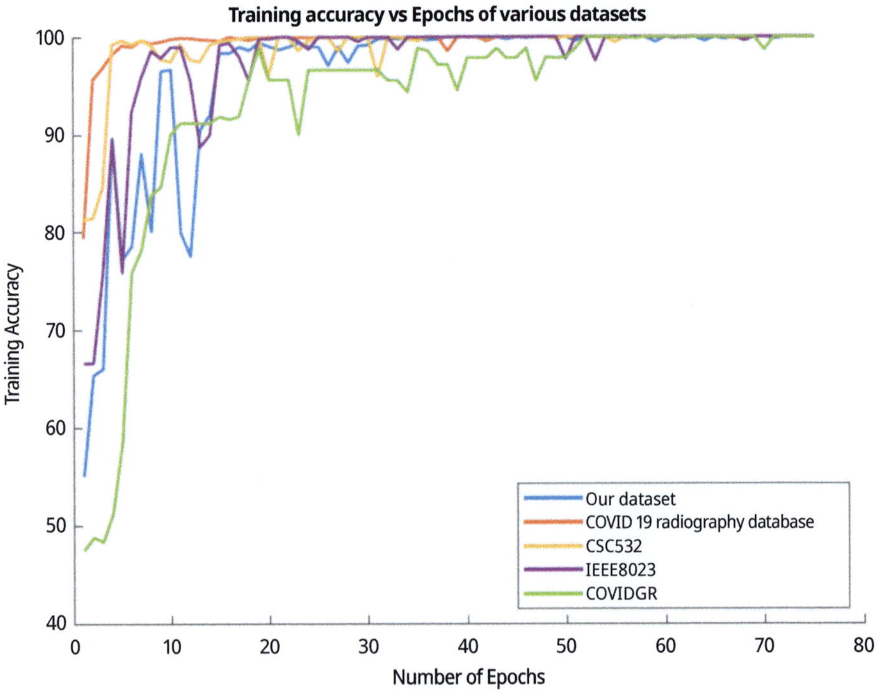

Figure 17: Training accuracy of stage 1 on various datasets.

This high value could be achieved by the right selection of filters, layers, and hyperparameters. The training and validation accuracy obtained over the epochs is demonstrated qualitatively in Figure 17. Table 3 gives the different performance metrics utilized

Table 3: Stage 1 performance measures' comparison of the proposed model.

Patient status	Recall	Precision	F_1-score
COVID negative	0.98	1.00	0.99
COVID positive	1.00	0.99	1.00

Table 4: Macro- and weighted average performance of the first stage.

	Recall	Precision	F_1-score
Macro-average	0.99	1.00	0.99
Weighted average	0.99	0.99	0.99

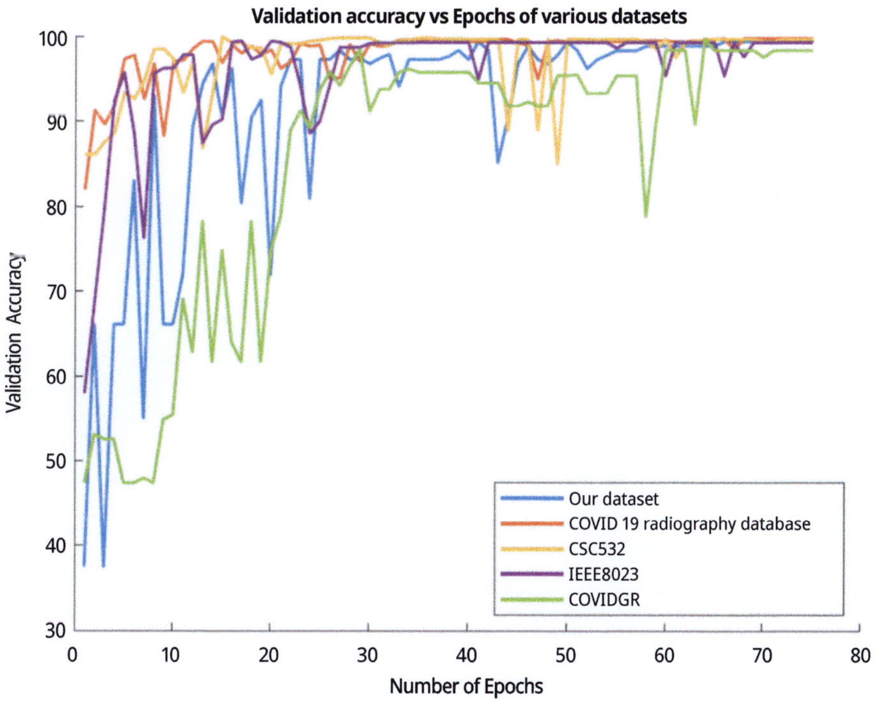

Figure 18: Validation accuracy of stage 1 on various datasets.

by the current algorithm and Table 4 demonstrates the Macro- and weighted average performance of the COVID-19 detection. From Table 3 it can be seen that precision of 1 on COVID-19-negative cases and 0.99 on COVID-positive cases have been obtained. A recall of 0.98 for COVID-19-negative and 1 for COVID-19-positive cases, respectively, has been observed. F_1-score has also been used as a parameter and the values of the F_1-score are 0.99 and 1 for negative and positive cases, respectively, for COVID-19-variant detection.

The training and validation losses obtained for the first stage concerning epochs can be visualized in Figure 16. A performance comparison with other recently proposed models is presented in Table 6. From Table 6 it can be seen that the first stage of the proposed model offers superior performances compared to other models. The comparison is also presented in Figure 23.

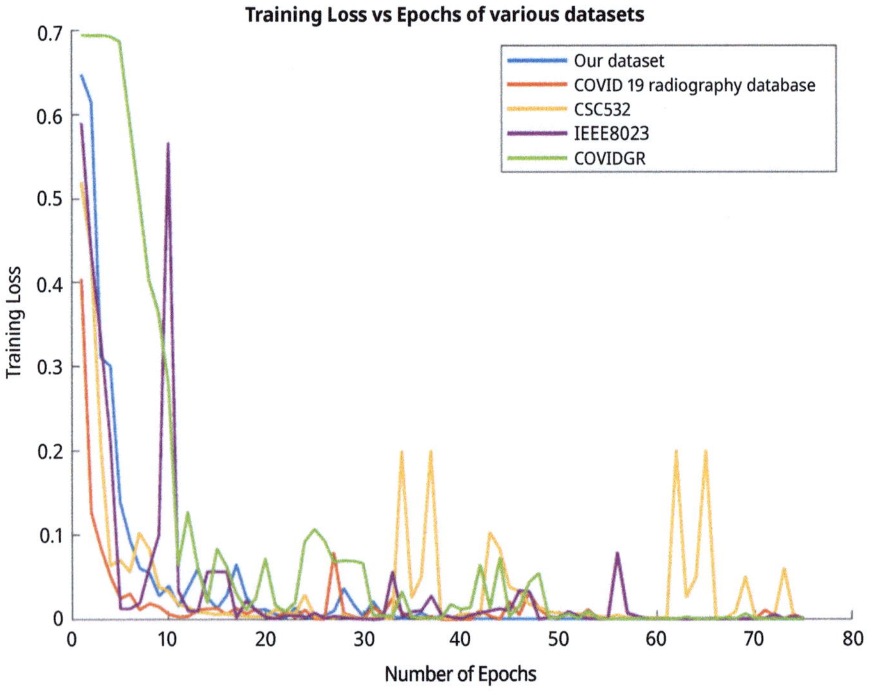

Figure 19: Training loss of stage 1 on various datasets.

Table 5: Stage 2 performance measures of the proposed model.

Variant	Precision	Recall	F_1-score
Alpha	1	1	1
Delta	1	0.96	0.98
Omicron	1	1	1

The confusion matrix for the second stage is given in Figure 21b. An accuracy of 98.46% for the multi-class classification task for this stage, that is, the variant classification stage has been obtained. The precision, F_1-score, and recall for the alpha, delta, and omicron variants are given in Table 5. A precision of 100% has been obtained for all the variants considered. The prediction accuracy can be increased further with more data for training. Here accuracy values are affected due to a lack of sufficient data.

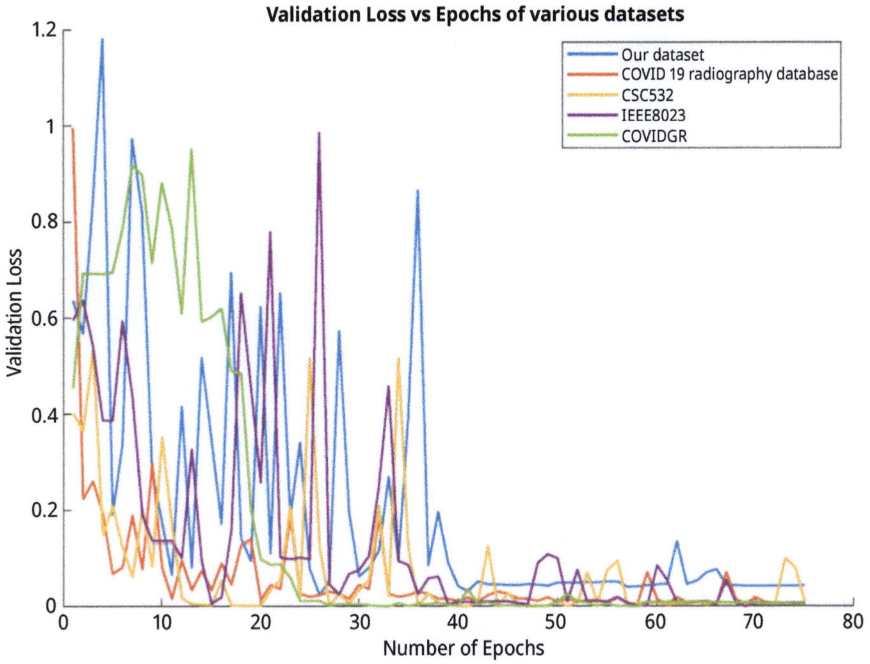

Figure 20: Validation loss of stage 1 on various datasets.

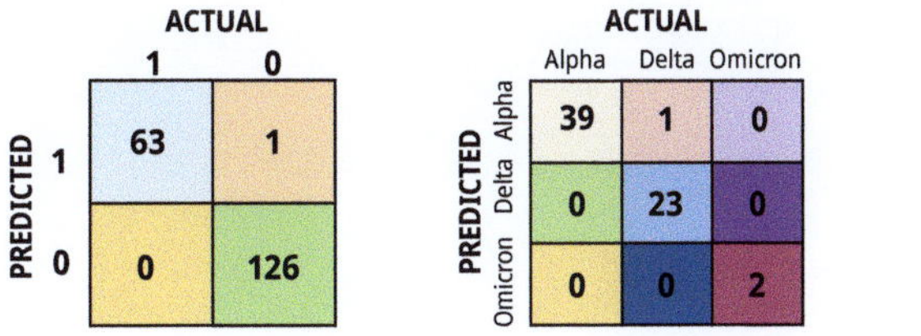

(a) Proposed model (b) Variant of concern classification

Figure 21: Confusion matrix.

9 Conclusions and scope of future works

In the present work a two-stage model to identify COVID-19 and classify it into different variants of concern from X-ray images has been proposed. The method proposed here achieved 99.47% and 98.46% accuracy of the COVID-19 detection stage and COVID-19 variant (alpha, delta, omicron) classification stage, respectively. The model proposed here has been demonstrated to achieve superior performance for COVID-19 detection along with its variant of concern detection in comparison to the existing works. The accuracy of variant detection can be improved by using a larger dataset. As the researchers could procure test and training images of limited variants of COVID-19 the suitability of the proposed algorithm to detect the other variants could not be tested. It is conjectured that the algorithm can be extended to detect other strains of COVID-19 like beta and gamma. With the advent of newer strains of COVID-19 almost periodically the application of the proposed algorithm to detect newer COVID-19 variants will be an interesting research area.

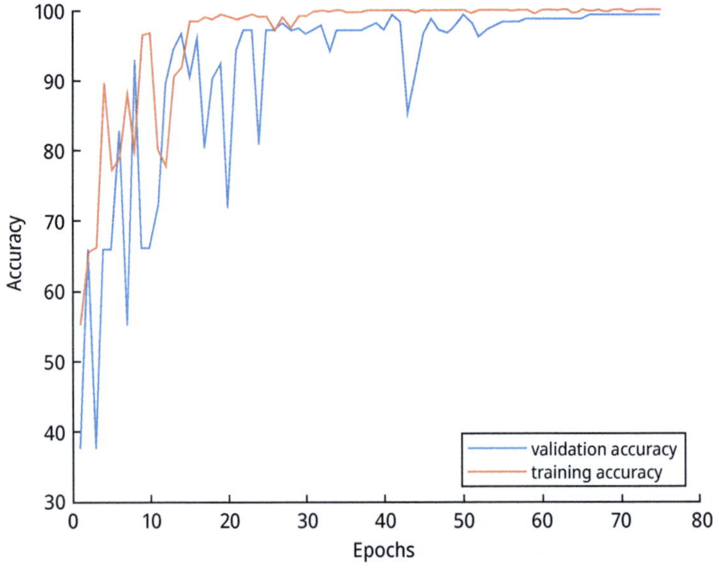

Figure 22: Training and validation accuracy of first stage.

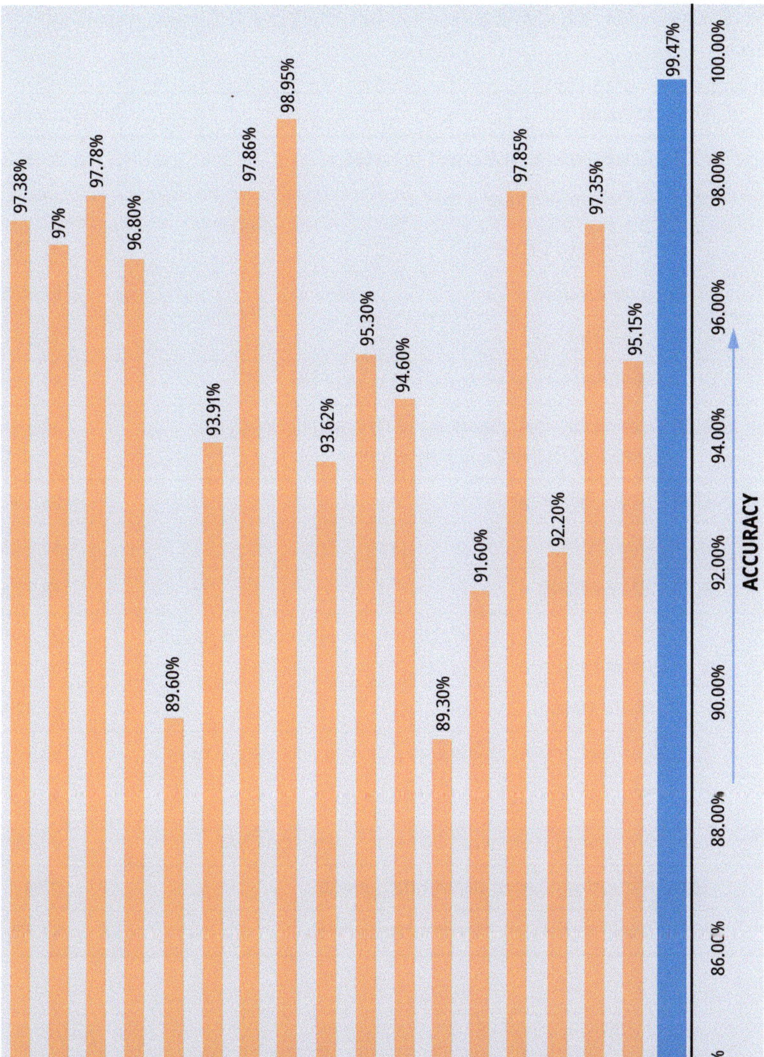

Figure 23: Other algorithms vs proposed algorithm.

Table 6: Comparison of various recent algorithms on our dataset of the COVID-19 detection stage with respect to performance.

Author	Year	Method	Accuracy (%)
Abbas et al. [20]	2021	Decompose, transfer, and compose	95.15%
Narin et al. [29]	2021	ResNet50 and ResNet101	97.35%
Albahli et al. [22]	2021	Pre-trained DenseNet	92.2%
Ozturk et al. [23]	2020	DarkCovidNet	97.85%
Wang and Wong [10]	2020	Covid-Net	91.6%
Xu et al. [41]	2020	Modified version of ResNet-18 using CNN	89.3%
Apostolopoulos et al. [42]	2020	transfer learning based on VGG19, MobileNetV2, Xception, ResNetV2, and Inception	94.6%
Sethy et al. [5]	2020	SVM + ResNet50	95.3%
Hemdan et al. [7]	2020	COVIDX-NET	93.62%
Hussain et al. [11]	2021	22-layer CNN	98.95%
Shankar et al. [28]	2021	barnacle mating optimization + cascade recurrent neural network	97.86%
Ahsan et al. [8]	2020	NasNetMobile	93.91%
Khan et al. [24]	2020	CoroNet: A DNN model based on Xception architecture	89.6%
Mahmud et al. [9]	2020	CovXNet: A multi-dilation CNN model	96.8%
Khasawneh et al. [25]	2021	Pre-trained customized DL models based on CNN	97.78%
Tuncer et al. [26]	2021	F-transform-based classification model	97%
Jamil et al. [31]	2021	Dual-stage vocabulary of features (VoF)	97.38%

References

[1] https://www.worldometers.info/coronavirus/

[2] Huang, G., Liu, Z., van der Maaten, L., Weinberger, K. Q. Densely connected convolutional networks. arXiv, 2016. https://doi.org/10.48550/ARXIV.1608.06993. https://arxiv.org/abs/1608.06993.

[3] Szegedy, C., Vanhoucke, V., Ioffe, S., Shlens, J., & Wojna, Z. (2016). Rethinking the inception architecture for computer vision. *2016 IEEE Conference on Computer Vision and Pattern Recognition (CVPR)*. https://doi.org/10.1109/cvpr.2016.308

[4] A diagnostic model for coronavirus disease 2019 (COVID-19) based on radiological semantic and clinical features: A multi-center study. https://doi.org/10.1007/s00330-020-06829-2

[5] Sethy, P. K., Behera, S. K. Detection of coronavirus disease (COVID-19) based on deep features. Preprints, 2020. 2020030300. doi: 10.20944/preprints202003.0300.v1.

[6] MZ, Che Azemin, et al. "COVID-19 Deep Learning Prediction Model Using Publicly Available Radiologist-Adjudicated Chest X-Ray Images as Training Data: Preliminary Findings." International Journal of Biomedical Imaging 2020 (2020): 8828855–8828855.
[7] Hemdan, Ezz El-Din, Marwa A. Shouman, and Mohamed Esmail Karar. "Covidx-net: A framework of deep learning classifiers to diagnose covid-19 in x-ray images." *arXiv preprint arXiv:2003.11055* (2020).
[8] Ahsan, M. M., Gupta, K. D., Islam, M. M., Sen, S., Rahman, M. L., Shakhawat Hossain, M. Covid-19 symptoms detection based on nasnet- mobile with explainable ai using various imaging modalities. Machine Learning and Knowledge Extraction, 2020, 2(4), 490–504. https://doi.org/10.3390/make2040027.
[9] Mahmud, T., Rahman, M. A., Fattah, S. A. Covxnet: A multi-dilation convolutional neural network for automatic covid-19 and other pneumo- nia detection from chest x-ray images with transferable multi-receptive feature optimization. Computers in Biology and Medicine, 2020, 122, 103869. https://doi.org/10.1016/j.compbiomed.2020.103869.
[10] Wang, L., Lin, Z. Q., Wong, A. Covid-net: A tailored deep convolutional neural network design for detection of covid-19 cases from chest x-ray images. SciRep, 2020, 10, 19549.
[11] Hussain, E., Hasan, M., Rahman, M. A., Lee, I., Tamanna, T., Parvez, M. Z. Corodet: A deep learning based classification for covid-19 detection using chest x-ray images. Chaos, Solitons Fractals, 2021, 142, 110495. https://doi.org/10.1016/j.chaos.2020.110495.
[12] https://github.com/agchung/Figure1-COVID-chestxray-dataset
[13] Cohen, Joseph Paul, et al. "Covid-19 image data collection: Prospective predictions are the future." *arXiv preprint arXiv:2006.11988* (2020).
[14] https://www.kaggle.com/khoongweihao/covid19-xray-dataset-train-test-sets
[15] https://github.com/agchung/Actualmed-COVID-chestxray-dataset
[16] https://github.com/UCSD-AI4H/COVID-CT
[17] https://www.kaggle.com/plameneduardo/sarscov2-ctscan-dataset
[18] https://www.kaggle.com/nabeelsajid917/covid-19-x-ray-10000-images
[19] https://www.kaggle.com/tawsifurrahman/covid19-radiography-database
[20] Classification of COVID-19 in chest X-ray images using DeTraC deep con- volutional neural network. https://doi.org/10.1007/s10489-020-01829-7
[21] Ucar, F., Korkmaz, D. COVIDiagnosis-Net: Deep Bayes-SqueezeNet based diagnosis of the coronavirus disease 2019 (COVID-19) from X-ray images. Medical Hypotheses, 2020, 140, 109761.
[22] Albahli, S., Ayub, N., Shiraz, M. Coronavirus disease (COVID-19) de- tection using X-ray images and enhanced DenseNet. Applied Soft Comput, 2021, 110, 107645.
[23] Ozturk, T., Talo, M., Yildirim, E. A., Baloglu, U. B., Yildirim, O., Rajendra Acharya, U. Automated detection of covid-19 cases using deep neural networks with x-ray images. Computers in Biology and Medicine, 2020, 121, 103792. https://doi.org/10.1016/j.compbiomed.2020.103792.
[24] Khan, A. I., Shah, J. L., Bhat, M. M. Coronet: A deep neural network for detection and diagnosis of covid-19 from chest x-ray images. Computer Methods and Programs in Biomedicine, 2020, 196, 105581. https://doi.org/10.1016/j.cmpb.2020.105581.
[25] Khasawneh, N., Fraiwan, M., Fraiwan, L., Khassawneh, B., Ibnian, A. Detection of covid-19 from chest x-ray images using deep convolutional neural networks. Sensors, 2021, 21(17), https://doi.org/10.3390/s21175940.
[26] Tuncer, T., Ozyurt, F., Dogan, S., Subasi, A. A novel covid-19 and pneumonia classification method based on f-transform. Chemometrics and Intelligent Laboratory Systems, 2021, 210, 104256. https://doi.org/10.1016/j.chemolab.2021.104256.
[27] Chandra, T. B., Verma, K., Singh, B. K., Jain, D., Netam, S. S. Corona virus disease (covid-19) detection in chest x-ray images using majority voting based classifier ensemble. Expert Systems with Applications, 2021, 165, 113909. https://doi.org/10.1016/j.eswa.2020.113909.

[28] Shankar, K., Perumal, E., Díaz, V. G., Tiwari, P., Gupta, D., Saudagar, A. K. J., Muhammad, K. An optimal cascaded recurrent neural network for intelligent COVID-19 detection using Chest X-ray images. Applied Soft Computing, 2021, 113, 107878.
[29] Narin, A., Kaya, C., Pamuk, Z. Automatic detection of coronavirus disease (covid-19) using x-ray images and deep convolutional neural networks. Pattern Analysis and Applications, 2021, 24(3), 1207–1220. https://doi.org/10.1007/s10044-021-00984-y.
[30] Szegedy, Christian, et al. "Inception-v4, inception-resnet and the impact of residual connections on learning." Proceedings of the AAAI conference on artificial intelligence. Vol. 31. No. 1. 2017.
[31] Jamil, S., Rahman, M. A dual-stage vocabulary of features (vof)-based technique for covid-19 variantsrsquo; classification. Applied Sciences, 2021, 11(24), https://doi.org/10.3390/app112411902.
[32] Ojala, T., Pietikainen, M., Maenpaa, T. Multiresolution gray-scale and rotation invariant texture classification with local binary patterns. IEEE Transactions on Pattern Analysis and Machine Intelligence, 2002, 24(7), 971–987. https://doi.org/10.1109/TPAMI.2002.1017623.
[33] Simonyan, Karen, and Andrew Zisserman. "Very deep convolutional networks for large-scale image recognition." *arXiv preprint arXiv:1409.1556* (2014).
[34] Howard, Andrew G., et al. "Mobilenets: Efficient convolutional neural networks for mobile vision applications." *arXiv preprint arXiv:1704.04861* (2017).
[35] He, Kaiming, et al. "Deep residual learning for image recognition." Proceedings of the IEEE conference on computer vision and pattern recognition. 2016.
[36] Bell, D. J. Covid-19: Radiology reference article. Radiopaedia.org, 2022. https://radiopaedia.org/ar ticles/covid-19-4?lang=us
[37] Rahman, T. Covid-19 radiography database, 2021. https://www.kaggle.com/tawsifurrahman/covid19-radiography-database
[38] Cohen, J. P., Morrison, P., Dao, L. Covid-19 image data collection. arXiv 2003.11597, 2020.
[39] Tabik, Siham, et al. "COVIDGR dataset and COVID-SDNet methodology for predicting COVID-19 based on chest X-ray images." IEEE journal of biomedical and health informatics 24.12 (2020): 3595–3605.
[40] https://www.kaggle.com/c/dlai3
[41] Xu, X., Jiang, X., Ma, C., Du, P., Li, X., Lv, S., Yu, L., Ni, Q., Chen, Y., Su, J., Lang, G., Li, Y., Zhao, H., Liu, J., Xu, K., Ruan, L., Sheng, J., Qiu, Y., Wu, W., Liang, T., Li, L. A deep learning system to screen novel coronavirus disease 2019 pneumonia. Engineering, 2020, 6(10), 1122–1129. https://doi.org/10.1016/j.eng.2020.04.010.
[42] Covid-19: automatic detection from X-ray images utilizing transfer learning with convolutional neural networks. doi: 10.1007/s13246-020-00865-4.

Kamarajan Rajagopalan, Aarya Senan Surasenan,
Aparna Ramakrishnan, Harsha Haridasan,
Johnson Retnaraj Samuel Selvan Christyraj*,
Jackson Durairaj Selvan Christyraj*

Computational genomic sequencing and its importance for identifying the emerging variants of COVID-19

Abstract: About 27 crores of people were affected worldwide by coronavirus disease, which was caused by novel severe acute respiratory syndrome coronavirus 2 (SARS-CoV-2). Understanding the evolutions and pathogenesis of virus is a key for the control of COVID-19, which can be accomplished by computational genome sequencing. The genome sequence of SARS-CoV-2 was instantly discovered and distributed on GenBank (MN908947.3). Many strains are evaluated because of the mutations in the genome of the virus. However, most of the exposed strains' (alpha, beta, gamma, delta, epsilon, zeta, eta, lambda, kappa, theta, omicron, and lota) sequences and lineages of concern resources were rapidly determined by next-generation sequencing (NGS) and shared on bioinformatics databases like BV-BRC BETA. Illumina NGS sequencing consists of four major steps such as sample preparation, cluster generation, sequencing, and data analysis. NGS presents an efficient unbiased way to classify the new strains of COVID-19 as well as provides an opportunity for the tracking of global transmission route of virus, detection of mutations to prevent the spread of new strains, reduce the use of molecular diagnostics assays, target screening for possible therapeutics, and characterization of co-infections, potent phenotype, therapeutic strategy, and genetic relatedness. In this chapter, we have covered advancements in technical aspects and the platforms for SARS-CoV-2 computational genome sequencing.

***Corresponding author: Jackson Durairaj Selvan Christyraj**, Regeneration and Stem Cell Biology Lab, Centre for Molecular and Nanomedical Sciences, International Research Centre, Sathyabama Institute of Science and Technology (Deemed to be University), Chennai, Tamil Nadu, India, e-mail: jacksondurairaj@sathyabama.ac.in

***Corresponding author: Johnson Retnaraj Samuel Selvan Christyraj**, Regeneration and Stem Cell Biology Lab, Centre for Molecular and Nanomedical Sciences, International Research Centre, Sathyabama Institute of Science and Technology (Deemed to be University), Chennai, Tamil Nadu, India, e-mail: johnnbt@sathyabama.ac.in

Kamarajan Rajagopalan, Regeneration and Stem Cell Biology Lab, Centre for Molecular and Nanomedical Sciences, International Research Centre, Sathyabama Institute of Science and Technology (Deemed to be University), Chennai, Tamil Nadu, India

Aarya Senan Surasenan, Aparna Ramakrishnan, Harsha Haridasan, Department of Human genetics, Bharathiar University, Coimbatore, Tamil Nadu, India

https://doi.org/10.1515/9783110767681-005

1 Introduction

1.1 Computational genomics

To discover the genome sequences of both DNA and RNA for the in-depth study of genomes, computational and statistical analysis is utilized in computational genomics [1]. Machine learning and statistical reasoning are essential for the study of large data like the genome, and it allows us to study the structure, function, and evolutionary relationship of large data sets in a smaller time. It is a branch of bioinformatics and computational biology but it focused on the whole genome [2].

Technical developments and the platforms for severe acute respiratory syndrome coronavirus 2 (SARS-CoV-2) computational genome sequencing have been addressed in this chapter. A technique to determine the complete genetic makeup of a certain organism or cell type is computational genomic sequencing. The two most popular genome sequencing techniques are clone-by-clone and whole-genome shotgun (WGS) sequencing. WGS approach is faster for sequencing but is not appropriate for bigger genomes like eukaryotic genomes. Over 90% of the worldwide sequencing data was produced by Illumina sequencing.

With no prior knowledge of the organisms, next-generation sequencing (NGS) offers a proactive, objective technique to identify new coronavirus strains and other infections. In order to stop the spread of novel strains, viral mutation identifications, and resistant strains, labs must swiftly uncover the track of transmission and detect mutations. NGS continues to provide public health officials, vaccine and medication manufacturers, and scientists with crucial signs. We can identify respiratory co-infections and antibiotic resistance alleles in therapeutic medicine and screen the precise correct targets for COVID-19.

1.2 Sequence alignment

Sequence alignment is a technique used in comparative genomics for the identification of homologous genes, mutations, structural and functional alterations within organisms by aligning homologous sequences or whole genome to find out the matches between sequences [3]. It can be pairwise alignment (compare two sequences) or multiple sequence alignment (compare multiple sequences at a time).

The terms "local alignment" and "global alignment" refer to two different sorts of alignments. Global alignment is called end–end alignment because it can able to align the entire sequence, and is suitable for aligning closely related sequences and homologous genes so the size should be equal. In local alignment, local regions of a sequence or a fragment of sequences with a high level of similarity are used for alignment. It is suitable for the alignment of more divergent and unrelated sequences, used to find out conserved patterns in DNA or protein sequences [4].

1.3 Dynamic programming

Finding the best matches in sequence alignment is a crucial step. In global alignment, the scoring scheme was used for the selection of best matches, but still, we cannot predict the deletion and insertions between sequences. Dynamic programming is introduced in 1953 by Richard Bellman [5]. In dynamic programming, we can solve a problem by breaking down into subproblems and adding the solutions at the end. It is a faster alignment algorithm and guarantees to find the best match between two sequences.

1.4 Needleman Wunsch algorithm

It was introduced in 1970 by Saul Needleman and Christian Wunsch as an application of dynamic programming. Two matrixes are required for this algorithm: score matrix and traceback matrix. Mainly three steps are involved:
- Setting up alignment matrix
- Scoring
- Identify the optimal path

Needleman–Wunsch algorithm is widely used for global alignment. It uses the tools EMBOSS and specialized BLAST [6].

1.5 High-performance computational biology

The introduction of computer technology into biology was a revolutionary step. During the beginning of the Human Genome Project, scientists faced a problem of availability of storage of data discovered and faster processing of data. It leads to the need for the introduction of high-performance computational biology. High-performance computation (HPC) can process large data and complex calculations at high speed. It can perform quadrillions of calculations per second. HPC is used in research labs, media, and entertainment, artificial intelligence, and machine learning [7].

1.6 Research contribution of computational biology

Biological concepts and information are made rigorous and accessible by computational biology. Additionally, it offers a reference framework that ties disparate individual insights together. When all the supporting data can be aggregated under one roof and a conclusion is arrived at, the research foundation is durable. By introducing statistics and data analytic techniques, computational biology transformed biology. Any research analysis needs large data collections, and thus the success of computational biology is therefore intimately correlated with the success of large-scale efforts to collect genotypes and phenotypes of model organisms and humans [8].

1.7 Comparative genomics

Comparative genomics aids in the conserved sequences identification and is a powerful tool for evolutionary study. It contributes to the development of drug designing, predicting unknown sequences by comparing with known sequences, finding genome evolutionary mechanisms, and early detection of genetic mutations in the embryonic stage.

1.8 What is genome made up of?

Genome is the genetic material of an organism made up of DNA or RNA. DNA is composed of nucleotides such as guanine, cytosine, adenine, and thymine (T). Thymine is replaced by uracil (U) in RNA and is single-stranded. The genetic material contains introns (nonexpressive sequence) and exons (expressive sequence) [9].

1.9 Which genomes are sequenced?

A total of 85,000 whole genomes are already sequenced. It includes mammals, birds, insects, other animals, and also bacteria and viruses. *Haemophilus influenzae* is the first organism to get a whole genome sequence, in 1995 [10]. The human genome project was an international project intended to map the complete genome of humans. It takes more than 13 years to complete [11].

1.10 How are genomes compared?

By global alignment, we can compare two genomes. Genomes were compared with one another based on their size, position of nucleotides, number of genes, and chromosomes [8].

1.11 Advancement in virus genome sequencing and application

The chances of getting mutations in the viral genome are higher in DNA viruses. The mutation ranges between 10^{-4} and 10^{-8} substitutions per nucleotide per cell infection (s/n/c), with DNA viruses occupying the 10^{-8}–10^{-6} range and RNA viruses the 10^{-6}–10^{-4} range [12]. So, the effective analysis of viruses is important for the identification of mutated viruses and their encoded functions. Computational tools are powerful for the identification of sequences and predict, annotate, and compare their functions. PCR amplicon sequencing, target enrichment sequencing, and metagenomic sequencing are the main viral genome sequencing methods. In metagenomics, the total DNA/RNA is collected from the host and sequenced by short gun sequencing. But in PCR amplicon enrichment, the viral DNA/RNA is amplified by PCR with primers. Target enrichment using whole viral genome is directly from a clinical sample [13].

1.12 SARS-CoV-2 genomics and evolutionary characteristics importance for genomic applications

SARS-CoV-2 is a virus from the *Betacoronavirus* genus, of the family Coronaviridae. It is a single-stranded positive-sense RNA virus [14]. Seven potential phylogenetic coronaviruses can infect humans who have been identified.

By sequencing, a total of 1,053 genomic sequences were found in 2020; after the filtration, 624 sequences were selected for multiple sequence alignment. They came to the conclusion that SARS-CoV, MERS-CoV, and SARS-CoV-2 evolved at a certain rate and took a certain amount of time to reach their most recent common ancestor [15]. The variants' evolved places and categories are given in Table 1.

Table 1: SARS CoV-2 variants' evolved places and categories (BV-BRC BETA).

S. no.	Variants	Countries	Category
1	B.1.1.7	Southeast England	Alpha
2	B.1.351	Nelson Mandela Bay, South Africa	Beta
3	B.1.427	Southern California, USA	Epsilon
4	B.1.429	Southern California, USA	Epsilon
5	B.1.526.1	New York	Epsilon
6	B.1.526	New York	Lota
7	B.1.617.1	India	Delta
8	B.1.617.2	United Kingdom	Delta
9	P.1	Brazil	Gamma
10	P.2	Brazil	Zeta
11	AY.1	Multiple countries	Delta
12	AY.2	USA	Delta
13	AY.3	USA	Delta
14	AY.3.1	USA	Delta
15	B.1.1.529	South Africa	Delta–omicron

2 Phylogenetics and phylodynamic studies

The phylogenetic study is the study of the evolutionary development of a species or an organism. Phylogenetic trees are a diagrammatic representation of evolutionary development [16]. By using phylogenetic trees, we can trace the pathway evolutionary development of a species and also find the common ancestors and closely related species. Phylodynamic studies are the interaction between epidemiological and pathogen evolutionary processes and relationships, including bacteria, fungi, and viruses. It helps in understanding the disease spreading frequency in populations and identification of influencing factors in disease spreading [17].

2.1 Computational genome sequencing for SARS-CoV-2

Metagenomic sequencing was used for the identification of causative viruses during the Covid-19 pandemic. It was identified within a week of the disease being reported, and took 6 months to sequence more than 60,000 near-complete viral genomes following the identification of SARS-CoV-2 [18]. Phylogenetic trees are used to understand the evolutionary rate and the mutation rate. Most mutations are deleterious, and the phylodynamic approaches were used for the investigation of reasons behind the outbreak. Phylogenetic study helps in the identification of population dynamics and virus lineage like SARS-CoV-2, which has six accessory proteins encoded by ORF3a, ORF6, ORF7a, and ORF8a [19].

2.2 Platforms for sequencing analysis of SARS-CoV-2: next-generation sequencing (NGS)

Understanding the origin, adaptive evolution, and transmission of SARS-CoV-2 depends on genome sequencing. Opting an ideal sequencing platform is therefore a crucial step. The sequencing data will help the scientific community in developing diagnostic tools for the detection of SARS-Cov-2. It will also help in identifying viral mutations that can affect vaccine potency [20].

2.3 Sequencing methods

Determine the order of nucleotides along the length of a DNA molecule using the genome sequencing method. This helps in identification of all or most of the genes and characterization of various structural features of the genome. The pioneering methods called first-generation sequencing were discovered by Maxam and Gilbert, and Sanger, during the 1970s [21]. The Maxam–Gilbert method or chemical sequencing method, although based on simple principles, lost its popularity because of the time-consuming process and extensive use of hazardous chemicals. In contrast to the few bases that can be sequenced by the Maxam–Gilbert method, Sanger sequencing was able to sequence 900 base pairs at a time [22]. Over the past few decades, a massive development has been seen in sequencing methods with emergence of second-generation sequencing which is supplemented by NGS. NGS is notable for its speed, high-throughput, and low-cost DNA sequencing. Compared to Sanger sequencing, NGS can detect variants such as DNA variants, including low-frequency variants and adjacent phased variants in less time and fewer hands-on steps. Various platforms available for NGS are Ion Torrent, 454 Pyrosequencing, Pacific Biosciences, Illumina (Solexa) sequencing, and SOLiD sequencing.

2.3.1 Sanger sequencing

Sanger method, despite its high cost and major drawback, is a popular method for sequencing until the emergence of high-throughput sequencing methods. It was developed by Frederick Sanger in 1977. It is based on the chain termination approach, in which the nucleotides in single-stranded DNA molecules are determined by complementary synthesis of polynucleotide chains. This method uses the DNA polymerase enzyme to drive the selective incorporation of chain-terminating dideoxynucleotides [23]. Modern Sanger sequencing uses fluorescently labeled dideoxynucleotides, which are detected by a laser after capillary electrophoresis. Sanger sequencing, despite its drawbacks, is still used in sequencing of specific genes or fragment of genes. It is able to determine substitutions and small deletions and insertions. Sanger sequencing can also be used along with NGS to confirm the variants determined by NGS and in backfilling NGS data.

2.3.2 Illumina sequencing

This is one of the most popular platforms of NGS. Illumina sequencing produced more than 90% of the global sequencing data. Genome analyzer, which was released by Solexa in 2006, was acquired by Illumina in 2008. Currently, Illumina owns platforms such as iSeq 100, MiSeq, NextSeq 550, NexSeq 1000, and NovaSeq 6000 producing 1.2 Gb, 15 Gb, 120 Gb, 360 Gb, and 6,000 Gb sequencing data per run, respectively.

This sequencing by synthesis method follows four basic steps: library preparation, cluster generation, sequencing, and data analysis. After being cut into single strands and grafted onto the flowcell, the library with fixed adaptors is denatured to create clusters that include clonal DNA fragments. Four different nucleotides (ddGTP, ddCTP, ddTTP, and ddATP), each of which contains a variety of cleavable fluorescent dyes and a detachable blocking group, would gradually add bases to the template before sequencing, and the signal could be caught by a charge-coupled device camera

[24]. Some of the limitations of Illumina sequencing are poor sequencing quality due to overlapping clusters and misincorporating DNA fragments, and lack of representation of GC-rich regions of heterogeneous genomes.

2.3.3 Comparative approach of Illumina sequencing

The iSeq 100 system, the smallest and most economical benchtop sequencing technology from Illumina, harnesses the potential of NGS. In one run, it can generate 1.2 Gb of sequencing data in 19 h. It is a quick and affordable solution for autonomous, small-scale NGS. The iSeq 100 system provides the power of NGS to almost any laboratory with almost any budget because of its low pricing and compact design. Targeted gene sequencing and small whole-genome sequencing can both be done using iSeq.

MiSeq can produce 540 Mb to 15 Gb sequencing data per run with 4–56 h running time. It has a read length of 1 × 36 bp to 2 × 300 bp. Targeted gene expression profiling, small genome sequencing, 16S metagenomics, miRNA, and small RNA analysis are all possible applications for miSeq.

NextSeq 550 produces an output of 90–150 Gb data per run with 35 h running time. It has a read length of 2 × 150 bp. NextSeq has a diagnostic and research mode, which provides the flexibility to do both diagnostic testing and clinical research on a single instrument. Transcriptome sequencing, targeted gene sequencing, small whole-genome sequencing, and chromatin analysis are some of the applications of NextSeq 550.

NextSeq 1000 and NextSeq 2000 have an output range of 30–360 Gb data per run with a maximum run time of 48 h. It has the latest advances in optics, instrument design, and reagent chemistry which minimizes the sequencing reaction volume and cost per run while increasing the output. Transcriptome sequencing spanning oncology, single-cell profiling, exome and large panel sequencing, genetic diseases, reproductive health, and agrigenomics are some of the applications of NextSeq 1000 and NextSeq 2000.

Up to 6 Tb and 20 B reads can be delivered by NovaSeq 6000 in less than 2 days. It has multiple flow cell types, two library loading workflows, and various read length combination which makes it the best in the business. It is used exclusively for research purposes. With its cutting-edge technology and clever design, NovaSeq offers high-throughput sequencing that is strong, easy to use, scalable, and dependable. It has a range of applications such as human whole-genome sequencing, tumor profiling, ultra-deep exome sequencing, chromatin analysis, and methylation sequencing.

2.3.4 Technologies by Oxford Nanopore (Flongle, MinION, GridION, and PromethION)

Nanopore sequencing is a third-generation sequencing technique. It was a method under development since 1995 for DNA sequencing. Oxford Nanopore Technologies has success with its commercialization [25]. Unlike other sequencing techniques, nanopore sequencing detects nucleotides without active DNA synthesis. It determines the nucleotide sequence by detecting the electric current variations when nucleic acids pass through the nanometer-sized protein channel, called nanopore. Different devices available under nanopore techniques are Flongle, MinION, GridION, and PromethION. The sequencing without DNA amplification eliminates PCR bias.

Some of the advantages of nanopore over alternatives are that they can produce ultralong reads. PromethION can yield 50–100 Gb data in a single flow cell, GridION can generate up to 250 Gb data, whereas the typical yield of MinION system is 5–10 Gb data. The ultralong reads have also made transcriptome analysis and direct RNA sequencing easier. It is also useful in reading highly repetitive sequences, nanopore sequencing is portable since it does not require any imaging device for nucleotide detection. Along with portability and its real-time nature, nanopore has become a quick and highly robust alternative. Even with all these advantages, nanopore has a major limitation of high error rates; it is not ideal for single nucleotide variations.

2.3.5 Ion Torrent

Toumazou et al. [26] created the Ion Torrent semiconductor sequencing method for the first time in 2006 and is generally referred to as sequencing by synthesis. When a nucleotide is integrated by a polymerase into a strand of DNA, hydrogen ions are produced as a byproduct. The Ion Torrent technology works on the principle of detection of this released hydrogen ion. During the process, H^+ ions are released, creating a strong positive voltage that alters the pH of the microenvironment. A transistor-based device that transforms this shift in current into a voltage signal can detect it [27]. The sequencing reaction occurs on a flow cell, a type of complementary metal-oxide semiconductor chip [28].

Ion PGM system has an output range of 600 Mb to 1 Gb. Ion Proton and Ion GeneStudio series system can generate an output of 10 Gb and 50 Gb data per run, respectively. The Ion Torrent sequencers generate read lengths of 200 bp which can be used to fill the gaps created in the assembly produced by other NGS platforms. Short read length and high error in sequencing data are some of the limitations of Ion Torrent technology. Ion Torrent also fails in interpreting homopolymer repeats of the same nucleotide as the signals generated from high repeat numbers cannot be differentiated properly.

2.3.6 Technical elements of SARS-CoV-2 genome sequencing analysis

Before sequencing SARS-CoV-2, some of the practical aspects which should be considered are the aims, expectations, and choice of the sequencing program. Technical considerations consist of determining the necessary amount of genomic sampling with respect to the defined aim, identifying the metadata required, choosing the appropriate sample and library preparation, bioinformatics, and analytical protocols.

2.4 Methods for genome sampling and the suggested study

The use of the sequencing data will determine the methods for genome sampling. Different applications have different sampling strategies such as investigation of transmission clusters, and small sample of all or most of the individuals within that cluster is considered. Evaluation of transmission driver's viral genome proportional to the cases should be sequenced. In order to investigate the local transmission, samples from the location of interest are enough.

2.4.1 Appropriate metadata

To increase the effectiveness of SARS-CoV-2 genomic data, appropriate metadata has to be collected along with samples. While collecting the metadata, it has to be ensured that the anonymity of patients is maintained. The unavoidable metadata include the date and location of the sample collection. Other information which can be used as metadata are age, gender, comorbid conditions, travel history, and symptoms. Sample and sequence-related metadata include specimen source, sample type, and sequencing technology. An ethical review should govern the sharing of metadata.

2.4.2 Logistic consideration

A very important phase in the process is sample collection. The availability of appropriate space and equipment for the isolation of sample has to be ensured. The samples for sequencing should be isolated with minimal contamination. Proper storage facility should be maintained for the collected samples. To avoid the transmission or contamination of SARS-CoV-2 material, a one-way flow of personnel and materials is strongly advised in the laboratory.

2.4.3 Peculiar material for sequencing

To make the sequencing data as efficient as possible, it is necessary to collect sufficient and high-quality SARS-CoV-2 RNA. Factors that might affect the quality and quantity of RNA samples are selection and handling of the clinical sample, the RNA isolation technique, and the degree of human error. It is advisable to choose the sample with high viral load and low amount of other genetic contamination. Sources of samples can be serum, naso-oropharyngeal swabs, sputum, oral fluids, fecal or anal swabs, and tissue samples isolated from cell culture or animal model. High viral loads are detected in nasal swabs, throat swabs, and saliva after the onset of symptoms.

2.4.3.1 Material choosing criteria

There may be different types of clinical samples available for sequencing; however, a sample which has high viral load and least contaminant of human or bacterial genome is preferred. The contamination can interfere with RNA extraction and hence may reduce sensitivity of sequencing.

2.4.3.2 Control samples

For an efficient sequencing, regulatory guidelines have to be followed. It is recommended in guidelines to use positive, negative, and sensitivity controls to ensure that all steps of the sequencing program are executed without contamination. Positive controls with known sequence can be used to verify the outcomes of the sequencing program. Negative control samples like water or buffer should be included in the run with multiple samples in order to eliminate the contamination during the sequencing run that can happen in a laboratory.

2.4.3.3 Logical considerations

Logistic considerations include deciding the location where the sequencing has to be conducted, it can be a diagnostic or academic laboratory. It has to be ensured that the appropriate funding, sufficient reagents, and computational resources are available for the sequencing program. Risk assessment is crucial while handling SARS-CoV-2. Biosafety and biosecurity have to be maintained at every step of sequencing. Sufficient skilled staff should be present to support all aspects of the sequencing program.

2.4.3.4 Biosafety and security

Biosafety establishes safe handling of infectious entity and hazardous materials in the guarded environment. It ensures the welfare of the health workers and halts the pathogen from entering the public space. It demands a risk assessment followed by containment abiding to principles. Risk assessment helps to resolve the crucial prospective steps and arrange accordingly. Establishments like Centers for Disease Control and Prevention (cdc.gov), International Society for Advancement of Cytometry, and the WHO have admonished that all the work pertaining to virus such as isolation and characteristic studies need to be carried out in BSL-3. However, diagnostic tests can be managed in BSL-2 by adhering to strict aerosol prevention measures [29].

2.4.3.5 Ethical consideration and human resources

Ethical consideration is a cluster of values and principles which should be abided to while doing human affairs. It ensures that any act carried out does not pose threat to the society or the individual. Covid-19 challenged the ethics followed until then. Healthcare leaders were asked to shift focus to the worst cases in order to mitigate the morbidity, mortality, and undesirable consequences of a pandemic [30]. On discovering a safe and effective vaccine, it should be administered in those at high risk, ensuring the equity. Ethical implications ought to be reviewed.

2.5 Ameliorating SARS-CoV2 genetic material prior to library construction

Samples were collected using swabs, which were then stored at 4 °C and analyzed by molecular diagnostic method and later stored at −80 °C. RT-qPCR was run following the WHO guidelines. RNA was extracted based on the guidelines of the CDC 2019-nCoV rRT-PCR Diagnostic Panel assay and then stored at −80 °C. SARS-CoV2 virus copy was quantified using SYBR green qRT-PCR [31].

2.6 Metagenomics studies of uncultured clinical samples

After the detection of organism by performing IDseq server-based pipeline, it was followed by quality control tests. Low-quality and low-complexity reads after the taxonomic identification were eliminated. An alpha- and beta-diversity analysis were effectuated to understand the sample diversity accompanied with a diversity analysis using SARS-CoV2 positive samples with Ct values above 30. Bulk mutations were noticed in the ORF1ab gene. Raw FASTA files were available for free [32].

2.7 Metagenomics strategies following cell culture

Metagenomics next-gene sequencing reveals whole viral genome and any coinfection. CLOMP (Clinically Okay Metagenomic Pipeline) results unearthed positive SARS-CoV2 samples which matched with the database of SARS-CoV-associated viruses. From the environmental datasets, varied beta coronavirus-like sequences together with SARS-CoV matches were observed. Future pandemics before emergence can be anticipated with the help of metagenomic strategy involving microbiome research and metagenomic profiling [32].

2.8 Approaches

Using the nucleic acid extract, reverse transcription was conducted. From this, multiple PCRs were carried out with primers enveloping entire genome of SARS-CoV2. Final products were collected in equimolar ratio. The amplicon balance, coverage metrics, and variant calls to the ARTIC v3 method were achieved using a fine-tuned amplicon technique.

3 Overview of bioinformatics for sequencing of SARS-Cov2

Significance of bioinformatics during the pandemic is indispensable from foreseeing possible biomolecules that aid in the treatment of infectious diseases and its prevention. With bioinformatics, it was able to spawn genomic sequences of SARS-CoV2 at an unprecedented rate.

Various curated data was made available for free in open sources to everyone to mitigate the condition and find solution. Reverse vaccinology is a vaccine developing process which involves detection of novel antigens through examination of an organism's genomic data, which relies on bioinformatics.

3.1 Archiving of raw data

Without metadata, genomic sequences are futile for applications. A group of people ensure that the metadata collected are rightly targeted for analysis for which they are intended. Some of the databases are Sequence Read Archive Repository, FASTA, GISAID, and Uniprot which features latest SARS-CoV2 proteins, host protein entries, receptors, and so on. These portals update the information regularly.

3.2 Genome assembly from raw data

Compressed FASTA files were being generated using tools. They were trimmed and aligned against a given reference genome. They were sorted, and final BAM files were indexed. VCF files were obtained from BAM files, and then using Jacquard program, VCF files were merged and produced a single VCF file which contained gleaned variants from all genomes.

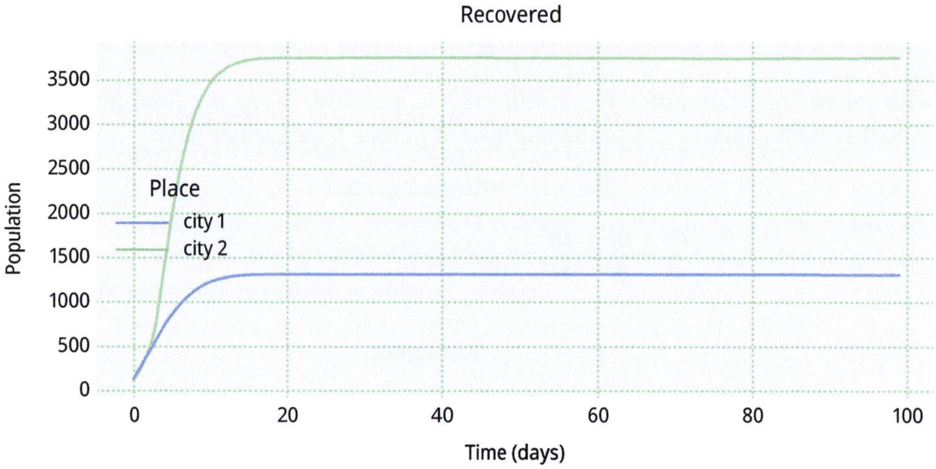

Figure 4: Variation of removed population with time in SIR model.

Figures 2–4 illustrate the effect of pandemic with time using SIR model.

2.2 SEIR model

In this model [9], population is divided into S, E, I, and R. Figure 5 demonstrates the model. Here, β is the transmission rate, δ is the rate of infection, and γ is the rate of recovery.

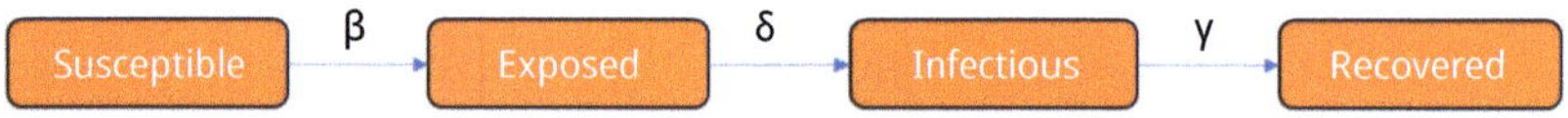

Figure 5: SEIR model.

Equations for modeling SEIR can be written as

$$\frac{dS}{dt} = \frac{-\beta SI}{N} \tag{6}$$

$$\frac{dE}{dt} = \frac{\beta SI}{N} - \delta E \tag{7}$$

$$\frac{dI}{dt} = \delta E - \gamma I \tag{8}$$

$$\frac{dR}{dt} = \gamma I \tag{9}$$

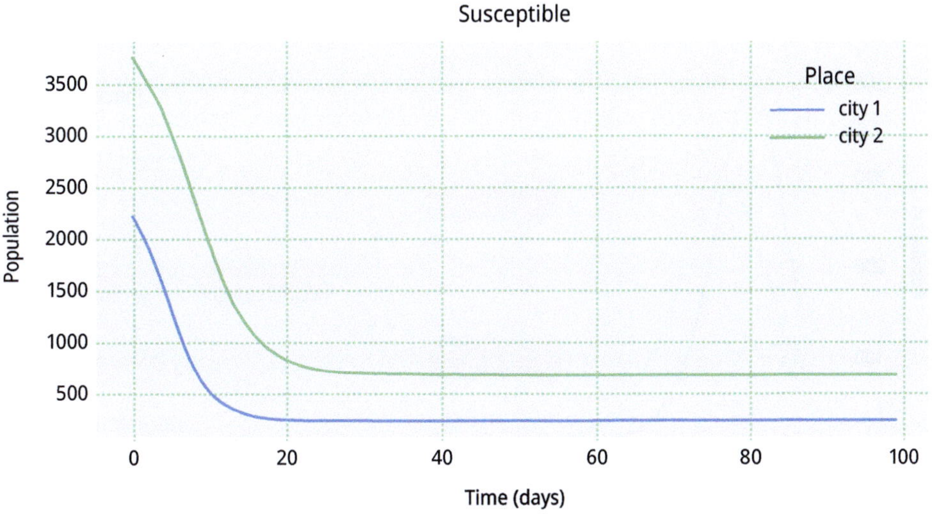

Figure 6: Variation of susceptible population with time in SEIR model.

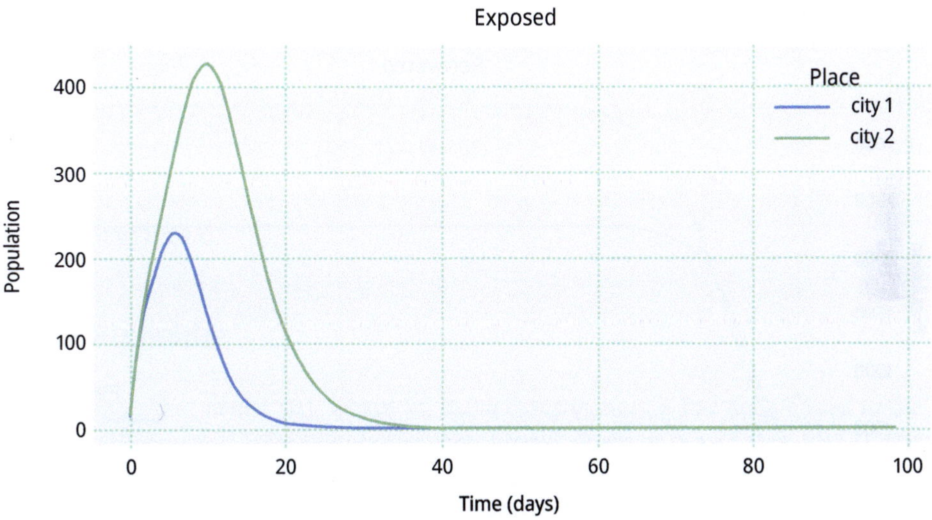

Figure 7: Variation of exposed population with time in SEIR model.

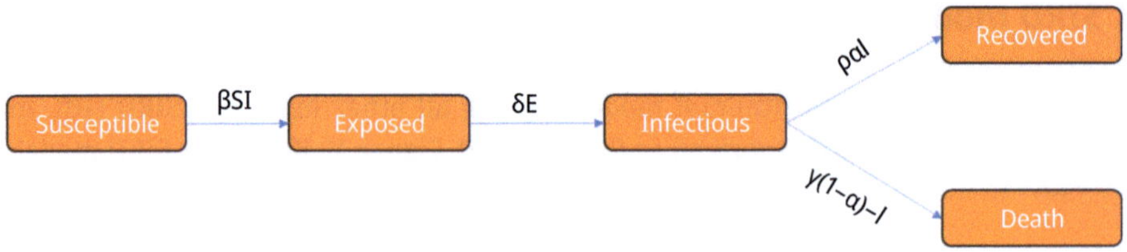

Figure 11: SEIRD model [11].

The differential equations of this model are:

$$\frac{dS}{dt} = \frac{-\beta SI}{N} \tag{14}$$

$$\frac{dE}{dt} = \frac{\beta SI}{N} - \delta E \tag{15}$$

$$\frac{dI}{dt} = \delta E - (1-\alpha).\gamma I - \alpha\rho I \tag{16}$$

$$\frac{dR}{dt} = (1-\alpha).\gamma I \tag{17}$$

$$\frac{dD}{dt} = \alpha\rho I \tag{18}$$

The above equations describe the proposed susceptible rate, exposed rate, rate of infection, recovery, and death, respectively. The parameters of the equations are: β is the transmission rate of disease, δ is the incubation period, α is fatality rate, γ is the recovery rate, and ρ is the death rate.

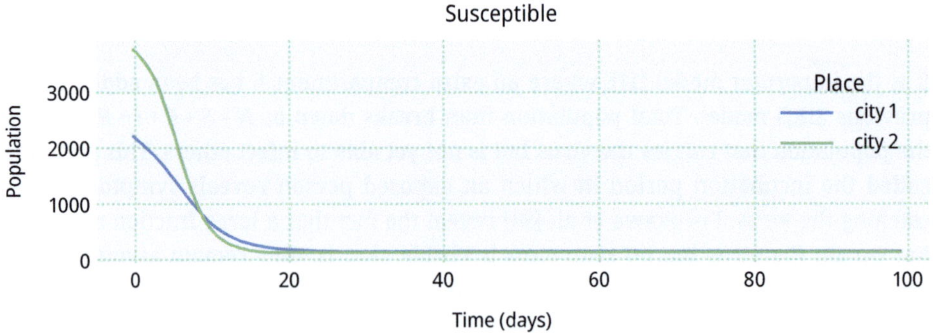

Figure 12: Variation of susceptible population with time in SEIRD model.

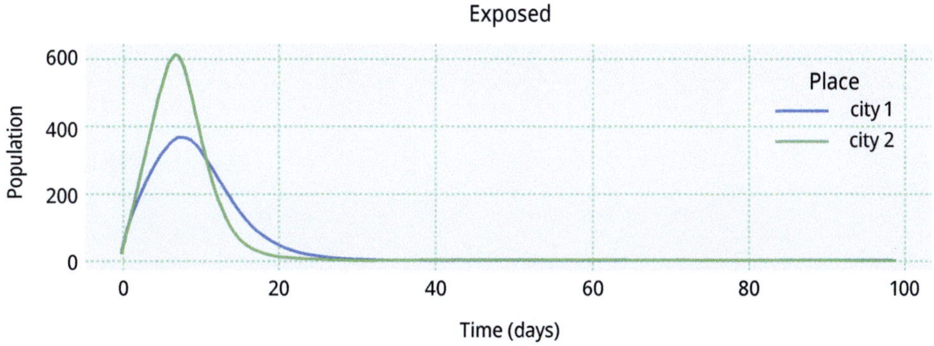

Figure 13: Variation of exposed population with time in SEIRD model.

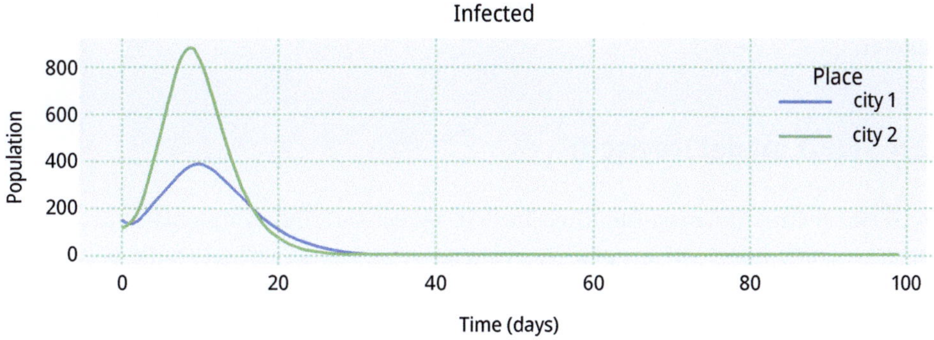

Figure 14: Variation of infected population with time in SEIRD model.

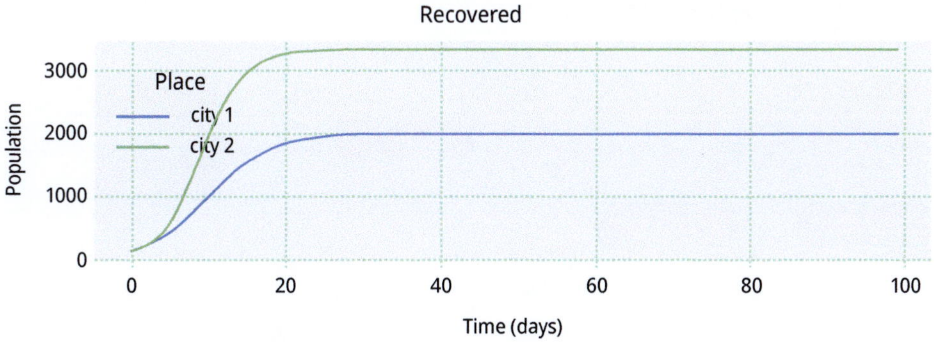

Figure 15: Variation of recovered population with time in SEIRD model.

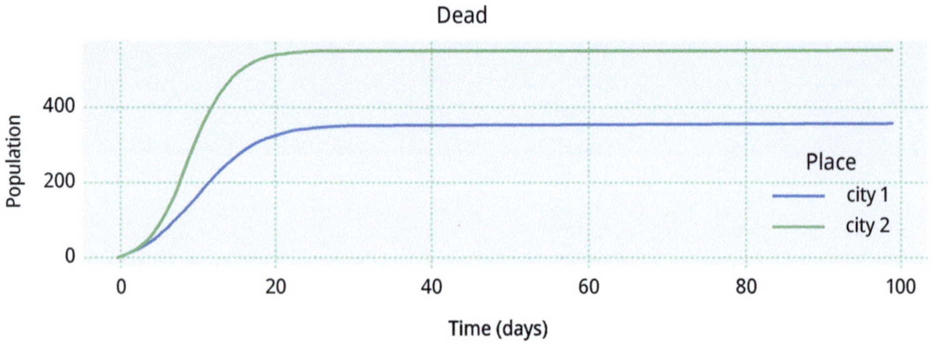

Figure 16: Variation of dead population with time in SEIRD model.

Figures 12–16 display the variation of S, E, I, R, and D with time using the SEIRD model.

2.5 SEIRD model (revised)

A SEIRD model has been modified in [35], by considering symptomatic as well as asymptomatic infectious people. This chapter reveals that asymptomatic population plays a significant role in the spread of COVID-19 infection. The infectious people compartment is categorized into symptomatic population and asymptomatic population. Similarly, the recovered compartment is also subdivided into a recovery from symptomatic infectious population and an asymptomatic infectious population. The authors consider that asymptomatic individuals will never enter into D compartment. The model is described in Figure 17:

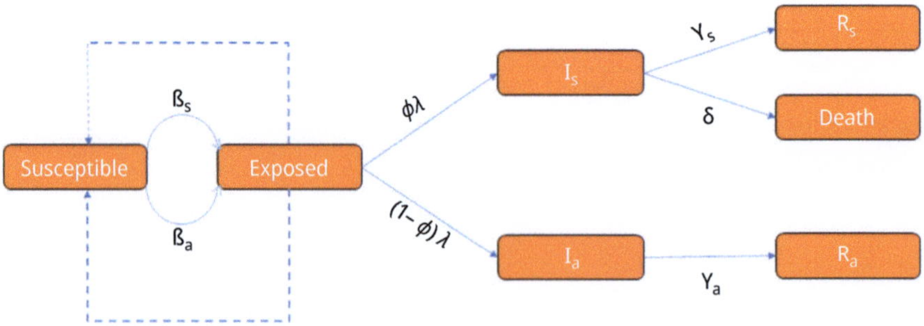

Figure 17: Modified SEIRD model.

2.6 SIRDV model

A model was proposed in [12], by considering two behavioral aspects of the population: level of caution and sense of safety. How the level of caution and sense of safety vary with the infection rate is determined by this model. The effect of vaccination and the behavioral aspect of population will determine the future scenario of the pandemic as predicted by the model. The model divides the population into *S, I, R, D*, and *V*. Figure 18 shows SIRDV model.

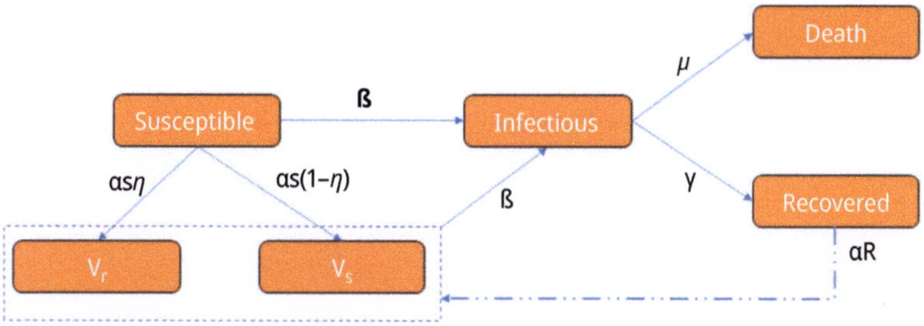

Figure 18: SIRDV model.

The population can get vaccine with rate α, and with the vaccine effectiveness (1–β), the part of the population (*Vs*) can become infected and then either recovers or not. Some other part of the vaccinated population (VR) will never be infected again:

$$\frac{dS}{dt} = -\beta SI - \alpha \tag{19}$$

$$\frac{dV}{dt} = -(1-\epsilon)VI + \alpha \tag{20}$$

$$\frac{dR}{dt} = \gamma I \tag{21}$$

$$\frac{dI}{dt} = (\beta S + \beta(1-\epsilon)V - \mu\gamma - \gamma) * I \tag{22}$$

$$\frac{dD}{dt} = \mu\gamma I \tag{23}$$

2.7 SEIAQRDT

It is very much required to classify infected people as symptomatic and asymptomatic for controlling the spread of infection. This model predicts the number of infected more precisely, which is surely helpful for designing the plan of action. The model in [34] is referred to as SEIAQRDT because it divides the population into eight compartments: *S*(*t*),

E(*t*), *I*(*t*) (symptomatic) population (that may infect others but not yet quarantined), *A*(*t*), infectious (asymptomatic) population (that can spread infection, but showing no symptoms), *Q*(*t*), the quarantined population (the confirmed population that is infectious), *R*(*t*) population, *D*(*t*) and *T*(*t*), the protected population. The differential equations of the model are as follows: Figure 19 shows SEIAQRDT model.

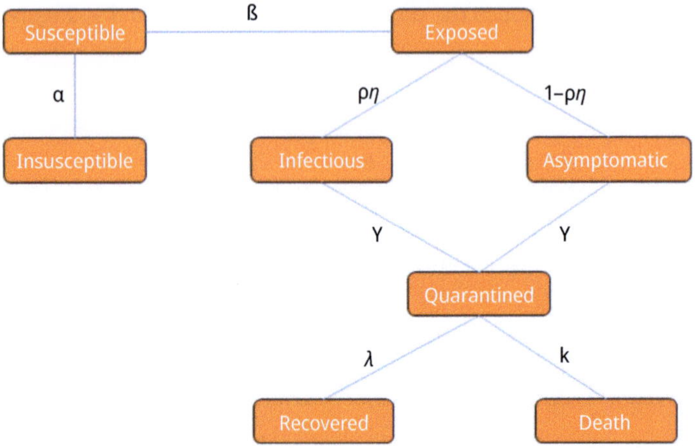

Figure 19: SEIAQRDT model.

$$\frac{dS}{Vdt} = -\frac{\beta S(t)(I(t) + q(A(t))}{N} - \alpha S(t) \tag{24}$$

$$\frac{dE}{dt} = \frac{\beta S(t)(I(t) + q(A(t))}{N} - \epsilon E(t) \tag{25}$$

$$\frac{dI(t)}{dt} = \rho E(t) - \gamma I(t) \tag{26}$$

$$\frac{dA(t)}{dt} = (1 - \rho)\epsilon E(t) - \gamma I(t) \tag{27}$$

$$\frac{dQ(t)}{dt} = \gamma(I(t) + A(t)) - \sigma(t)Q(t) - V(t)Q(t) \tag{28}$$

$$\frac{dR(t)}{dt} = \sigma(t)Q(t) \tag{29}$$

$$\frac{dD(t)}{dt} = V(t)Q(t) \tag{30}$$

$$\frac{dT(t)}{dt} = \sigma S(t) \tag{31}$$

2.8 SIDARTHE

To predict the course of pandemic, a new model was proposed in [5], which divides infected individuals as diagnosed or nondiagnosed. Diagnosed individuals are quarantined and ensure less chance of spreading the virus The model SIDARTHE divides the population into *S*, *I*, diagnosed (*D*), ailing (*A*), recognized (*R*), threatened (*T*), healed (*H*), and extinct (*E*). Figure 20 shows SIDARTHE model.

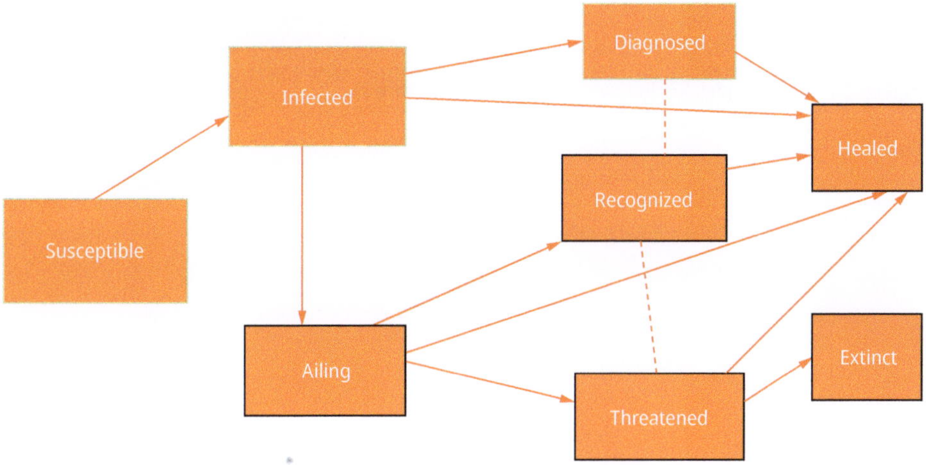

Figure 20: SIDARTHE model.

2.9 SEIHRD

The population is divided into several compartments again in [37]. *S*, *E*, *I*, Iu, HR, HD, RU, RD, and *D*. *Iu* is infectious but undetected (*Iu*): In this compartment, the infected people cannot be detected with disease.

Hospitalized or in quarantine at home: After detection of the disease, the person is in quarantine under the supervision of doctor. Hospitalized (HU): In this compartment, hospitalized persons will stay. Some are stuck in home and they can spread infection. At the end of this state, they enter into the recovered compartment.

Hospitalized person with chance of death (denoted by HD): The person is hospitalized and can infect others. After HD compartment, people enter into the *D* compartment.

RU denotes the population who is recovered from disease but undetected previously. RD indicates the population who is recovered and previously detected as infected. SEIHRD model is illustrated in figure 21.Comparison among models is illustrated in table 2. Table 3 and 4 discuss the comparison among different strains.

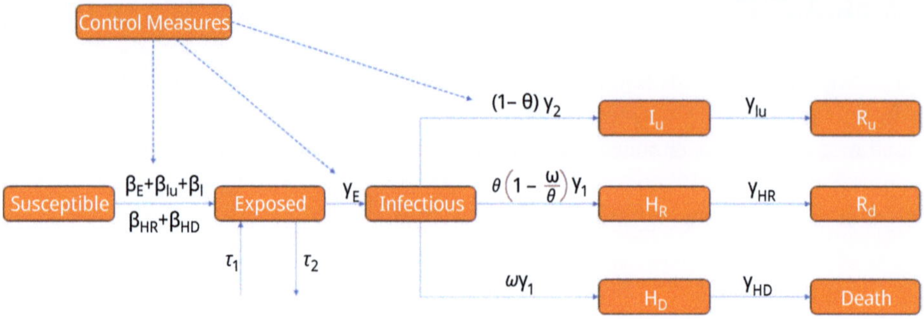

Figure 21: SEIHRD model. SEIHRD model is illustrated in figure 21.

3 Comparative analysis of multiple models

Table 2: Comparison among models.

Model name	Number of compartments	Name of compartments	Name of parameters	Assumptions	Technique	Contribution	Drawback
SIR [7]	3	$\{S, I, R\}$	β-Transmission coefficient, γ-recovery rate	Total population remains constant. Birth and death rates are not considered. After recovery from disease, immunity has been assured	Solving differential equations	To predict the number of susceptible, I, and recovered person	It does not consider the latent time between exposed and I.
eSIR [8]	3	$\{S, I, R\}$	β-Transmission coefficient, γ-recovery rate	Transmission rate is not constant	Markov chain Monte Carlo methods are used	To adopt different types of time-varying quarantine protocols and isolation policies	The model combines removed and dead in a single compartment
SIRD [10]	4	S, I, R, D	β-Transmission coefficient, γ-recovery rate, death rate	May be delay in reporting of new cases and also initially new case detection rate is low.	Feeding data into models	Prediction on infectious, recovered, and dead	From susceptible class to I class is considered. No exposed compartment has been designed in this model

(continued)

Table 2 (continued)

Model name	Number of compartments	Name of compartments	Name of parameters	Assumptions	Technique	Contribution	Drawback
SEIR [9]	4	S, E, I, R	β-Transmission coefficient, γ-recovery rate	Total population remains constant. The recovered individual is immune from the disease	Feeding data into models	Prediction on infectious and recovered is achieved	Death compartment is not considered here
SEIRD [11]	4	S, E, I, R, D	β-Transmission coefficient, γ-recovery rate, δ-death rate	They assume that population is homogeneously mixed	Feeding data into models	Future prediction on infectious, recovered, and dead	A compartmental SEIRD model considers that the population is homogeneously mixed
SEIJR [38]	5	S, E, I, confirmed (J), R, and D	α is average spreading velocity, β is diagnosed rate, γ_1 and γ_2 are death rates, μ is cure rate, t_1, t_2, and t_3 are time delays	Number of death in exposed compartment is negligible	Mathematical model using differential equation. Particle swarm optimization	Reliable prediction of future infection trend. Important discussion regarding future precautionary actions	I to D and J have the same delay time and J to R and D have the same delay due to unavailability of data

SEIAR [39]	5	*S*, *E*, *I*, asymptomatic (*A*), *R*	8	Existence of asymptomatic infectious people and migration of population is considered	Mathematical model	Impact of asymptomatic patients in spreading the disease is studied and also calculate the curve of the number of infectious based on the Euler numerical method	Dead compartment is not considered here
R-SEIRD [40]	5	*S*, *E*, *I*, *R*, *D*		Knowledge of initial state of population is not required	Certainty-equivalent expectation-maximization (CE-EM) technique is used	1. The model relaxes the assumptions of the standard SEIRD model 2. The model fits well with available data 3. Experimentally exhibits that this model is able to express the diversity of behavior observed in the United States, and that the methodology performs better than the standard methods	The asymptomatic person is not considered in this model
SEIR-P [41]	5	*S*, *E*, *I*, *R*, *P*	There are 17 parameters	Parameters are nonnegative	For integer-order epidemic model, multistage method is used. Numerical simulation is performed	Qualitative analysis is carried out for integer as well as fractional model	Acuteness of disease and death is not being considered. Initial value of the parameters is recorded which may change at later time

(continued)

Table 2 (continued)

Model name	Number of compartments	Name of compartments	Name of parameters	Assumptions	Technique	Contribution	Drawback
SEPIR [42]	5	S, E, presymptomatic-I, R	6	Spatially varying density of people	Mathematical modeling	Predict the effect of different quarantine levels imposed in different areas, providing a unified framework for heterogeneous spread of the epidemic	Death compartment is not considered
SIRDV [12]	6	S, I, R, D, VR, VS	Mortality rate, recovery rate, sense of caution, transmission rate, vaccination rate, vaccine effectiveness, and sense of safety	Population behavior remains same throughout the pandemic. Uniform rate of vaccination is considered	Mathematical modeling	Provides future Covid trend considering vaccination integrated with population behavior. Level of caution and sense of safety	Rate of death is considered as constant. Proper test case data is not available
SIDARTHE [5]	8	S, I, diagnosed, ailing, recognized, threatened, healed, extinct	16	This model differentiates between I individuals depending on whether they have been diagnosed and on the acuteness of their symptoms	Mathematical modeling	In this model, fractional order is considered	Population is considered as constant

SEIAQRDT [36]	8	S, E, I, asymptomatic, quarantined, R, D, and insusceptible	8	In this model, asymptomatic and symptomatic patients are treated differently. The lockdown measure and other precautionary measures are also considered	Inputting data into mathematical model. The relative squared error analysis is used to calculate the relative error of the model	The output data with SEIARQDT model is very close to actual data	Transmission of disease, effect of vaccination, medication strategies, impact of withdrawal of lockdown, etc., have not been addressed in this model
θ-SEIHRD [43]	9	$\{S, E, I, H, R, D\}$	14 parameters	Population is homogeneously distributed. Movement between territories is not considered	Mathematical modeling	Effect of total detected case with the real number of infected case is considered. The impact of control measures is also analyzed	Not considered the effect of humidity and temperature on COVID-19. Incomplete information

Table 3: Comparison among strains.

Variant	Scientific name	Country in which first evolve	Date of trace	Date of designation	VOI/VOC	Mutation	Features
Alpha	B.1.1.7	UK	September 2020	18 December 2020	VOC:18-DEC-2020	23	50% more transmissible compared to SARS-CoV-2 variants
Beta	B.1.357	South Africa	May 2020	18 December 2020	18-DEC-2020	21	50% more transmissibility. Efficacy of some monoclonal antibody treatment. Less neutralization by convalescent and post vaccination antibodies
Gamma	P.1	Brazil	November 2020	11 January 2021	11-JANUARY-2021	21	Low efficacy of monoclonal antibody treatment. Low neutralization by convalescent and post vaccination antibodies
Delta	B.1.617.2	India	October 2020	4 April 2021	VOI: 4-APRIL-2021 VOC: 11-MAY-2021	32	Contagious and cause acute illness. Less potential efficacy of some monoclonal antibody treatment. Low neutralization by convalescent and post vaccination antibodies
Omicron	B.1.1.529	Multiple countries	November 2021	24 Nov 2021	VOI: 24-NOV-2021 VOC: 26-NOV-2021	32	Much more contagious but less fatal compared to delta

Table 4: Comparison among strains-2.

Variant	Number of countries affected	Impact of vaccine	Impact of vaccine against hospitalization	Transmissibility	Immune evasiveness	Features
Alpha	172	Two doses of Pfizer were 93% effective. Two doses of AstraZeneca were 66% effective. For both the vaccines, after one dose, it is 50% effective [45]	The Pfizer vaccine was 94% effective against hospitalizations for the alpha variants after one dose and 96% effective after two doses. The AstraZeneca vaccine was 71% effective against hospitalizations after one dose and 92% effective after two [45]	+++	–	50% more transmissible compared to existing SARS-CoV-2 variants
Beta	120	Two doses of Pfizer were 75% effective. Two doses of AstraZeneca were 60% effective. For both the vaccines, after one dose it is 33% effective [45]		+	++++	50% more transmissibility. Efficacy of some monoclonal antibody treatment. Less neutralization by convalescent and postvaccination antibodies
Gamma	72	November 2020		++	++	Significantly low efficacy of monoclonal antibody treatment Low neutralization by convalescent and postvaccination antibodies

(continued)

Table 4 (continued)

Variant	**Number of countries affected**	**Impact of vaccine**	**Impact of vaccine against hospitalization**	**Transmissibility**	**Immune evasiveness**	**Features**
Delta	100	Two doses of Pfizer were 88% effective. Two doses of AstraZeneca were 60% effective. For both the vaccines, after one dose it is 33% effective [45]	The Pfizer vaccine was 94% effective against hospitalizations from the delta variants after one dose and 96% effective after two doses. The AstraZeneca vaccine was 71% effective against hospitalizations after one dose and 92% effective after two [45]	++++	++++	Contagious and cause severe illness. Less potential efficacy of some monoclonal antibody treatment Low neutralization by convalescent and postvaccination antibodies
Omicron	South Africa	–		++++	++	Much more contagious but less fatal compared to delta

4 Comparative analysis of multiple strains of SARS-CoV-2

Due to mutations, different variants or strains of viruses evolve. Mutations in the SARS-CoV-2 virus have been causing the disease COVID-19 since December 2019, with the virus mutating regularly so that there are several versions of it today. Mutation is a normal phenomenon that a virus goes through as it is spreading. When these mutations are significantly different from the original one, the mutated version is called a variant. However, from among the thousands of variations, only a few mutations are likely to be significant. A variant is called "variant of interest" (VOI) if it has several mutations with significant changes and they are spreading widely. As of December'21 only four variants have been declared as "variants of concern" (VOC). A VOI becomes VOC when it becomes either more resistant to vaccines, or when its mortality rate is higher. VOCs are strains of SARS-CoV-2 that have super spreading capability as well as fatal [44]. It can escape body's immune system and cause severe illness. There are four VOCs till now. They are called alpha, beta, gamma, delta, and omicron.

5 Impact of vaccination against COVID-19

Vaccination has substantial impact on mitigating the outbreak of Covid-19, not only preventing deaths but also helping to maintain the economy of country. In the past, vaccine development has typically taken several years, but for SARS-CoV-2, the progress of vaccine development happens within a year. Twenty-three vaccines against SARS-CoV-2 have been approved for use and many more are under development. More than 47% of scientific papers published in 2021 have been related to vaccines and their development [46]. It has been shown that 470,000 deaths had been prevented by vaccination in [45]. But inequity in access to vaccination creates much adverse effects on vaccine [47].

More than 1,650 million doses of two vaccines have been injected in India. More than 50.8% of population in India has received vaccines. Effectiveness of vaccination against symptomatic infection, hospitalization, and death have been demonstrated in [48]. From [48], it is found that vaccine effectiveness against hospitalization and death is more than 80% for AstraZeneca, Pfizer-BioNTech, and Moderna.

From Table 5, it is observed that with the increasing rate of vaccination, death of 7 days average data decreased till August 2021. After August 2021, death toll increased. In January 2022, the infected as well as death toll increased abruptly. Figure 22 displays the variation of death with time. Seven days average data on infected declined from January 2021 till May 2021. Figure 23 shows the variation of Infected with time. Vaccine effectiveness against alpha, beta, and gamma has been highlighted in [45], where it is seen that for alpha strain the vaccine is highly effective, but for beta and

Table 5: Infected–death–vaccinated.

Date	I average (7 days)	Total death average (7 days)	Vaccinated partly	Percentage	Vaccinated fully	Percentage	Buster dose percentage
24.3.2020	8,603	95	0	0%	0	0%	0%
24.04.2020	29,427	2,093	0	0%	0	0%	0%
09.05.2020	28,553	1,764	0	0%	0	0%	0%
19.08.2020	46,022	1,020	0	0%	0	0%	0%
04.10.2020	44,027	715	0	0%	0	0%	0%
13.12.2020	220,908	2,341	22,143	0%	4,771	0%	0%
30.01.2021	159,760	3,147	29,369,127	8.9%	7,166,492	2.2%	0%
20.03.2021	54,876	1,083	90,070,122	27.3%	50,006,478	15.2%	0%
26.5.2021	33,840	586	172,672,442	52.4%	143,459,806	43.5%	0%
07.08.2021	106,677	506	197,243,853	59.9%	170,327,491	51.7%	0%
31.10.2021	72,707	1,350	222,656,343	67.6%	194,179,891	58.9%	6.5%
10.12.2021	118,565	1,292	238,825,412	72.5%	202,793,637	61.5%	17.2%
25.01.2022	619,958	2,441	251,518,114	76.3%	210,084,897	63.8%	25.8%

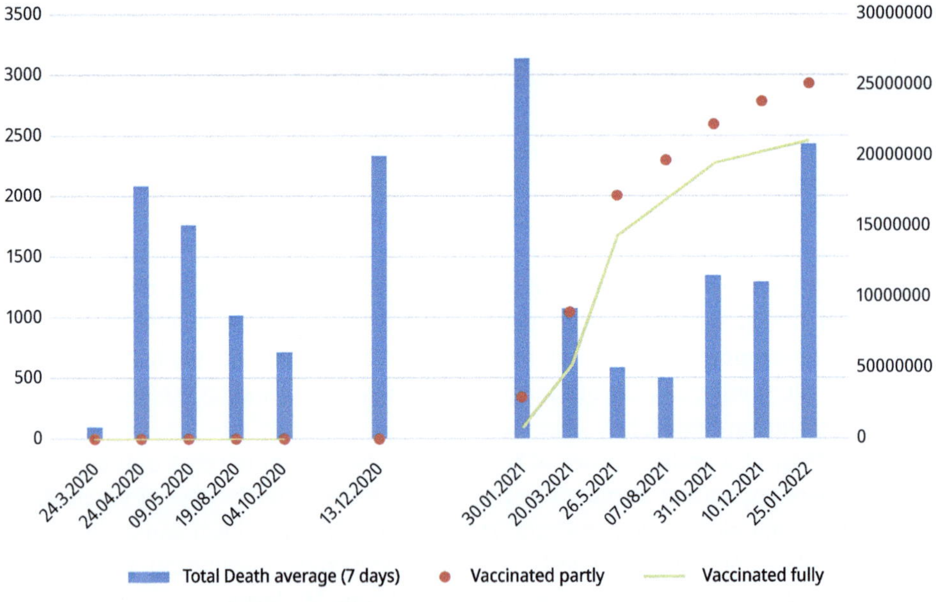

Figure 22: Variation of death with vaccination.

gamma strain, the effectiveness is lesser. It is found in [22] that after second dose of vaccination, approximately 27 (for interquartile range 18–43)–42 days (for interquartile range 26–63) gap is seen for positive result in RT-PCR for alpha strain, whereas for delta strain, the gap is 51 (for interquartile range 35–70) and 90 days (for interquartile range 69–110).

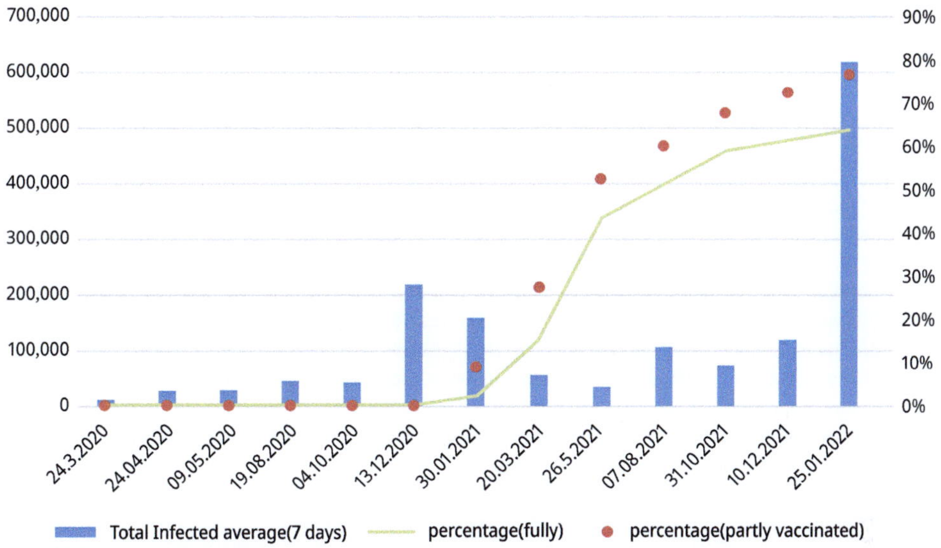

Figure 23: Variation of infected with vaccination.

6 Conclusion

COVID-19 causes a huge socioeconomic challenge to mankind. Mathematical modeling has contributed much for predicting the effect of any pandemic. This chapter focuses on a comparative analysis of deterministic epidemic models. The objective is to analyze different compartmental epidemic models: SIR, ESIR, SEPIR, SEIR, SEIJR, SEIAR, SEIR-P, SIRD, SEIRD, R-SEIRD, SEIRDH, SEIQARDT, SIDARTHE, θ-SEIHRD, and SIRDV, and study the involved parameters in the mathematical modeling of COVID-19. Comparative analysis of multiple strains of SARS-CoV-2 with respect to their features like date of trace, date of designation, and VOI/VOC is also explained in this chapter. Strains of SARS-COV-2 are compared with respect to transmissibility and immune evasiveness. The impact of vaccination on different strains is much more relevant to discuss. From the collected data, it is inevitable that with the increasing rate of vaccination, death of 7 days average data decreased till August 2021. Approximately 470,000 deaths had been prevented by vaccination. But inequity in access to vaccination creates much adverse effects on the success story of the vaccine. After August 2021, death and infected increased though infected data remained constant from October 2021. In January 2022, the infected as well as death toll increased abruptly.

References

[1] Li, Q. Early transmission dynamics in Wuhan, China, of novel coronavirus-infected pneumonia. The New England Journal of Medicine, 2020, 382(13), 1199–1207.

[2] WHO COVID-19 Dashboard. Geneva: World Health Organization, 2020. Available online: https://covid19.who.int/.

[3] Saha, J., Barman, B. B., Chouhan, P. Lockdown for COVID-19 and its impact on community mobility in India: An analysis of the COVID-19 community mobility reports. Children and Youth Services, 2020, 2020, Article 105160. doi: 10.1016/j.childyouth.2020.105160.

[4] Florindo, H. F., Kleiner, R., Vaskovich-Koubi, D., et al. Immune-mediated approaches against COVID-19. Nature Nanotechnology, 2020, 15, 630–645. https://doi.org/10.1038/s41565-020-0732-3.

[5] Giordano, G., Blanchini, F., Bruno, R., Colanary, P., Filippo, A. D., Matteo, A. D., Colaneri, M. Modelling the COVID-19 epidemic and implementation of population-wide interventions in Italy. Nature Medicine, 2020, 26, 855–860. https://doi.org/10.1038/s41591-020-0883-7.

[6] Kermark, W. O., McKendrick, A. G. Contributions to the mathematical theory of epidemics. Proceedings of the Royal Society A, 1927, 115(772), 700–721.

[7] Cooper, I., Mondal, A., Antonopoulos, C. G. A SIR model assumption for the spread of COVID-19 in different communities. Chaos, Solitons & Fractals, 2020, 139, 110057.

[8] Xiang, Z. Y., Li, Y. F., Song, X. Y. Dynamic analysis of a pest management SEI model with saturation incidence concerning impulsive control strategy. Nonlinear Analysis: Real World Applications, 2009, 10(4), 2335–2345.

[9] He, S., Peng, Y., Sun, K. SEIR modeling of the COVID-19 and its dynamics. Nonlinear Dynamics, 2020, 101(3), 1667–1680.

[10] Matadi, M. 2014. The SIRD epidemial model. 89. 1–14

[11] Korolev, I. Identification and estimation of the SEIRD epidemic model for COVID-19. Journal of Econometrics, 2021, 220(1), 63–85.

[12] Usherwood, T., LaJoie, Z., Srivastava, V. A model and predictions for COVID-19 considering population behavior and vaccination. Scientific Reports, 2021, 11, 12051. https://doi.org/10.1038/s41598-021-91514-7.

[13] Mehdaoui, M. A review of commonly used compartmental models in epidemiology. arXiv preprint arXiv:2110.09642, 2021.

[14] Sturniolo, S., Waites, W., Colbourn, T., Manheim, D., Panovska-Griffiths, J. Testing, tracing and isolation in compartmental models. PLoS Computational Biology, 2021, 17(3), e1008633. https://doi.org/10.1371/journal.pcbi.1008633.

[15] Li, M.-T., Cui, J., Zhang, J., Sun, G.-Q. Transmission analysis of COVID-19 with discrete time imported cases: Tianjin and Chongqing as cases. Infectious Disease Modelling, 2021, 6, 618–631. ISSN 2468–0427. https://doi.org/10.1016/j.idm.2021.03.007.

[16] Potluri, R., et al. Impact of prophylactic vaccination strategies on Ebola virus transmission: A modeling analysis. PLoS ONE, 2020, 15.

[17] Lee, B. Y., Haidari, L. A., Lee, M. S. Modelling during an emergency: The 2009 H1N1 influenza pandemic. Clinical Microbiology and Infection, 2013, 19, 1014–1022.

[18] Nuraini, N., Sukandar, K. K., Hadisoemarto, P., Susanto, H., Hasan, A. I., Sumarti, N. Mathematical models for assessing vaccination scenarios in several provinces in Indonesia. Infectious Disease Modelling, 2021, 6, 1236–1258. ISSN 2468–0427. https://doi.org/10.1016/j.idm.2021.09.002.

[19] Matrajt, L., Eaton, J., Leung, T., Brown, E. R. Vaccine optimization for COVID-19: Who to vaccinate first? medRxiv2020.08.14.20175257, 2020.

[20] Bubar, K. M., et al. . Model-informed COVID-19 vaccine prioritization strategies by age and serostatus. MedRxiv, 2020.09.08.20190629, 2020.

[21] Arruda, E. F., Das, S. S., Dias, C. M., Pastore, D. H. Modelling and optimal control of multi strain epidemics, with application to COVID-19. PLOS ONE, 2021, 16(9), e0257512. https://doi.org/10.1371/journal.pone.0257512.

[22] Eyre, D. W., Taylor, D., Purver, M., Chapman, D., Fowler, T., Pouwels, K. B., Walker, A. S., Peto, T. E. A. Effect of Covid-19 vaccination on transmission of alpha and delta variants. New England Journal of Medicine, 2022.

[23] Davies, N. G., Kucharski, A. J., Eggo, R. M., Gimma, A. CMMID COVID-19 working group, Edmunds WJ. The effect of non-pharmaceutical interventions on COVID-19 cases, deaths and demand for hospital services in the UK: a modelling study, 2020. https://doi.org/10.1101/2020.04.01.20049908.

[24] Shao, N., Zhong, M., Yan, Y., Pan, H., Cheng, J., Chen, W. Dynamic models for coronavirus disease 2019 and data analysis. Mathematical Methods in the Applied Sciences, 2020, 43(7), 4943–4949. https://doi.org/10.1002/mma.6345. PMID: 32327866.

[25] Jia, J., Ding, J., Liu, S., Liao, G., Li, J., Duan, B., et al. Modeling the control of COVID-19: Impact of policy interventions and meteorological factors. Electronic Journal of Differential Equations, 2020, 2020(23), 1–24.

[26] Tarrataca, L., Dias, C. M., Haddad, D., Arruda, E. F. Flattening the curves: On-off lock-down strategies for COVID-19 with an application to Brazil. Journal of Mathematics in Industry, 2021, 11(1), 2. https://doi.org/10.1186/s13362-020-00098-w.

[27] Kantner, M., Koprucki, T. Beyond just "flattening the curve": Optimal control of epidemics with purely nonpharmaceutical interventions. Journal of Mathematics in Industry, 2020, 10, 23. https://doi.org/10.1186/s13362-020-00091-3.

[28] Allen, L. J. S., Bolker, B. M., Lou, Y., Nevai, A. L. Asymptotic profiles of the steady states for an SIS epidemic patch model. SIAM Journal on Applied Mathematics, 2007, 67(5), 1283–1309.

[29] Wang, W., Ruan, S. Simulating the SARS outbreak in Beijing with limited data. Journal of Theoretical Biology, 2004, 227(3), 369–379.

[30] Ding, D. Q., Wang, X. P., Ding, X. H. Global stability of multigroup dengue disease transmission model. Journal of Applied Mathematics., 2012, 12, 11–20.

[31] Levin, M. W., Shang, M., Stern, R. Effects of short-term travel on COVID-19 spread: A novel SEIR model and case study in Minnesota. PLoS ONE, 2021, 16(1), e0245919. https://doi.org/10.1371/journal.pone.0245919.

[32] Bhaduri, E., Manoj, B. S., Wadud, Z., Goswami, A. K., Choudhury, C. F. Modelling the effects of COVID-19 on travel mode choice behaviour in India. Transportation Research Interdisciplinary Perspectives, 2020, 8, 100273. ISSN 2590–1982. https://doi.org/10.1016/j.trip.2020.100273.

[33] Sattenspiel, L., Dietz, K. A structured epidemic model incorporating geographic mobility among regions. Mathematical Biosciences, 1995, 128(1–2), 71–91.

[34] Furukawa, N. W., Brooks, J. T., Sobel, J. Evidence supporting transmission of severe acute respiratory syndrome coronavirus 2 while presymptomatic or asymptomatic. Emerging Infectious Diseases, 2020, 26(7), e201595. doi: 10.3201/eid2607.201595.

[35] Chatterjee, S., Sarkar, A., Karmakar, M., Chatterjee, S., Paul, R. SEIRD model to study the asymptomatic growth during COVID-19 pandemic in India. Indian Journal of Physics Proceedings of the Indian Association for the Cultivation of Science, 2020, 2004, 1–13. doi: 10.1007/s12648-020-01928-8. Epub ahead of print. PMID: 33250600; PMCID: PMC7678779.

[36] Kumari, P., Singh, H. P., Singh, S. SEIAQRDT model for the spread of novel coronavirus (COVID-19): A case study in India. Applied Intelligence, 2021, 51, 2818–2837, https://doi.org/10.1007/s10489-020-01929-4.

[37] Ivorra, B., Miriam, R. F., Vela, M., Ramos, A. M. Mathematical modeling of the spread of the coronavirus disease 2019 (COVID-19) taking into account the undetected infections. The case of China. Communications in Nonlinear Science and Numerical Simulation, 2020, 88, 105303. doi: 10.1016/j.cnsns.2020.105303.

[38] Sun, S., Zheng, Y. The research of SEIJR model with time-delay based on 2019-nCov. IEEE Access, 2021, 9, 117949–117956. doi: 10.1109/ACCESS.2021.3107521.
[39] Chen, M., Li, M., Hao, Y., Liu, Z., Hu, L., Wang, L. The introduction of population migration to SEIAR for COVID-19 epidemic modeling with an efficient intervention strategy. Information Fusion, 2020, 64, 252–258. doi: 10.1016/j.inffus.2020.08.002. Epub 2020 Aug 6. PMID: 32834796; PMCID: PMC7406520.
[40] Menda, K., Laird, L., Kochenderfer, M. J., et al. Explaining COVID-19 outbreaks with reactive SEIRD models. Scientific Reports, 2021, 11, 17905. https://doi.org/10.1038/s41598-021-97260-0.
[41] Akindeinde, S. O., Okyere, E., Adewumi, A. O., Lebelo, R. S., Fabelurin, O. O., Moore, S. E. Caputo fractional-order SEIRP model for COVID-19 Pandemic. Alexandria Engineering Journal, 2022, 61(1), 829–845. ISSN 1110–0168. https://doi.org/10.1016/j.aej.2021.04.097.
[42] Tsori, Y., Granek, R. Epidemiological model for the inhomogeneous spatial spreading of COVID-19 and other diseases. PLOS ONE, 2021, 16(2), e0246056. https://doi.org/10.1371/journal.pone.0246056.
[43] Nave, O., et al. . Θ-SEIHRD mathematical model of Covid19-stability analysis using fast-slow decomposition. Peer Journal, 2020, 8, e10019. doi: 10.7717/peerj.10019–31.
[44] Otto, S. P., Day, T., Arino, J., Colijn, C., Dushoff, J., Li, M., Mechai, S., Van Domselaar, G., Wu, J., Earn, D., Ogden, N. H. The origins and potential future of SARS-CoV-2 variants of concern in the evolving COVID-19 pandemic. Current Biology: CB, 2021, 31(14), R918–R929. https://doi.org/10.1016/j.cub.2021.06.049.
[45] Duong, D. Alpha, Beta, Delta, Gamma: What's important to know about SARS-CoV-2 variants of concern? CMAJ: Canadian Medical Association Journal = Journal de l'Associationmedicalecanadienne, 2021, 193(27), E1059–E1060. doi: 10.1503/cmaj.1095949.
[46] Mallapaty, S., Callaway, E., Kozlov, M., Ledford, H., Pickrell, J., Van Noord En, R. How Covid vaccines shaped 2021-in eight powerful charts. Nature, 2021, 600, 580–583. doi: https://doi.org/10.1038/d41586-021-03686-x.
[47] Chen, Z., et al. Global diversity of policy, coverage, and demand of COVID-19 vaccines: a descriptive study Preprint at https://doi.org/10.1101/2021.10.25.21265504, 2021.
[48] Bernal, J., et al. Early effectiveness of COVID-19 vaccination with BNT162b2 mRNA vaccine and ChAdOx1 adenovirus vector vaccine on symptomatic disease, hospitalisations and mortality in older adults in England. https://doi.org/10.1101/2021.03.01.21252652

Aparajita Bhattacharya, Arindam Mitra*

Development and repurposing of drugs against COVID-19 using artificial intelligence

Abstract: Severe acute respiratory syndrome coronavirus 2 (SARS-CoV-2), a lineage of Betacoronavirus, is the causative agent of COVID-19, which has caused millions of deaths and crippled economies around the world. Early detection and treatment of COVID-19 cases are crucial for containment and reduction in disease transmission. During an emergency such as a pandemic like COVID-19, when there is a lack of available treatment against a new disease, drug repurposing or repositioning can be an effective strategy to control the disease. Drug repositioning is cost-effective, minimizes failure in clinical trials, and obtains relatively speedy approval from regulatory authorities. Artificial intelligence (AI)-mediated drug repositioning treatment of COVID-19 patients can speed up the management and medical care for the patients. AI, which includes cognitive computing, deep learning, convolutional neural networks, and machine learning, can identify potential antiviral drugs for treating a disease. The time frame for extracting essential facts, statistics, and evaluation of the existing preapproved and approved drugs using molecular descriptors can be reduced by AI technology. Based on experimental data, different supervised machine learning and deep learning algorithms are implemented as a part of AI strategies to identify the repurposable drug effectively. Screening of presently available drugs and the existing library of natural compounds or novel drug candidates for the treatments against COVID-19 can be based on protein–ligand or protein–peptide interactions, which are facilitated through machine learning and deep learning. Such screening reduces the frequency of failures that might occur in clinical trials. This chapter focuses on repurposing existing drugs using AI strategies, particularly in the context of SARS CoV 2.

1 Introduction

The Coronavirus genome contains a positive-sense single-stranded RNA and belongs to the family Coronaviridae, subfamily Coronavirinae, and the order Nidovirales [1]. In general, birds and mammals are infected by Coronavirus, which constitutes one of the

***Corresponding author: Arindam Mitra**, Department of Biological Sciences, School of Life Science and Biotechnology, Adamas University, Kolkata, West Bengal, India,
e-mail: arindam.mitra@adamasuniversity.ac.in, ORCID ID: 0000-0002-1591-6164
Aparajita Bhattacharya, Department of Biological Sciences, School of Life Science and Biotechnology, Adamas University, Kolkata, West Bengal, India

https://doi.org/10.1515/9783110767681-007

diverse groups of virus families. Spike proteins, a major surface protein of Coronavirus, differ widely among genera of Coronavirus and confers specificity for the attachment to host cell surface receptors. Severe acute respiratory syndrome coronavirus 2 (SARS-CoV-2) is the causative agent of the disease COVID-19. The two subfamilies of the Coronaviridae family are Letovirinae and Orthocoronavirinae. Alphaletovirus, Alphacoronavirus, Betacoronavirus, Gammacoronavirus, and Deltacoronavirus are the five genera of the coronavirus [2, 3]. Studies in the characterization of various strains of SARS-CoV-2 have revealed the existence of gastrointestinal and respiratory issues with COVID-19 [4]. Tiredness, dry cough, respiratory problems, and fever are the commonly observable symptoms of COVID-19. According to the CDC guidelines, the incubation period of COVID-19 is between 2 and 14 days. Generally, in most cases, the symptoms appear 5 days post-infection [4]. The death rate indicates the disease's extreme outcomes and is constantly monitored and updated by global health organizations and agencies. The morbidity of Coronavirus is 3–4%. It has caused mounting infections and caused incalculable devastation to the world economy [5–8]. The four structural proteins of spike, envelope, membrane, and nucleocapsid show similarity among the Betacoronavirus. Betacoronavirus has three lineages such as SARS-CoV, SARS-CoV-2, and Middle East respiratory syndrome, and have infected over 100 million people worldwide [9]. All three lineages could be transmitted to humans via zoonosis. SARS-CoV-2 encodes at least 29 proteins, including 4 structural proteins, 16 nonstructural proteins, and 9 accessory proteins [10, 11]. SARS-CoV-2 binds to the ACE-2 receptor of the human epithelial cells in the lungs.

Antiviral drugs against SARS-CoV-2 frequently target surface and other proteins. Some drugs have been approved initially via emergency authorization for treatment against COVID-19. Remdesivir, developed by Gilead Sciences, targets RNA-dependent RNA polymerase (Rdrp) and received emergency authorization from Food and Drug Administration, USA (FDA) [1, 2]. Hydroxychloroquine, an angiotensin inhibitor, also received approval from FDA and is employed for high-risk COVID-19 patients [3, 4]. Several drugs have been repurposed for the treatment of SARS-CoV-2. In times of pandemic, there is an immediate requirement for drugs to treat COVID-19 patients. However, conventionally drug discovery and testing processes can take several years, and some can take even decades. In a global pandemic, there is an immediate need for drugs for treatment; hence, an existing approved drug for one condition can be used or repurposed to meet the urgent need to address a global pandemic like COVID-19. Such drug repurposing can enhance the speed of drug discovery and reduce costs associated with drug development, particularly in clinical trials.

Furthermore, as the safety profile of the repurposed drug is known, it would also get speedy approval from regulatory agencies once other criteria of the intended drug are established. Artificial intelligence (AI) can facilitate drug discovery, repurposing and development, and even combination therapy. Such technology can be beneficial when there is an urgent need for treatment or when there is no available treatment for a given ailment or disease. In the COVID-19 situation, AI-empowered drug repurposing can be of immense benefit, especially with technological progress in AI and enhanced computational power. Having the credibility of being an evidence-based medical tool, AI has been utilized in drug discovery or repurposing to treat COVID-19 patients at the right time. The technology can even be called a lifesaver in the health sector as it broadens the perspective of a drug that has been repurposed or developed. The benefits of drug repurposing are summarized in Figure 1.

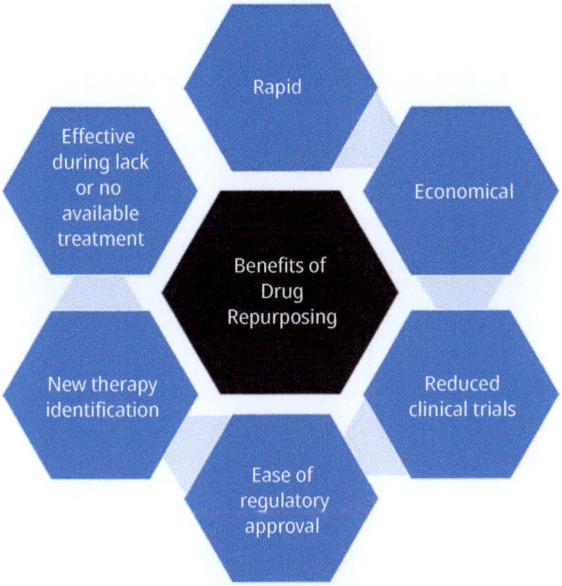

Figure 1: Benefits of drug repurposing or repositioning.

AI simulates human intelligence and makes machines programmed to think like humans and mimic actions such as problem-solving and data interpretation. AI-based approaches are machine learning (ML) and deep learning (DL). The drug repurposing approaches for COVID-19 are based on network, structure, and ML or DL approaches. This chapter reviews the strategies for repurposing and discovering drugs against COVID-19 using AI. This review shows the contribution of AI in the application of a way to prevent COVID-19.

1.1 Drugs repurposed for the treatment of COVID-19

In the current scenario, doctors use antiviral drugs to treat COVID patients because of the lack of related SARS-CoV-2 medicines. These drugs inhibit various biochemical pathways and proteins, and thus they help prevent viral growth. Many of these drugs have been repurposed for COVID-19 and used with varying efficacy and safety. Among them, antimalarial drugs, chloroquine, and hydroxychloroquine are widely used.

1.1.1 Hydroxychloroquine ($C_{18}H_{26}ClN_3O$)

Hydroxychloroquine is an aminoquinoline. R and S enantiomers constitute this medicine. Like chloroquine, it elevates the endosome's pH and prevents virus particles' formation and entrance.

SARS-CoV-2 is effectively treated with hydroxychloroquine [5]. It has a preference for cross-linking human DNA. It is also a TLR 7 and 9 competitor, influencing the function of angiotensin-converting enzyme 2 in humans.

1.1.2 Lopinavir ($C_{37}H_{48}N_4O_5$)

Gag polyprotein, along with its proteolytic products, controls the different events of the life cycle of human immunodeficiency virus (HIV), such as assembly, budding, and maturation. It is primarily used to treat HIV-1 patients, but in this pandemic, it was found that it can be used in combination with ritonavir [6]. However, lopinavir's bioavailability and biotransformation are very poor. Ritonavir inhibits the metabolism of lopinavir by inactivating the enzyme responsible for its metabolism. The hydroxy ethylene scaffold in lopinavir helps mimic the peptide linkage cleaved by HIV protease and thus reduces the action of the HIV-1 protease enzyme [6]. Darunavir ($C_{27}H_{37}N_3O_7S$) is also used to treat HIV-1. It also inhibits the activity of the protease. This compound is now under clinical trial to treat COVID-19 patients [7]. The mode of action of darunavir is related to that of lopinavir as it also reduces the proteolysis of Gag protein. Darunavir mainly interacts with two amino acids of the primary chain in protease (Asp-29 and Asp-30). This compound is effective for the treatment of resilient strains of HIV1 [8].

1.1.3 Ritonavir ($C_{37}H_{48}N_6O_5S_2$)

It is an HIV protease inhibitor. P-glycoprotein and MRP efflux channels help ritonavir to control the protease inhibitors.

1.1.4 Favipiravir ($C_5H_4FN_3O_2$)

Pyrazine is an analog of favipiravir and is employed to treat influenza by targeting the RNA-dependent RNA polymerase [9]. These enzymes are mainly used for the replication and transcription of viral genomes. Favipiravir inhibits the replication of influenza A and B [10]. This drug is used for the treatment of the Lassa and Ebola virus. Favipiravir can restrict the entry and exit of viruses from cells; thus, they are used to treat patients with COVID-19 [11]. The active form of favipiravir, ribofuranosyl-5′-triphosphate, RTP, prevents viral genome replication by blocking the RNA polymerase enzyme.

2 AI-mediated process of drug discovery against COVID-19

Traditional drug discovery could take more than 10 years to complete. However, AI uses an in silico approach in the drug discovery and pharmacogenomics process and reduces the time for both in vitro and in vivo assays. Drug discovery starts with a hypothesis, validating the idea by selecting lead candidates from the database and optimizing parameters such as binding to the target, therapeutic effect, bioavailability, and toxicity. Identification of lead molecules is made by AI algorithms such as neural networks, omics analysis, protein fold prediction, and homology modeling. Some web-based tools like Deep Tox, PADME, and Lim tox predict toxicity associated with the lead molecules. Some AI tools for drug discovery include PADME, PREDICT, XenoSite, and ORGANIC.

During the COVID-19 pandemic, many studies utilized AI/ML-based approaches to develop novel drugs against COVID-19. The approaches are the discovery of targets and small molecules and the prediction of clinical trials' outcome. AI/ML-based generative chemistry pipeline has been designed to predict the novel drug-like inhibitors of COVID-19. The approach uses homology modeling and crystal structure of target proteins. The deep Q-learning approach utilizes drug design based on fragments using medicinal chemistry knowledge to develop novel molecules to target SARS-CoV-2 3C-like (3CL) protease. Another study explored the deep docking model from the ZINC library and selected some thousand potential 3CL protease inhibitors. CogMol, a deep generative model (DGM), can generate thousands of drugs targeting a given protein sequence. The AI-based platform has successfully designed targets to inhibit several targets of SARS-CoV-2, including 3CL protease, RBD of S protein, NSP9, and replicase. Another DGM has successfully found inhibitors of 3CL protease, which used transfer and reinforcement learning for developing molecules with drug-like attributes. Another study explored the development of an AI-based model for creating broad-spectrum drugs for SARS-CoV-2 by using a deep massage passing neural network. In vitro studies have further demonstrated that the selected compounds have a strong affinity to bind to 3CL protease. Using a combination of search algorithm and multi-neural network has further identified new drug candidates by using a strategy of re-training and search. All these approaches are in Figure 2.

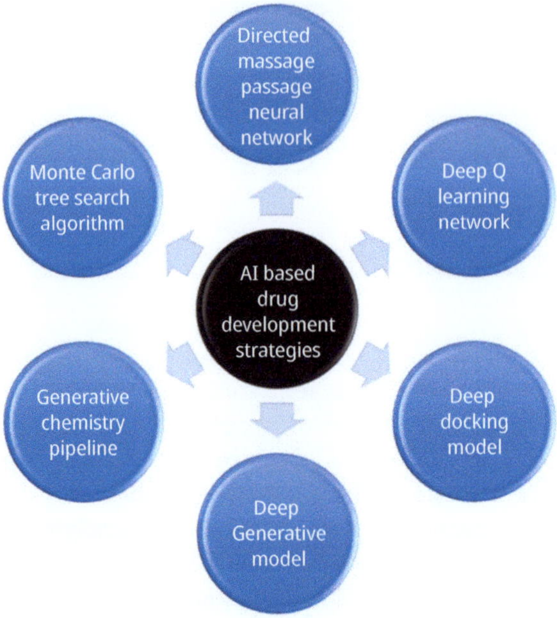

Figure 2: The AI-mediated strategy of drug development against COVID-19.

3 AI-based drug repurposing approaches against COVID-19

The drug repositioning process differs from conventional medicine development against COVID-19. Often, computational approaches can be used for drug repurposing, including network-based, structure-based, and AI-based approaches or a combination of these approaches [12–14].

3.1 Network-based approach

For repurposing the drugs, the objective is to rapidly predict and manipulate related biological pathways and the off-target biology from existing safe drugs that can be subjected to clinical trials via wet-lab approaches; network-based model simulation. AI helps to screen the new targets using existing drugs and even facilitates the identification of chemical entities. For virus–host interactome analysis, it has been proved to be the primary computational approach [15].

The UK-based benevolent AI leveraged the knowledge graph derived through artificial technology, which combines biomedical data from structured and unstructured sources [16]. It inhibits the host protein AAK1, and the drug has been approved for treating rheumatoid arthritis [17]. The DL derived based on the drug–target interaction (DTI) model forecasts economically available drug that inhibits viral infection. It can target protease and helicase that is related to SARS-CoV-2. Deep convolutional neural network technology can target various SARS-CoV-2 protein-binding sites of different coronaviruses and assist in developing novel broad-spectrum antiviral medicines. The identification of existing drugs targeting the main viral proteins, especially the main protease ($3CL^{pro}$) and spike protein, can be accomplished by other multitask DL model applications. The mining of PolypharmDB, a known platform of drugs and their predicted binding site, can be cited as an example.

The network-based approach is crucial for drug repurposing because it combines many databases [18, 19]. Networks can represent the molecular interaction in the biological pathways or systems [20]. In this approach, nodes represent drugs, diseases, or proteins, and the edges denote the connection among the nodes [21, 22]. The interaction of drugs with targets, diseases, proteins, and other drugs can be generated using a network approach. Such interactive patterns and connections can speed up the identification of potential new biological targets and can be helpful in drug discovery and repurposing [23]. Two network-based approaches can benefit COVID-19 management, including clustering and propagation approaches.

The network-dependent clustering approach attempts to find the drug–target relationship [24]. Several methods employed using clustering algorithms according to the topological structure of networks is the aim of the network-established clustering approach.

3.2 Network-established propagation approach

The human protein interactome model measures network closeness between therapeutic targets and HCV-associated proteins to select worthy potential medicines for HCV. A pan-HCV protein subnetwork is produced by combining human Coronavirus with a host protein found in the literature. The network-based approach aids in the examination of several key patterns that may be used to classify proteins that are functionally related to HCV. A networking technique may be used to investigate several practical and essential methods to classify protein functionally connected with HCVs across the human system network. It can also mimic proteins for therapeutic targeting of specific ailments [15, 25].

3.3 Structure-based approach

Viral screening can help identify small chemical compounds associated with molecular targets with their 3D structure. The structure-established approach helps screen many compounds quickly, reducing the cost of developing a new disease. Structural biology approaches include efforts to decipher the structure of proteins essential to infection, reproduction, and spread of the virus. A molecular docking-based process involves a computational technique to know the relationship between chemical and biological components, which helps drug repurposing [26]. Drugs have been repurposed against COVID-19 following structure-based medicine, and the results were out even before the availability of three-dimensional structures. The findings can be used for the structure prediction of several target viral proteins, all essential for virus activity [27]. Such an approach can conduct virtual screenings of chemical libraries, including authorized drugs and natural compounds.

The Protein Data Bank, a repository of the three-dimensional structures of proteins, now has a section dedicated to COVID-19 proteins [28]. A computer-aided drug design identified the SARS-CoV-2 Mpro complexed along with an inhibitor [29]. Over 500 SARS-CoV-2 proteins linked with ligand structures and their target cell receptors were solved and made available (up to October 14, 2020). X-ray crystallography can solve the structures with a good resolution. These computer simulations tried to predict the capacity of existing drugs to either limit their activity or impede their identification and alliance interaction with cell counterparts, which is required for viral entry and multiplication. The standard methodology is followed for the thorough virtual scanning of drug databases. Different docking procedures, including molecular dynamics simulations, are typically done in more sophisticated ways. The free energy prediction and the top hits with the specified target protein are used to achieve this [30].

3.4 Artificial intelligence-based approach

Another field of ML is DL. This approach is proposed for attempting to find drugs that are potential for antiviral activity against the Coronavirus [31]. This approach actively combats the effects of COVID-19. The assigned learning facilitates screening of an excessive number of compounds and finding the actions that have the potential to inhibit SARS-CoV-2 [32]. In addition, DTI based on DL is called molecule transformer DTI, commonly referred to as MT-DTI. The viral components of SARS-COV-2, like proteinase and helicase, may be disintegrated by the commercially available antiviral drugs, which are predicted with the help of this model (MT-DTI). Applying the MT-DTI forecast, raw prediction of FDA-approved antiviral medications and target viral proteins is evaluated. MT-DTI also predicted a comparison of binding affinities of three drugs approved by the FDA to those measured by AutoDock Vina might not precisely match and can require validation by other experimentation [33].

4 AI/ML-based algorithms for drug repurposing against COVID-19

There are many approaches for drug repositioning against COVID-19. They are network-based, integrated docking-based, and expression-based approaches, as shown in Figure 3.

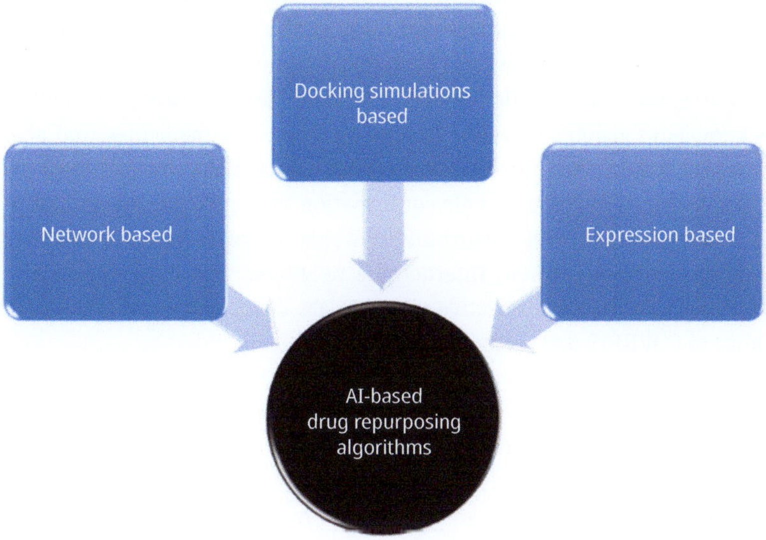

Figure 3: AI-based approaches for drug repositioning against COVID-19.

4.1 Network-based algorithms

The knowledge graphs connect various medical elements, such as diseases, drugs, and proteins. Applying network-related algorithms to knowledge graphs can identify target proteins or specific regions of the interactome of the host [34, 35]. Human proteins that belong to a complex or part of the signaling are often considered excellent targets for inhibition of viruses in the virus–host network. A combination of network and learning approaches can further identify other targets of SARS-CoV-2. Several studies have used protein–protein interactome network-based techniques to forecast therapeutic prospects [36].

A convolutional neural network-based DL model employed a protein–ligand network and used SARS-CoV-2 3CL protease as a seed for identifying targets for COVID-19. This model identified various chemical ligands, including meglumine, vidarabine, adenosine, and possible peptide ligands, including isoleucine, lysine, and proline amino acids, as a potential therapy [9]. Molecular transfer DTI, a pretrained language model, is also used to evaluate FDA-approved antivirals. Atazanavir, an antiretroviral drug predicted by MT-DTI, targets HIV and has also been found to have an inhibitory effect against the 3CL protease [37]. A convolutional neural network has been created to identify potential targets against SARS-CoV-2 ligands that predicted 33 ligands that can bind strongly to spike protein of the SARS-CoV-2. With the combination of multiple network-based strategies [38] and a combining DL approach, CoV-KGE has been developed to detect drugs for COVID-19 after comprehensively captivating the links between medicines, diseases, and protein-gene pathway expression, systematic analysis of transcriptions, and proteomic data. Human cells infected with SARS-CoV-2 are the sources of these. The trials have successfully identified 41 drug candidates for the treatment of COVID-19, including dexamethasone, indomethacin, niclosamide, and toremifene [39]. It generates a large knowledge graph connecting host genes, pathways, medicines, and phenotypes. The awareness about candidate drugs' resemblance to biological relationships came from deep graph embedding. Large-scale confirmation through experimentation finally represented 22 drug candidates. By fusing different module forms while considering virus–host interactions, protein–protein interactome networks, and drug–target networks, these algorithms can discover effective, appropriate drugs and combinations of drugs in the instance of COVID-19 drug remodeling.

4.2 Expression-based algorithms

The expression of defense genes in the diseased conditions can be used to repurpose drugs against COVID-19. The drugs that reverse the expression of defense genes in a diseased state can be an effective strategy for controlling the disease [40]. Feeding the data from transcriptomics in an AI-based platform has led to an insight into the effectiveness of approved drugs or natural compounds. Combining data from transcriptomic, proteomic, structural, and aging markers creates a computational drug repurposing strategy [41]. Aged patients, in particular, are vulnerable to SARS-CoV-2 infections; hence, gene expression changes in such population and when combined with AI was effective in finding drugs such as clemastine and quinapril. Extraction of typical features from omics data is also possible by anticipated data augmentation strategy, which has outperformed advanced methods. The model's validity is tested by screening chemical compounds from the drug bank against the clinical profile of COVID-19.

4.3 Integrated docking simulation algorithms

ML-aided molecular docking is very important for virtual screening. Molecular docking can determine how a drug would interact with a specific biological target in the pathogen, hence, its potential for drug repurposing. Docking simulations can be combined with AI/ML techniques to speed up the drug repurposing processes. Using a

MathPose and a CNN, termed MathDL, could predict the binding sites for 3CL protease. Similarly, another random forest aggression model predicted potential candidate ligands, of which the FDA approves many. Other approaches involve combining end-to-end neural networks with docking algorithms to evaluate the approved list of drugs. Screening the drugs further in various databases such as ZINC enabled the identification of Amprenavir, a drug that has already received approval for the treatment of HIV.

5 Conclusions

The spread of COVID-19 has disrupted the economy of the world. This chapter discussed how AI technology has helped scientists repurpose existing drugs against COVID-19 patients in this pandemic. It has been used to protect healthcare professionals and can be used to shield against the next pandemic. AI will continue to repurpose existing drugs and help to develop new drugs against COVID-19 to prevent such a situation due to the outbreak of new diseases. ML approaches have been used to reposition the drugs, while DL-based methods have been used to generate novel drugs or candidates for targeting SARS-CoV-2.

The emergency of the COVID-19 pandemic has shifted drug discovery and drug repurposing research at an unprecedented pace to find a drug for the containment of SARS-CoV-2. However, this immediate requirement of drug candidates may not serve science as proper clinical trials and evaluations are needed to ensure the safety and efficacy of any drug. Computational studies on the same host target have often identified different drugs. A major setback in these studies is the lack of experimental support or evidence to support the results. In many cases, the drugs identified were not successful in clinical trials. In many instances, experiments were not carefully designed, or the interpretation of the results was not made adequately. Besides, some scientific studies were not adequately peer-reviewed before publishing, which adds to the existing data pool lacking rigor.

One primary reason of AI-based approaches in drug discovery or repurposing has not been practical is that initially the pathogen information was not substantial or enough. Basic research on pathogens like SARS-CoV-2 could strengthen knowledge and mechanisms regarding highly pathogenic microorganisms. AI technology has the potential to speed up the process of COVID-19 and other infectious disease management and medical care. The COVID-19 pandemic is expected to continue shortly to the evolution of SARS-CoV-2 strains, which might pose additional challenges. The existing drug or a vaccine may not be practical due to mutation or change in the sequence of the virus. As a result, drugs screened or repurposed for one strain of SARS-CoV-2 may not be as effective with other strains. Hence, the results of newer studies should be continued to feed into relevant databases for proper AI-based training or search. This

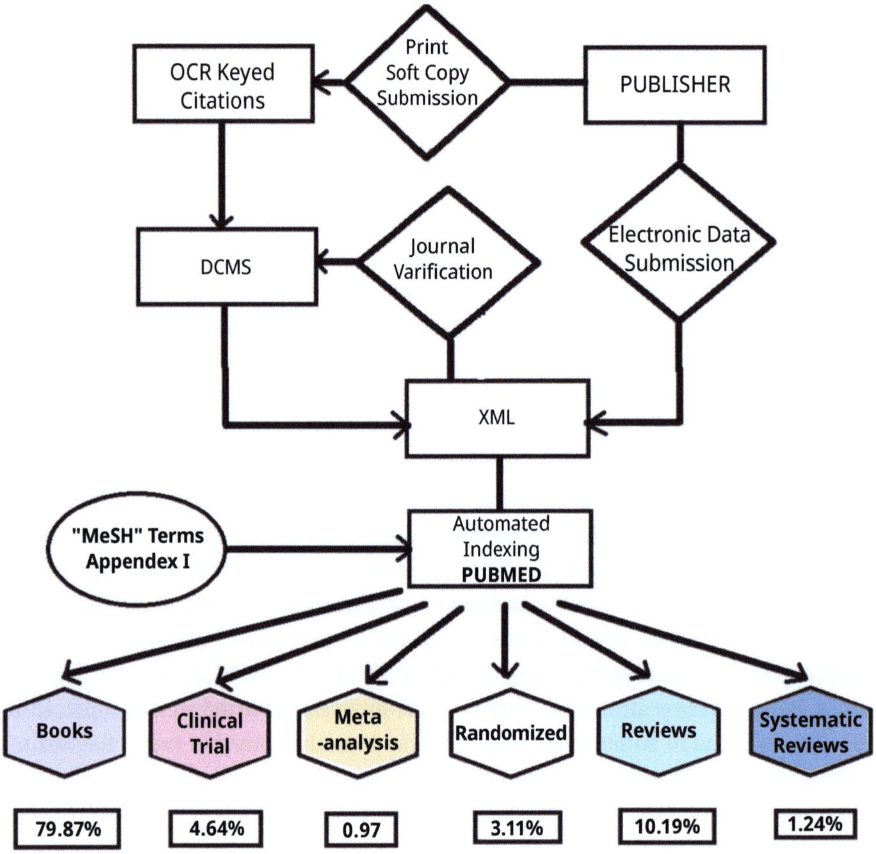

Figure 3: Data flow process and number of entries available for psychological diseases in the PUBMED database.

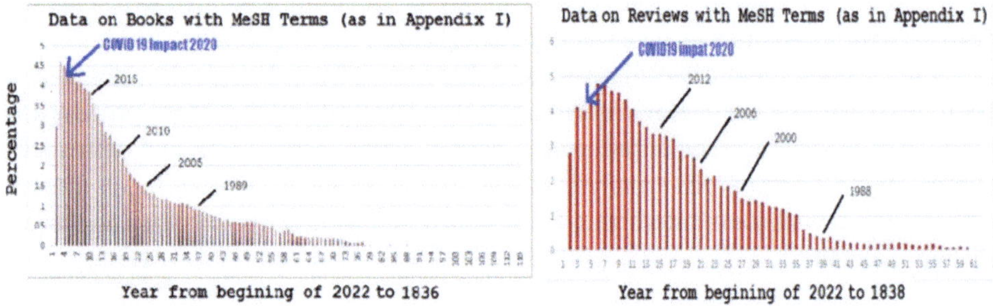

Figure 4: Data of descriptive research (books and reviews published) on psychological disorders in the PUBMED database.

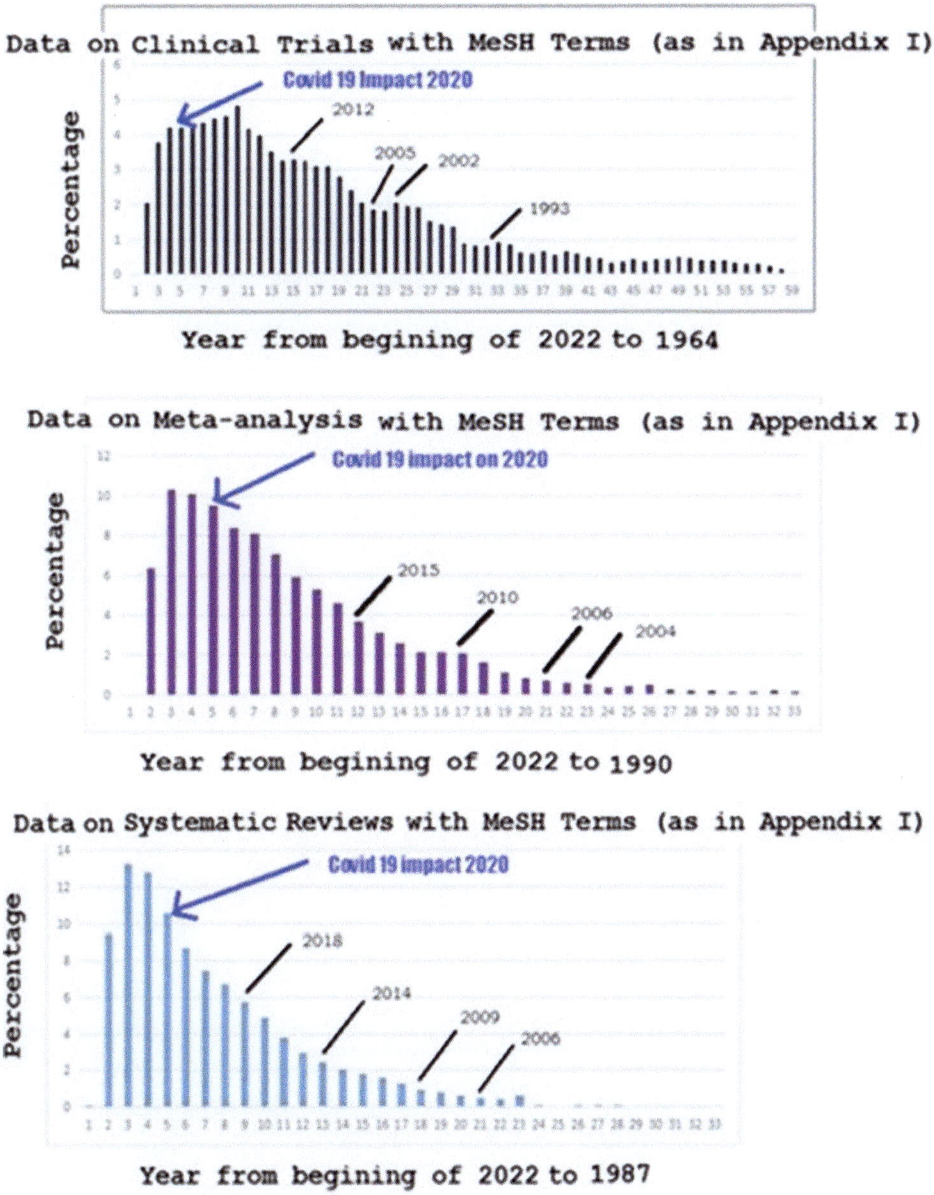

Figure 5: Data of analytical research (clinical trials, systematic reviews, and meta-analysis published) on psychological disorders in the PUBMED database.

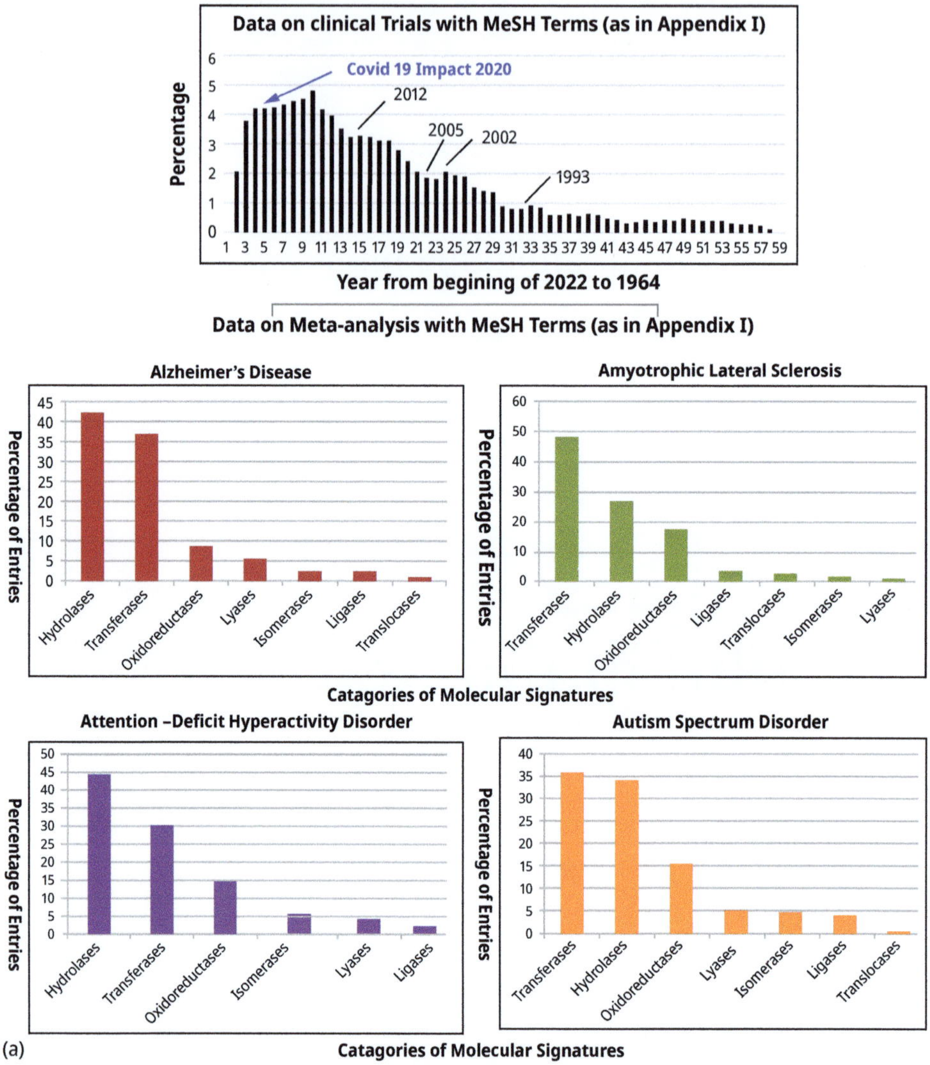

(a)

Figure 6: (a)–(d) Molecular signatures and entries in the RCSB-PDB databases and relative numbers and types of molecules related to some psychological disorders identified.

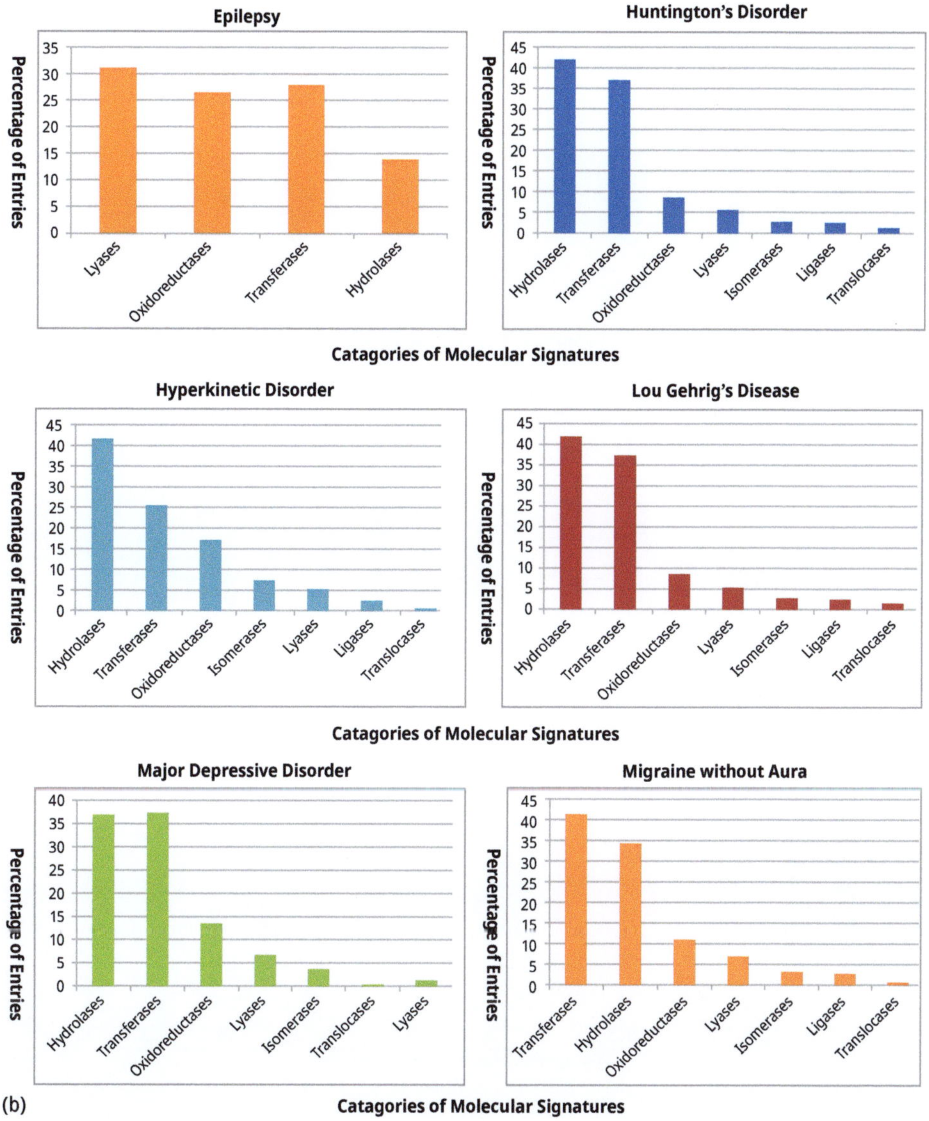

(b)

Figure 6 (Continued)

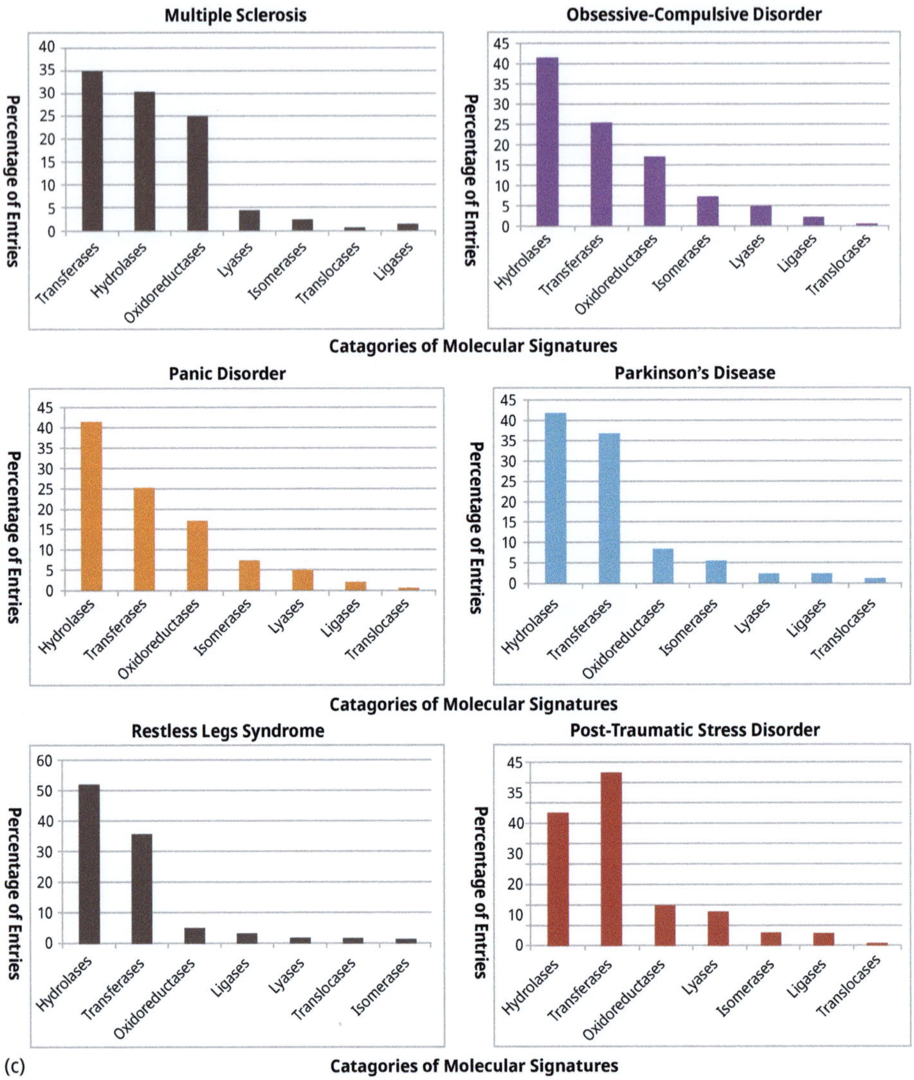

Figure 6 (Continued)

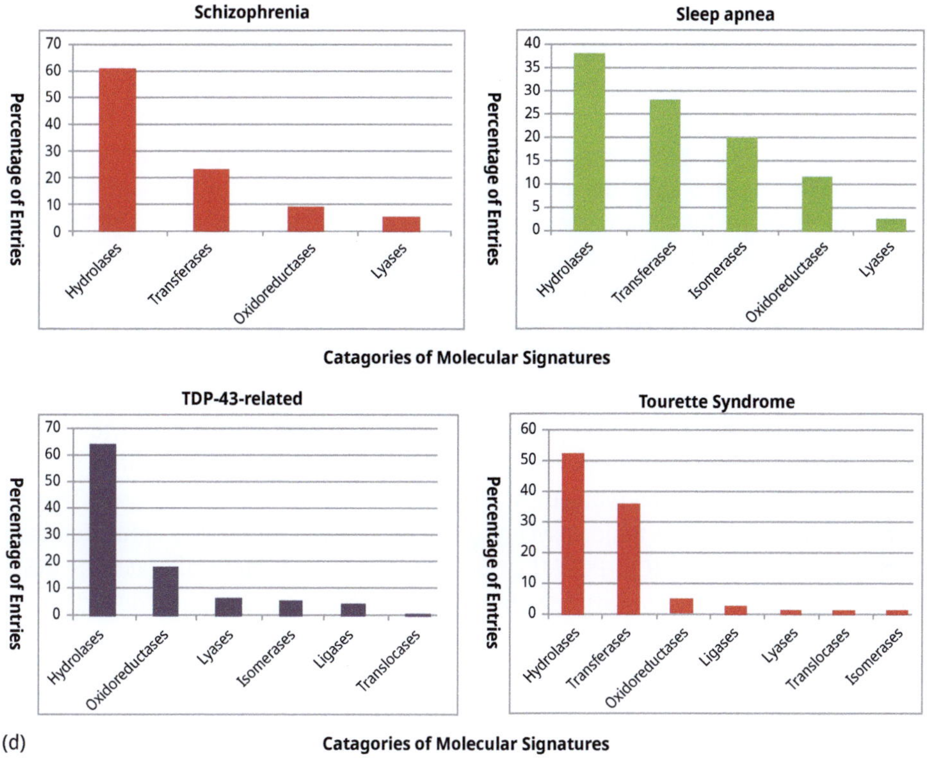

(d)

Figure 6 (Continued)

4 Discussion

Mental well-being is indispensable for productivity, and in this chapter, the goal is to identify the major psychological disorders for which significant amount of published research is available in scientific bibliographic databases. NCBI-PUBMED is the most superior database of peer-reviewed health-care research, and it has aid to identify the major psychological disorders that have been recorded scientifically in quantitative terms. While RSB-PDB assisted to find the biomolecular cause of the identified psychological disorders that hinders human productivity significantly. These databases authenticate data by their in-house quality control protocols and scientific review. This approach is simple and straightforward and can be replicated for identification of subtypes of any diseases and can aid to identify their causes. In order to provide accurate information on health-care and allied aspects, simple and easily deploy strategies should be developed. For categorizing major psychological disorders and to have an overview of biomolecular aspects of these syndromes, a straightforward approach harnessing the biomolecular computational databases has been attempted in this study. This would aid to prioritize target groups that are in utmost need of therapeutic intervention during and beyond the pandemic. Psychological disorders and syndromes are large group of ailments with often interconnected manifestation. Several biomolecular entities have been identified, which are vital for maintaining a sound mental health. In this chapter, the computational databases and their architecture with respect to various biomolecules such as catalytic proteins and enzymes that maintain optimum mental faculty have been analyzed in a data-driven machine learning environment. Moreover, the databases of biomolecular entities and small molecules have been reviewed. Finally, a meta-analytic approach attempted to figure out some current trends in the interventions for maintaining sound mental health. This interdisciplinary study would aid to give an overview of developments that aims toward preserving a productive and sound mental health with respect to a data-driven biomedical and machine learning ecosystem. This chapter describes a novel strategy to utilize advanced biomedical databases for mental health research. This research not only identifies major psychological disorders from bibliographic database of health information (NCBI-PUBMED) but also focus on bimolecular targets (RSB-PDB) which may serve as a starting point to mitigate these psychological disorders.

5 Limitations

The role of optimization for query formation during accessing biomedical data is of prime importance. In this chapter, the goal is to identify major psychological disorders reported during or before the COVID pandemic. The goal was not biased in terms of some handful of scientific reports but to rely on the whole database that would reduce false-positive or false-negative entries (Figure 7).

The limitations of the databases are that it takes so much of filtering before the user gets certain query resolved. For example, if the user desires to have the "list of psychological disorders reported most frequently in peer-reviewed scientific literature during and before the pandemic," the NCBI database cannot generate the list. Rather, the user needs to establish a most suitable query using Boolean operators and subsequently manually mine the most relevant scientific reports to able to generate the list. Similarly to identify the most important biological entity responsible for the group of psychological disorders, RCSB-PDB database cannot find out the single most important entity responsible for these disorders. In this background, the strategy described here stands good to generate relevant and user-friendly biomedical information. The novelty of this work lies in the fact that this exercise has identified the crucial points that may be automated to make a program for generating the point and authentic information from biomedical databases.

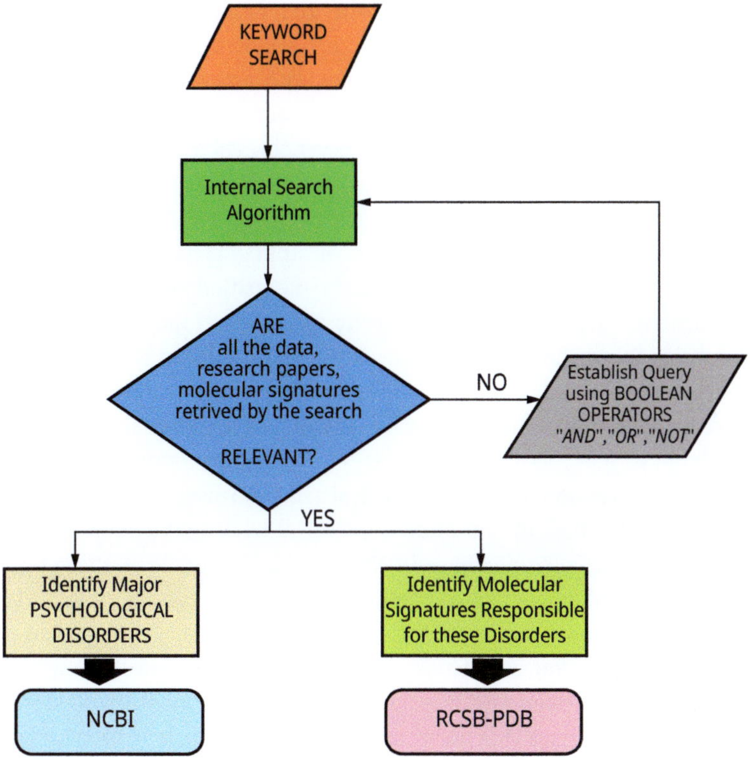

Figure 7: Reducing bias using the robustness of the full database rather than a handful of research studies.

6 Conclusion

Having accurate information of various aspects of psychological conditions would aid to ensure medical care to those who are in utmost need [2, 3]. Moreover, certain group of population may have limited access to accurate information and facts during the onset of natural disasters and crisis [4]. According to the reports of detailed studies, it has been found that organizing or enabling health-care infrastructure to address the effects of the pandemic would aid to take psychologically informed interventions [1].

There has been renewed interest in the relationship between "psychological factors" and manifestation of various diseases. For example, psychiatric morbidity has been examined at all levels of severity of respiratory diseases like asthma. This is seen in both adults and children, and higher rates of psychiatric disorder compared to nonasthmatic populations have been reported [29, 30]. In today's rapidly changing scenarios, psychological stress may lead to other systemic complications. For example, several authors have reviewed the possible mechanisms of interaction between anxiety, depression, and asthma. Studies [31] suggest that recent advances in the understanding of interactions between the central nervous system, immune system, and endocrine function provide plausible biological pathways linking psychosocial stress with asthma. Environmental impact on psychological and mental condition is also prominent. Therefore, in this complex scenario it becomes imperative to identify major psychological conditions that are clinically significant.

The aim of this study was to enumerate the major psychological ailments and disorders through a database approach and data mining of bibliographic database. Subsequently, to examine the molecular signature of the identified diseases from a scientific database is attempted. According to this study, there are 22 major psychological disorders or conditions that should be monitored. The data mining strategy identified 22 major illness of mental origin in the PUBMED database. It is also indicated that initially there were much descriptive research regarding psychological conditions that were published from as early as 1836. However, more technical studies in terms of meta-analysis, systematic review, as well as clinical trials on psychological disorders started later. According to the current analysis, clinical trials on various aspects of psychological conditions started somewhere in 1964. From 1993 onward, there was significant increase in the number of clinical trials. Therefore, this work successfully enumerated the major lineal conditions related to mental and psychological condition from data mining. Moreover, the characteristics of scientific reports regarding mental disorders and related conditions have also been categorized. Subsequently, the study harnessed another scientific database that accumulates and stores various biomolecular data. RSB-PDB database analysis indicated that there are more or less six categories of catalytic entities that are involved in the molecular mechanism of these clinical disease conditions. Among the molecular entities, hydrolases are the most frequent molecular device that is associated with 17 out of 22 identified mental disorders. In more than 65% cases, the identified molecular entities in TDP-43-related disorder are hydrolases. Oxidoreductases and transferases are the molecular entities that are also related to many of the psychological disorders identified.

Moreover, in this study, it is also revealed that the cases of epilepsy and schizophrenia are different in their molecular mechanism. These two diseases are well characterized and only four classes of enzymes are related to these conditions instead of usual six molecules in varied degrees of association. This preliminary study has successfully identified major psychological conditions through data mining. This study also indicates the immediate need for more and more clinical trials. It is recommended that more systematic reviews and meta-analysis are needed to explore more crucial details of different psychological conditions. Moreover, the revelation of biomolecular entities that are associated with different psychological diseases would aid to prioritize therapeutic interventions needed to handle such psychological conditions.

References

[1] Inchausti, F., et al. Psychological intervention and COVID-19: What we know so far and what we can do. Journal of Contemporary Psychotherapy, 2020, 50, 243–250.

[2] Killgore, W. D. S., et al. Psychological resilience during the COVID-19 lockdown. Psychiatry Research, 2020, 291, 113216.

[3] Serafini, G., et al. The psychological impact of COVID-19 on the mental health in the general population. QJM: An International Journal of Medicine, 2020, 113(8), 531–537.

[4] Kontoangelos, K., Economou, M., Papageorgiou, C. Mental health effects of COVID-19 pandemia: A review of clinical and psychological traits. Psychiatry Investigation, 2020, 17(6), 491.

[5] Martin, A., Leone, L., Fries, W., Naccarato, R. Quality of life in inflammatory bowel disease. The Italian Journal of Gastroenterology, 1995, 27, 450–454.

[6] Walker, E. A., Gelfand, M. D., Gelfand, A. N., et al. The relationship of current psychiatric disorder to functional disability and distress in patients with inflammatory bowel disease. General Hospital Psychiatry, 1996, 18, 220–229.

[7] Debnath, S. Characterization of extracellular proteins to explore their role in bio-flocculation for harvesting algal biomass for wastewater treatment. In: The Role of Microalgae in Wastewater Treatment, Springer, Singapore, 2019, 229–266.

[8] Debnath, S., Addya, S. Structural basis for heterogeneous phenotype of ERG11 dependent Azole resistance in C. albicans clinical isolates. Springerplus, 2014 3(1), 1–16.

[9] Debnath, S., Addya, S. Mis-sense mutations in Tafazzin (TAZ) that escort to mild clinical symptoms of Barth syndrome is owed to the minimal inhibitory effect of the mutations on the enzyme function: In-silico evidence. Interdisciplinary Sciences: Computational Life Sciences, 2015, 7(1), 21–35.

[10] Castellani, B., Castellani, J. Data mining: Qualitative analysis with health informatics data. Qualitative Health Research, 2003, 13(7), 1005–1018.

[11] Liu, L., Özsu, M. T. (eds.). Encyclopedia of database systems, Vol. 6, New York, NY, USA, Springer, 2009.

[12] Haux, R., Frank, J., Knaup, P. The IMIA WGI database on health and medical informatics programs and courses: A call for participation. Methods of Information in Medicine, 1997, 36(03), 233–234.

[13] Blak, B., Thompson, M., Dattani, H., Bourke, A. Generalisability of the Health Improvement Network (THIN) database: Demographics, chronic disease prevalence and mortality rates. Journal of Innovation in Health Informatics, 2011, 19(4), 251–255.

[14] Kimura, S., Sato, T., Ikeda, S., Noda, M., Nakayama, T. Development of a database of health insurance claims: Standardization of disease classifications and anonymous record linkage. Journal of Epidemiology, 2010, 20(5), 413–419.

[15] Suinesiaputra, A., Medrano-Gracia, P., Cowan, B. R., Young, A. A. Big heart data: Advancing health informatics through data sharing in cardiovascular imaging. IEEE Journal of Biomedical and Health Informatics, 2014, 19(4), 1283–1290.

[16] Saheb, T., Saheb, M. Analyzing and visualizing knowledge structures of health informatics from 1974 to 2018: A bibliometric and social network analysis. Healthcare Informatics Research, 2019, 25(2), 61–72.

[17] Witham, M. D., Frost, H., McMurdo, M., Donnan, P. T., McGilchrist, M. Construction of a linked health and social care database resource–lessons on process, content and culture. Informatics for Health and Social Care, 2015, 40(3), 229–239.

[18] Moen, A., Knudsen, L. M. M. Nursing informatics: Decades of contribution to health informatics. Healthcare Informatics Research, 2013, 19(2), 86–92.

[19] Rocha, B. M., Filos, D., Mendes, L., Vogiatzis, I., Perantoni, E., Kaimakamis, E., Natsiavas, P., Oliveira, A., Jácome, C., Marques, A., Paiva, R. P. A respiratory sound database for the development of automated classification. In: International Conference on Biomedical and Health Informatics, Singapore, Springer, 2017, November, pp. 33–37.

[20] Harris, S., Shi, S., Brealey, D., MacCallum, N. S., Denaxas, S., Perez-Suarez, D., Ercole, A., Watkinson, P., Jones, A., Ashworth, S., Beale, R. Critical Care Health Informatics Collaborative (CCHIC): Data, tools and methods for reproducible research: A multi-centre UK intensive care database. International Journal of Medical Informatics, 2018, 112, 82–89.

[21] Lu, J. et al. (2015). Data Mining Techniques in Health Informatics: A Case Study from Breast Cancer Research. In: Renda, M., Bursa, M., Holzinger, A., Khuri, S. (eds) Information Technology in Bio- and Medical Informatics. ITBAM 2015. Lecture Notes in Computer Science(), vol 9267. Springer, Cham. https://doi.org/10.1007/978-3-319-22741-2_6

[22] Rocha, B. M., Filos, D., Mendes, L., Serbes, G., Ulukaya, S., Kahya, Y. P., Jakovljevic, N., Turukalo, T. L., Vogiatzis, I. M., Perantoni, E., Kaimakamis, E. An open access database for the evaluation of respiratory sound classification algorithms. Physiological Measurement, 2019, 40(3), 035001.

[23] Kurniati, A. P., Rojas, E., Hogg, D., Hall, G., Johnson, O. A. The assessment of data quality issues for process mining in healthcare using Medical Information Mart for Intensive Care III, a freely available e-health record database. Health Informatics Journal, 2019, 25(4), 1878–1893.

[24] del Mar García-Gil, M., Hermosilla, E., Prieto-Alhambra, D., Fina, F., Rosell, M., Ramos, R., Rodriguez, J., Williams, T., VanStaa, T., Bolíbar, B. Construction and validation of a scoring system for the selection of high-quality data in a Spanish population primary care database (SIDIAP). Journal of Innovation in Health Informatics, 2011, 19(3), 135–145.

[25] Navin, K., Krishnan, M. M., Lavanya, S., Shanthini, A. A mobile health based smart hybrid epidemic surveillance system to support epidemic control programme in public health informatics. In: 2017 international conference on IoT and application (ICIOT), IEEE, 2017, May, pp. 1–4.

[26] Shwetha, G., Lakshmi, P. V., Raja, N. S. M. Analysis of medical image and health informatics using big data. In: 2017 Third International Conference on Science Technology Engineering & Management (ICONSTEM), IEEE, 2017, March, pp. 1005–1009.

[27] Liu, F., Liu, C., Zhao, L., Zhang, X., Wu, X., Xu, X., Liu, Y., Ma, C., Wei, S., He, Z., Li, J. An open access database for evaluating the algorithms of electrocardiogram rhythm and morphology abnormality detection. Journal of Medical Imaging and Health Informatics, 2018, 8(7), 1368–1373.

[28] Canese, K., Weis, S. PubMed: The bibliographic database. The NCBI Handbook, 2013, 2, 1.

[29] Campbell, D. A., Yellowlees, P. M., McLennan, G., et al. Psychiatric and medical features of near fatal asthma. Thorax, 1995, 50, 254–259.

[30] Mrazek, D. A. Psychiatric complications of pediatric asthma. Ann Allergy, 1992, 69, 285–293.

[31] Wright, R. J., Rodriguez, M., Cohen, S. Review of psychosocial stress and asthma: An integrated bio-psychosocial approach. Thorax, 1998, 53, 1066–R1.

Lam Oanh Ha, Trung Hieu Nguyen, Van Chien Nguyen*

Developing financial inclusion in the context of Covid-19 pandemic: the case of a developing country

Abstract: Technology revolution 4.0 has brought e-banking financial products and services to development because it helps to increase transparency, ensure privacy, speed up transaction processing, thereby creating trust and maintaining loyalty to the customers. Financial inclusion has made important contributions to economic growth in many countries. In the context of Covid-19 pandemic, countries that have continuously maintained a state of social distancing have changed the consumption habits of people and businesses. Through empirical research of an emerging country in Southeast Asia, the research results show that financial inclusion has greatly supported basic financial products and services such as mobilizing and lending capital at a reasonable cost. In addition, the research results also confirm that Internet banking or mobile banking, Fintech services are most commonly used while other services such as securities investment, technology insurance are not yet developed. The research believes that the Covid-19 pandemic could lead to a faster development of financial inclusion due to people's changing habits and the increasing use of financial technology in transactions.

1 Introduction

Financial inclusion plays an important role in the economic development of every country. Overall, financial inclusion aims to provide formal financial services in a convenient and low-cost way to all citizens [1, 2]. For low-income people, financial inclusion enhances access to finance, contributing to livelihoods, thereby promoting economic growth. The question that many authors raise is whether digital finance will continue to thrive in times of crisis [3, 4].

Financial inclusion has evolved toward providing individuals and organizations having access to financial services at reasonable prices. Financial inclusion is determined by three criteria: (1) access to financial services, (2) use of financial services,

***Corresponding author: Van Chien Nguyen,** Institute of Graduate Studies, Thu Dau Mot University, Binh Duong, Thu Dau Mot City, Vietnam, e-mail: chiennv@tdmu.edu.vn
Lam Oanh Ha, Department of Finance and Banking, Thu Dau Mot University, Binh Duong, Thu Dau Mot City, Vietnam, e-mail: oanhhl@tdmu.edu.vn
Trung Hieu Nguyen, Banking University Ho Chi Minh City, Ho Chi Minh City, Vietnam, e-mail: hieunt@buh.edu.vn

https://doi.org/10.1515/9783110767681-009

and (3) quality of products and delivery services. According to a study by Sarma and Pais [1], helping people have access to financial and banking services at reasonable costs and with quality are the main goal of financial inclusion. Therefore, financial inclusion makes a great contribution to promoting stable and sustainable economic growth by contributing to reducing poverty, reducing income inequality in the economy. Furthermore, Singh and Prasad [5] asserted that in addition to supporting the financial system to increase the savings rate, promoting financial inclusion also helps individuals and organizations to access financial resources with reasonable costs, thereby promoting economic growth.

With important contributions to the economy, financial inclusion is a topic of interest to researchers and policy makers but has also become a target of development at financial institutions and banks. These organizations have applied 4.0 technology platforms to their products and services with the goal of diversifying financial and banking utilities for customers [6–8]. Products such as Fintech, electronic money, digital finance, digital financial inclusion, digital payments, digital technologies, mobile banking, besides noncash payment services, and other services such as online savings, online loans, and online investments have been considered worldwide, contributing to perfecting the comprehensive financial system.

Vietnam is located in Southeast Asia and is considered to have a fast-growing economy and more trade openness into the regional economy. With its geographical location bordering China, Vietnam benefits from China's economic growth. However, the Covid-19 pandemic originated in China, and Vietnam was also one of the countries first affected by the pandemic [9, 10]. Under the influence of the COVID-19 pandemic, especially in 2020 and 2021, many localities across the country implemented social distancing, leading to some changes in payment activities in the banking system [11, 12]. Therefore, it leads to an explosion in the number of Vietnamese people using electronic banking and financial services. According to the statistics of the State Bank of Vietnam [13] on domestic payment transactions via Internet and mobile banking, the second quarter of 2021 increased by 15.55% in quantity and 172.56% in value compared to the first quarter of 2021. And this number is 112,127.33% and 2,025.60%, respectively, over the same period last year (Q2/2020). Specifically, customers not only use these services for payment purposes but also to access financial and credit grants from the government and credit institutions without leaving their homes. Therefore, we have carried out this research to evaluate financial inclusion through the use of e-banking financial products and services in Vietnam in the pandemic as well as proposed some recommendations of developing financial inclusion in the future.

In that context, comprehensive financial development in the context of the Covid-19 pandemic in order to maintain the provision of full-fledged services and products to people and businesses is necessary and is the basis for financial development in the near future. The research analyzes a case study in Vietnam, an emerging country with great achievements in economic development. Through this research, it provides some suggestions on the development of financial inclusion in developing and emerging countries around the world. In fact, the research results demonstrate that the development of financial inclusion has contributed to the development of basic financial products and services such as capital mobilization and lending or payment services at a reasonable cost. Moreover, the results also confirm that Internet banking/mobile banking and Fintech services are most commonly used in Vietnam, while other services such as securities investment and technology insurance have not yet developed.

In addition to the introduction discussed, the study consists of the following sections: Section 2 discusses previous studies, and Section 3 discusses data sources and research methods. Section 4 deals with the results, and finally conclusions and future research.

2 Previous studies

Financial inclusion ensures that all actors in the economy can access and use the formal financial system [1, 14]. There are three main characteristics of a comprehensive financial system: (1) a financial system that facilitates efficient allocation of productive resources, thereby reducing the cost of capital; (2) a financial system that reduces the time and cost of financial management through access to formal financial services; and (3) an inclusive financial system increases the transparency of capital markets, reduces inequality with the disadvantaged in society, and reduces the proliferation of informal sources of credit. Thus, a comprehensive financial system provides a path to safe savings methods, establishes synchronization between financial services, and is the basis for increased welfare in the economy.

Ozili [4] demonstrates that digital finance through Fintech providers is having a positive impact on financial inclusion in emerging economies. Low-income individuals prefer digital finance because the benefits are similar to banking services and they only need to pay a lower cost. This research also points out the negative impact of digital finance on financial inclusion that providers will discriminate against customers based on differences in income, risk, and their level of education.

Demirgüç-Kunt and Klapper [15], Demirgüç-Kunt et al. [16], and Ozturk and Ullah [17] argue that the development of financial inclusion gives the economy the opportunity to access financial products and services at a reasonable cost. The development of financial markets has brought more opportunities for people and businesses in the economy to access many financial benefits and economic development, in which financial institutions are one of the key factors for promoting financial inclusion. Financial inclusion contributes to reducing poverty, reducing income inequality, and informal finance, as well as increasing access to formal banking and financial services. Another possibility is in the meta-analysis of research on financial inclusion. Gálvez-Sánchez et al. [18] find that the financial system is becoming more efficient, accessible, and sustainable, thanks to the explosion in technology, especially financial technology – Fintech. Furthermore, Aziz et al. [19] show that digital banking has a positive impact on the development of financial inclusion in each country between 1994 and 2020.

As suggested by Sarma and Pais [1] and Singh and Prasad [5], it is evident that helping people having access to financial and banking services at reasonable costs is the goal of financial inclusion. Through the above analysis, the evidence shows that the development of digital banking has a positive impact on financial inclusion in most countries. Financial inclusion is also capable of giving people and businesses the opportunity to access financial services and products at low cost, especially digital banking that connects payments. Without interruption in all circumstances, even in the context of the Covid-19 pandemic that has disrupted supply chains, many countries implemented social distancing.

3 Data and methodology

We use the qualitative method through in-depth interviews on the Google Meet platform with 10 experts having knowledge in the banking and finance industry, especially with in-depth knowledge of financial inclusion to achieve the following objectives: (1) identifying e-banking financial services products in Vietnam; (2) positioning the role of e-banking financial products and services in the development of financial inclusion; and (3) identifying the impact of the pandemic on human behavior and the trend of financial inclusion. The research methodology can be written in Figure 1:

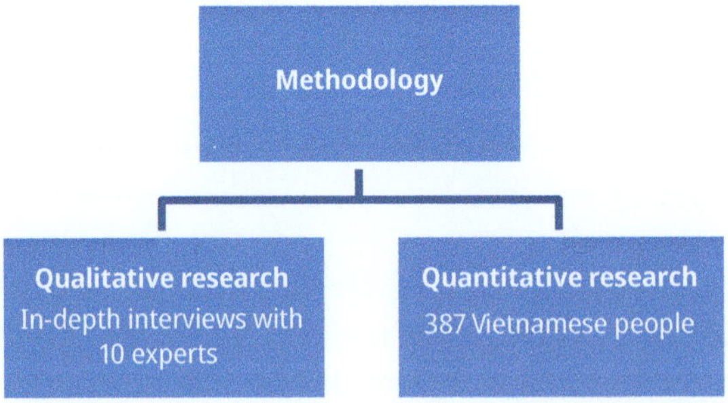

Figure 1: Research methodology (source: drawn by authors).

In addition, we also use a quantitative research method, which is conducted through an online survey using Google docs. The results obtained from the responses of 387 Vietnamese people were used to assess the formal financial system on the technology platform with e-banking financial products and services.

4 Results

4.1 Qualitative research results

Vietnam's domestic payment demand in recent years has been improved to meet the development of the economy. In the context of the Covid-19 pandemic, the demand for payment continues to increase, thereby requiring the financial system to implement digital transformation faster in order to meet the needs of people and businesses. Table 1 shows that the number of domestic payment transactions via Internet and mobile banking in the second quarter of 2021 increased sharply compared to the second quarter of 2020. This is also a period of intense pandemic in Vietnam; therefore, many transactions transferred from traditional transactions to technology-based transactions.

Table 1: Domestic payment transactions via Internet and mobile banking.

Indicator	Number of transactions	Transaction value (billion Vietnam dong)
Q2/2020	567,568	697,879
Q1/2021	551,270,258	5,442,600
Q2/2021	636,966,391	14,834,150
Changes of Q2/21 with Q1/21	15.55%	172.56%
Changes of Q2/21 with Q2/20	112,127.33%	2,025.60%

Source: Government [20] and MBBank [21].

Through in-depth interviews with 10 experts who are PhDs in finance and banking, leaders of MBBank Binh Duong, leaders of Vietinbank Binh Duong, leaders of HDbank Binh Duong, Techcombank in Ho Chi Minh City, as well as leader of Viettel pay and Viettel post in Binh Duong clarify more about comprehensive financial development in Vietnam. The survey sample characteristics are presented in Table 2.

Table 2 shows that the percentage of men and women interviewed is 60% and 40%, respectively. The interviewees are mainly working in the financial and banking sector, and having knowledge of digital banking and finance. All experts are over 25 years old, and approximately 60% experts are over 40 years old.

According to the survey results, we find that all experts agree that financial inclusion has an impact on measuring the access to the formal banking and financial system of entities in the economy. Therefore, financial conclusion in recent years has helped people and businesses access to financial and banking products and services, such as mobilizing capital, borrowing capital to payment services at the most reasonable cost. In addition, the findings indicate that the financial conclusion that increases its transparency is consistent with a greater contribution of the state management in the monetary policies.

Table 2: Characteristics of in-depth interview samples.

Indicator		Quantity	Percentage
Gender	Male	6	60%
	Female	4	40%
Age	Under 25	0	0%
	Between 25 and 40	4	40%
	Over 40	6	60%
Position	Vice President of Banking University of Ho Chi Minh City	2	20%
	Director of MBBank Binh Duong	1	10%
	Deputy Director of MBBank Binh Duong	1	10%
	Head of Customer Relations Department Vietinbank	1	10%
	Director of HDBank Binh Duong	1	10%
	Head of HDBank individual customer department	1	10%
	Deputy Director of Techcombank Ho Chi Minh City	1	10%
	Deputy Director of Viettel pay	1	10%
	Director of Viettel post Binh Duong	1	10%

Source: Author's analysis.

The results of the discussion on the impact of digital banking on financial inclusion received mixed opinions from experts. The results of these opinions in Table 3 suggested two directions such as (1) opportunities and (2) threats, and are divided into four groups of financial actors in the Vietnamese economy, including state, businesses, financial institutions, and individuals–households.

Table 3: Impact of digital banking on financial inclusion.

Party	Opportunities	Threats
Government	Development of cashless payments Minimizing informal credit (black credit) Reducing tax revenue loss contributes to ensuring revenue for the state budget Anti-money laundering Increasing welfare for all subjects	Investing in infrastructure and building a legal corridor for digital banking and finance People's capacity for understanding and acceptance
Business	Business development toward e-commerce and online payment Saving sales costs, office costs, and brand promotion	Competition from domestic and foreign competitors Infrastructure and technology investment costs are high Operations and management personnel know the technology

Table 3 (continued)

Party	Opportunities	Threats
Financial institutions	Expanding customer network Diversifying products and services Trade promotion and global brand promotion	Insufficient legal provisions Attack of malicious software People's preference to use cash Customers create virtual accounts for fraud
Individuals–households	Access to official capital sources at reasonable interest rates Save money and travel time Needs are met anytime, anywhere, conveniently, and quickly	Risk of loss of information and data Unable to control personal finances (borrowing beyond ability to pay, addiction to online shopping) Fraud (transfer money to virtual accounts, lured into investment, lured to borrow money)

Source: Author's analysis.

A majority of experts participating in the in-depth interview are leaders of organizations providing digital banking and financial services. The author also receives their opinions summarized in Table 4 as follows:

Table 4: Digital banking and financial services products.

Products	Manufacturers	Customers
Pay and shop online	Commercial bank, Fintech company	All customers
Sending savings online		
Transfers		
Granting credit online	Some commercial banks and some Fintech companies	Business customers or individual customers with proof of income
Stock investment	Securities company	All investors
Technology insurance	Insurtech company	All customers

Source: Author's analysis.

Table 4 shows that online credit granting and technology-based insurance sales have begun to appear in Vietnam. Consumers do not need to go to the bank, and insurance company can still use these products. However, these products are only sold by a few suppliers because Vietnamese people still do not have the habit of buying insurance proactively and are afraid of debt [21]. These could be the remaining pieces of digital banking and finance to help perfect the comprehensive financial system in Vietnam. Through this assessment, it can be seen that the financial inclusion has really been developed in Vietnam in recent years, and the pandemic has made financial inclusion more developed. This is consistent with the statement of Sarma and Pais [1] and Singh and Prasad [5], who both believe that helping people have access to financial and banking services at reasonable costs is the important goal of financial inclusion.

4.2 Quantitative research results

The quantitative study received 387 responses via Google docs, in which the number of men and women participating in the survey is 186 and 201, respectively. The majority of survey participants are aged from 36 to 45 years old with 129 people, accounting for 33.33%. In terms of respondents' occupations, students accounted for the highest proportion at 21.96% with 85 respondents, followed by retired people (61 people or 15.76%). In addition, bankers and teachers ranked the third and the fourth with 55 respondents (14.21%) and 38 people (9.82%), respectively. There are 132 survey participants living in Binh Duong, accounting for 34.11%, followed by Ho Chi Minh City and Hanoi with the number of 107 people (27.65%) and 52 people (13.44%), respectively. Detailed information about the survey sample characteristics is shown in Table 5.

Table 5: Survey sample characteristics by sex, age, occupation, and place of residence.

Characteristics		Quantity	Percentage
Gender	Male	186	48.06%
	Female	201	51.94%
Age	Under 25	57	14.73%
	From 26 to 35	101	26.10%
	From 36 to 45	129	33.33%
	From 46 to 55	43	11.11%
	Over 55	57	14.73%
Occupation	Banker	55	14.21%
	Student	85	21.96%
	Teacher	38	9.82%
	Worker	30	7.75%
	Software engineer	16	4.13%
	Construction engineer	11	2.84%
	Real estate business	15	3.88%
	Self-employed	23	5.94%
	Public administrative officer	11	2.84%
	Doctor	9	2.33%
	Insurance business	10	2.58%
	Stockbroker	7	1.81%
	Lawyer	5	1.29%
	Retirer	61	15.76%
	Others	11	2.84%

Table 5 (continued)

Characteristics		Quantity	Percentage
Place of living	Hanoi Capital	52	13.44%
	Ho Chi Minh City	107	27.65%
	Binh Duong province	132	34.11%
	Dong Nai province	19	4.91%
	Can Tho City	15	3.88%
	Da Nang City	22	5.68%
	Others	40	10.34%

Source: Author's analysis.

When asked about the digital banking and financial applications, the majority of answers received are Internet banking, mobile banking, and/or Fintech services. While other services such as stock investment, technology insurance is not really popular. Especially Fintech is being developed strongly in recent times based on payments on Momo wallet, Viettel pay, Zalo pay, Airpay, Payoo, but has not become the most popular application in Vietnam. Specific applications of digital banking and finance are presented in Table 6:

Table 6: Digital banking and finance applications.

Applications	Quantity	Percentage
Internet banking	251	64.86%
Mobile banking	324	83.72%
Fintech (Momo wallet, Viettel pay, Zalo pay, Airpay, and Payoo)	237	61.24%
Stock investment	179	46.25%
Technology insurance	36	9.30%

Source: Author's analysis.

Regarding the purpose of using these applications, Table 7 shows that 387 (100%) survey respondents use e-banking financial applications for money transfer, payment, and online shopping purposes. These are relatively simple activities and have become popular in many countries. However, only 47.29% (183 people) deposited savings on these applications. The number of people who borrow money from e-banking financial applications is 106 people (27.39%), while using electronic applications for the purpose of investing in securities and buying insurance has the rate of 46.25% (179 people) and 9.30% (36 people).

With the question "When did you start using e-banking financial applications?" Most of the respondents said that the impact of the COVID-19 pandemic has had the strongest impact on the use of e-banking applications. Due to the long-term social distancing policies of the Government of Vietnam, it has changed the shopping and payment habits of the people, and the number of people using e-banking financial services has increased strongly in 2021. The results suggested are in Table 8.

Table 7: Purpose of using e-banking financial applications.

Using	Quantity	Percentage
Transfers	387	100%
Pay and shop online	387	100%
Saving	183	47.29%
Borrowing capital	106	27.39%
Stock investment	179	46.25%
Insurance	36	9.30%

Source: Author's analysis.

Table 8: Time to start using e-banking financial applications.

Year	Quantity	Percentage
Pre-2019	93	24.03%
2019	42	10.85%
2020	87	22.48%
2021	165	42.64%

Source: Author's analysis.

Through the research, we also recorded the opinions of some survey subjects as follows:

Recommending banks to consider integrating securities investment and insurance features in the same e-banking application.
Needing more online loan instructions or enable this feature on the application. I have seen it for a long time but still can't use it.
Banks need to strengthen measures to secure customer and investment information to speed up transaction processing.
There should be more promotions for customers using e-banking services.
Considering adding investment advice and personal financial management utilities integrated in the e-banking application.

5 Future trends of financial inclusions in the new context

Through interviews with experts participating in in-depth interviews, the study discussed the future trend of financial inclusion in Vietnam in the context of the Industrial Revolution 4.0 and especially in the epidemic situation lasting in the future. After synthesizing the opinions of experts, the results are summarized in Table 9.

Table 9: Expert opinion on future trends of financial inclusion.

Trends	Comments of experts
Adoption to the pandemic	When implementing the "new normal," Vietnam has accepted to live with the pandemic, which means that all industries, including banking and finance, must accompany the epidemic. It considers that a challenge for the entire economy could be existed. In addition, it also provides an opportunity to develop e-banking products and services because people will continue to maintain the habit of using this service to limit exposure. At the same time, all actors in the economy will easily access the official financial system through this channel.
Developing technological revolution 4.0	With technology platforms such as blockchain, IoT, AI, and cloud computing, e-banking financial service providers will step by step integrate traditional products into applications to better serve customers. Therefore, comprehensive finance is promoted at the best because users will be able to choose financial and banking products with reasonable costs.
Changes in people's behavior	Vietnamese people will reduce face-to-face communication to limit the spread of the disease. Therefore, customers will prioritize choosing products and services provided on the Internet such as e-banking, Fintech.
Other factors	The Government of Vietnam promotes the project of developing noncash payments in Vietnam for the period of 2021–2025 [20]. According to this project, Vietnam will actively participate in the Industrial Revolution 4.0, giving priority to perfecting the legal framework, building an ecosystem for digital economic development, digital transformation, development of e-commerce, digital banking and finance, and promotion of financial inclusion.

Source: Author's analysis.

It can be concluded that the Industrial Revolution 4.0 not only brings advantages in developing financial inclusion but also creates competitive pressure forcing financial institutions to change continuously. The results of the Industrial Revolution 4.0 on blockchain, digital banking, digital finance, and cryptocurrencies are being adopted and significantly impact the business of the banking and financial sector [3]. These technological breakthroughs have made significant contributions to promoting financial inclusion amid the COVID-19 pandemic. Inheriting the research results of scientists around the world and the comments of experts in the banking sector, it can be affirmed that the application of Industrial Revolution 4.0 on products and services in the financial and banking sector will promote financial inclusion in Vietnam. This evidence has been reinforced by the work of Gálvez-Sánchez et al. [18], who argue that the financial system is becoming more efficient, accessible, and sustainable. Similarly, Aziz et al. [19] show that digital banking has had a positive impact on the development of financial inclusion in many countries recently. The evidence is similar to Vietnam, which shows the positives in financial inclusion development, and the COVID-19 pandemic is likely to accelerate this development.

6 Conclusions

Technological revolution 4.0 has brought e-banking financial products and services to development because it helps to increase transparency, ensure privacy, speed up transaction processing, thereby creating trust and maintaining loyalty to the customers. The pandemic occurred on a global scale, requiring people to protect themselves, and governments implementing social distancing and isolation had a significant impact on changing the consumption habits of each person in the economy. Research conducted in Vietnam through qualitative research and quantitative research shows that financial inclusion in recent years has helped subjects use banking and financial products and services, such as mobilize capital and borrow capital to payment services at the most reasonable cost. Moreover, e-banking services such as Internet banking or mobile banking and Fintech services are most commonly used, while other services such as securities investment and technology insurance are not really popular. In addition, the study also said that the Covid-19 pandemic made financial inclusion develop faster, and policies to adapt to the pandemic such as social distancing and isolation have changed people's habits. It is imperative to use a variety of financial technologies in transactions, thereby promoting inclusive financial development. However, the study also poses some challenges for future research. Future research proposals should assess the relationship between digital finance and economic crises.

References

[1] Sarma, M., Pais, J. Financial inclusion and development. Journal of International Development, 2011, 23(5), 613–628. https://doi.org/10.1002/jid.1698.

[2] Tay, L.-Y., Tai, H.-T., Tan, G.-S. Digital financial inclusion: A gateway to sustainable development. Heliyon, 2022, 8(6), e09766. https://doi.org/https://doi.org/10.1016/j.heliyon.2022.e09766.

[3] Mehdiabadi, A., Tabatabeinasab, M., Spulbar, C., Karbassi Yazdi, A., Birau, R. Are we ready for the challenge of Banks 4.0? Designing a roadmap for banking systems in Industry 4.0. International Journal of Financial Studies, 2020, 8(2), 32.

[4] Ozili, P. K. Impact of digital finance on financial inclusion and stability. Borsa Istanbul Review, 2018, 18(4), 329–340.

[5] Singh, V. K., Prasad, R. Diffusion of banking products in financial inclusion linked savings accounts: A case study based on Pradhan Mantri Jan Dhan Yojana in India. Global Business Review, 2021. https://doi.org/10.1177/09721509211006866.

[6] Frame, W. S., White, L. J. Technological change, financial innovation, and diffusion in banking. NYU Working Paper No. 2451/33549, 2014, Available at SSRN: https://ssrn.com/abstract=2380060.

[7] Peters, G.W., Panayi, E. Understanding Modern Banking Ledgers Through Blockchain Technologies: Future of Transaction Processing and Smart Contracts on the Internet of Money. In: Tasca, P., Aste, T., Pelizzon, L., Perony, N. (eds) Banking Beyond Banks and Money. New Economic Windows. Springer, Cham, 2016. https://doi.org/10.1007/978-3-319-42448-4_13

[8] Ha, L. O., Nguyen, V. C., Tien, D. D. T., Ngoc, B. T. B. Factors affecting the intention of using fintech services in the context of combating of fake news. In: Combating Fake News with Computational

Intelligence Techniques, Studies in Computational Intelligence, Vol. 1001, Lahby, M., Pathan, A. S. K., Maleh, Y., Yafooz, W. M. S. (eds.), Cham, Springer, 2022. https://doi.org/10.1007/978-3-030-90087-8_14.

[9] Nguyen, D. T., Tran, V. D., Ghafoor, A. The impact of Covid-19 lockdown on intention to follow preventive measures in Vietnam: Integrated protection motivation theory and theory planned behavior. Cogent Business & Management, 2022, 9(1), 2054502. https://doi.org/10.1080/23311975.2022.2054502.

[10] Nguyen, V. C., Nguyen, T. T. The effect of covid 19 pandemic on the financial market's performance: evidence from top ASEAN stock markets. In: Finance, Law, and the Crisis of COVID-19, Contributions to Management Science, Mansour, N., M. Bujosa Vadell, L. (eds.), Cham, Springer, 2022. https://doi.org/10.1007/978-3-030-89416-0_9.

[11] Government Directive No. 15/CT-TTg on the implementation of urgent measures to prevent and control the COVID-19 epidemic. 2020, Available at https://moh.gov.vn/documents/176127/356256/31.3.2020+16+CT-TTg.pdf/ce106212-59de-4093-bfcc-47f50a9044f2 (accessed on 3rd April 2022).

[12] Tran, V. D. Using mobile food delivery applications during the COVID-19 pandemic: Applying the theory of planned behavior to examine continuance behavior. Sustainability, 2021, 13(21), 12066. MDPI AG. Retrieved from http://dx.doi.org/10.3390/su132112066.

[13] State Bank of Vietnam Domestic payment transactions via Internet and Mobile Banking. 2021, Available at https://www.sbv.gov.vn/webcenter/portal/vi/menu/trangchu (accessed on 3rd April 2022).

[14] Kouladoum, J.-C., Wirajing, M. A. K., Nchofoung, T. N. Digital technologies and financial inclusion in Sub-Saharan Africa. Telecommunications Policy, 2022, 102387. https://doi.org/https://doi.org/10.1016/j.telpol.2022.102387.

[15] Demirgüç-Kunt, A., Klapper, L. Measuring financial inclusion: Explaining variation in use of financial services across and within countries. Brookings Papers on Economic Activity, 2013, 2013(1), 279–340.

[16] Demirgüç-Kunt, A., Klapper, L., Singer, D., Ansar, S., Hess, J. The Global Findex Database 2017: Measuring financial inclusion and opportunities to expand access to and use of financial services. World Bank Economic Review, 2020, 34, S2–S8. https://doi.org/10.1093/wber/lhz013.

[17] Ozturk, I., Ullah, S. Does digital financial inclusion matter for economic growth and environmental sustainability in OBRI economies? An empirical analysis. Resources, Conservation and Recycling, 2022, 185, 106489. https://doi.org/https://doi.org/10.1016/j.resconrec.2022.106489.

[18] Gálvez-Sánchez, F. J., Lara-Rubio, J., Verdú-Jóver, A. J., MeseguerSánchez, V. Research advances on financial inclusion: A bibliometric analysis. Sustainability, 2021, 13(6), 3156. https://doi.org/10.3390/su13063156.

[19] Aziz, M. R. A., Jali, M. Z., Noor, M. N. M., Sulaiman, S., Harun, M. S., Mustafar, M. Z. I. Bibliometric analysis of literatures on digital banking and financial inclusion between 2014–2020. Library Philosophy and Practice, 2021, 2021, 1–31.

[20] Government Decision No. 1813/QD-TTg approving the project on developing non-cash payment in Vietnam for the period of 2021–2025. 2021, Available at https://datafiles.chinhphu.vn/cpp/files/vbpq/2021/10/1813.signed.pdf (accessed on 3rd April 2022).

[21] MBBank. Fintech & digital bank in 10/2021, 2021. Available at: https://mbbank.com.vn/resources/files/Tin-MB/MB-voi-bao-chi/2021/BAO-CAO-NGANH/BC-THANG-10/mbb-quarter-oct2021.pdf.

Mehtab Alam*, Ihtiram Raza Khan, M. Afshar Alam, Farheen Siddiqui, Safdar Tanweer

Role of AI, IoT, and IoD in avoiding and minimizing risks of future pandemics

Abstract: Pandemics have been affecting our societies from time to time. The 1918 Spanish flu, also known as influenza pandemic, took away the life of more than 500 million people. In 1957, East Asia saw the emergence of the Asian flu which took a toll on the human civilization with the loss of around 1.1 million people. The year 1968 saw the rise of H3N2 virus causing the Hong Kong flu and decreasing the population by 4 million.

The latest pandemic Corona virus-19 (COVID-19) affected the whole world and reduced the world population by 5.4 million. It is evident that with the enormous advancement of the field of technology and medicine, humans are not fully safe. These advancements are not enough to protect humans from disasters. It is an old saying "prevention is better than cure." It implies that we, with those advancements, still have to be well prepared for such types of drastic events. Artificial intelligence (AI), machine learning (ML), Internet of things (IoT), and Internet of drones (IoD) are the current technologies which can help us in the future to predict, counter, and minimize the effects of pandemics. In this chapter, the authors have discussed how AI, IoT, and IoD technologies can assist and aid humans in overcoming as well as minimizing the consequences of such pandemics.

1 Introduction

Pandemics and epidemics leave huge burdens on our societies, economies, and our lives. The current coronavirus (COVID-19) pandemic has led to loss of a large number of human lives. It led to massive income and productivity losses, more than 81 million jobs were lost, and large number of startups and small business were shut down apart from the unprecedented loss to the global as well as national gross domestic product (GDP) [1]. Earlier pandemics also had implications on the society. Pandemics are defined as an unknown disease or vector that spreads rapidly across the communities which ranges from a number of countries or continents or sometimes throughout the globe. Pandemics, in its weakest form, can lead to the death of a several million people [2].

We have seen a number of pandemics in the last 100 years or so. The year 1918 pandemic was an influenza pandemic, caused by H1N1 virus, called Spanish flu, which

***Corresponding author: Mehtab Alam**, Department of Computer Science and Engineering, Jamia Hamdard, New Delhi, India
Ihtiram Raza Khan, M. Afshar Alam, Farheen Siddiqui, Safdar Tanweer, Department of Computer Science and Engineering, Jamia Hamdard, New Delhi, India

https://doi.org/10.1515/9783110767681-010

took more than 500 million human lives. The 1957 pandemic, caused by H2N2 virus, also known as Asian flu, led to the death of 1.1 million people. In the 1968 pandemic, caused by H3N2 virus, known as Hong Kong flu, 4 million people lost their lives. In the 1977 pandemic, caused by H1N1 virus, also known as the Russian flu, led to the death of around 0.7 million people around the globe. The most recent 2009 pandemic, caused by H1N1 virus, known as swine flu, saw a death of around 284,000 people [1]. The current COVID-19 pandemic, is known to have come in the era of technology, which has seen the death of around 21.5 million people.

In this chapter, we first discuss the latest smart technologies, that is, artificial intelligence (AI), Internet of things (IoT), and Internet of drones (IoD), in detail. In the next section, we discuss the pandemics in the last 100 years in detail. The next section includes the role of the smart technologies in preventing or reducing the effects of these pandemics on the society and the people. We have concluded our paper in the next section. References are listed at the last.

2 Smart technologies

The twenty-first century has seen the unprecedented rise in technology and advancements. The smart city paradigm is taking lifestyles to unprecedented heights. People are sitting in driverless cars which map their own routes, stop and start as per the traffic and street signals, without any human interventions [3]. At their homes, they have smart lights, which switch themselves on when the natural light becomes dim and switch themselves off when the Sun rises or there is no one at home. They get their coffee ready at the stroke of 9 without any delay or the coffee being cold. With the help of smart transportation system, passengers do not need to wait for the public transport for hours; they receive alerts on their phones when their desired transport is near to them. At their offices, the smart air conditioners maintain comfortable working conditions in the cabins and chambers. All these smart devices and smart technologies have made the life easier and comfortable [4]. In this section, we have discussed three smart technologies, namely, AI, IoT, and the latest IoD in detail.

2.1 Artificial intelligence (AI)

AI is the field of science which deals with providing the digital computers or computer-controlled robots to carry out tasks which require intelligence and are associated with the intelligent beings. AI provides the computers with the ability to learn from past experiences, ability to reason things, discover meanings from different unrelated objects and things, generalize meanings, and so on [5]. Since the development of the computers in the 1940s, it has been understood that the computers are capable of carrying out complex tasks such as playing games involving humans like chess and finding proofs to unsolved mathematical theorems – that too with great efficiency. Even after such advancements in the computing speeds and huge memory capacity, matching the human capabilities is still an achievement very far away. But, still in today's world, AI has found its way in almost every sector of business and society. AI is being used extensively in healthcare in medical diagnosis and early detection of diseases, voice recognition (smart assistants) and hand writing recognition, online search engines, self-driving cars, robotics, ad-hoc networks, and so on [6]. AI is being used in almost every industry and business nowadays [7].

2.1.1 How does AI work?

Working of AI can be explained under two processes: big data and AI. In the big data part, the data being generated on daily basis from various sources and devices is collected and then sent to the server or the cloud for further processing. Noise and unwanted data is removed from this structured or unstructured data and stored in databases and servers. This data is then processed using single or multiple CPU/GPU and AI algorithm to detect patterns and inferences for further use. Once the data is processed, the model is ready to make predictions and helping out business and industries in making profits [8]. AI is able to carry out a great deal of tasks as of now, but making predictions is one of the most common and first use of AI. Figure 2 shows the working of AI.

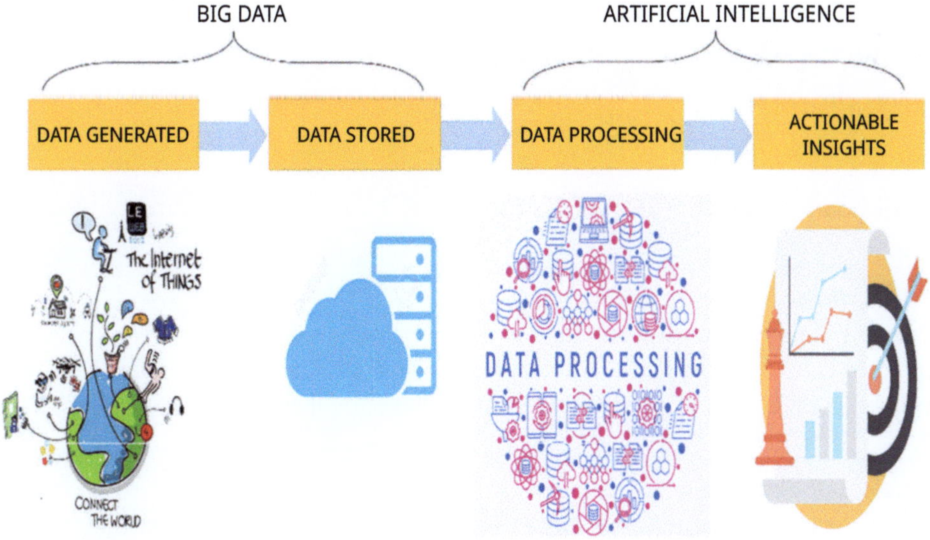

Figure 1: Working of AI.

2.1.2 Types of AI

We can broadly classify AI in the following seven types. Figure 2 depicts the types of AI:

2.1.2.1 Reactive machines

This is the oldest type of AI system having very limited capabilities. They only have the ability to respond to different kinds of stimuli. They do not have any memory of their own, that is, they cannot use previously gained experience in taking present actions [9]. Examples of reactive machines are IBM's Deep Blue and Google's AlphaGo.

2.1.2.2 Limited memory

These machines have the abilities of a reactive machine with the capabilities of learning from the historical data to make decisions [10]. This is the most widely used type of AI. Examples of limited memory machines are chatbots, virtual assistants, and self-driving cars.

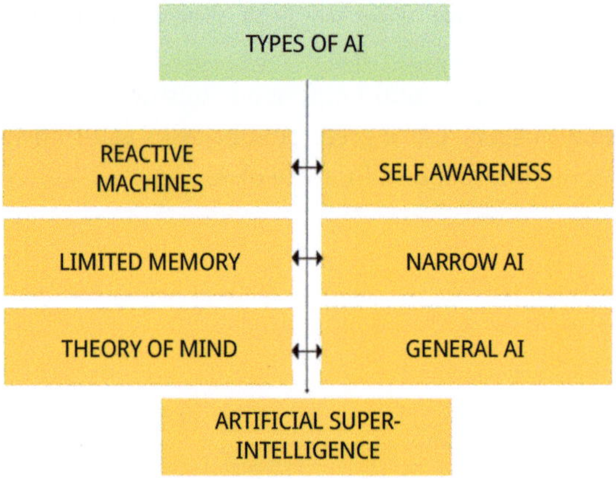

Figure 2: Seven types of AI.

2.1.2.3 Theory of mind

Currently, this type of AI exists either as a concept or as a work in progress. Theory of mind AI is the next level of AI systems that is currently under innovation. These machines are thought to be able to understand humans and their emotions and needs [11].

2.1.2.4 Self-awareness

This is believed to be the final stage of AI and also a work in progress and is only hypothetical. This AI possesses human-level consciousness and understands the world

2.1.3.3 Robotics

Robotics help in designing and
nating or reducing the human e
are capable of substituting hum
adapting to it. Robots consist o
which is working underneath in
the help of AI, humans have bee
on a daily basis and/or tasks wh

Below we have listed some
also depicted in Figure 5.

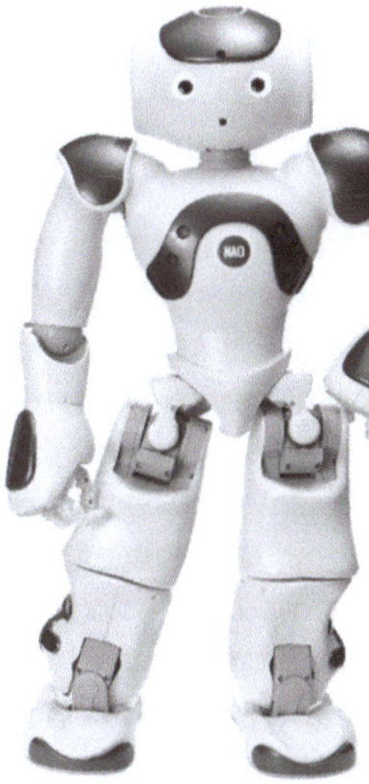

Power supply
Actuators
Electric motors
Pneumatic air muscles
Muscle wires
Piezo motors
Sensors

Some of the applications of an
exploration, and transportation.

2.1.3.4 Image/visual recognitio

Image recognition with the help
tic segmentation of the results

around it. Self-awareness in AI depends on how researchers understand the consciousness of humans and how they replicate it into the machines [12].

2.1.2.5 Narrow AI

These are the AI systems that have the ability to perform a specific task autonomously using human-like capabilities. They perform only the task that they are programmed to do, thus having a very limited or narrow range of competencies. All the AI systems working nowadays fall in this category [13].

2.1.2.6 General AI

General AI is the ability of an AI system to learn, perceive, understand, and function completely like a human. These systems are not yet implemented and will be able to teach themselves from connections and generalizations across domains. This will make the AI system just as capable as humans [14].

2.1.2.7 Super AI (artificial superintelligence)

The development of artificial superintelligence will be the peak of AI research [15].

2.1.3 AI technologies

Currently, there are a number of AI technologies [16]. Figure 3 depicts some AI technologies.

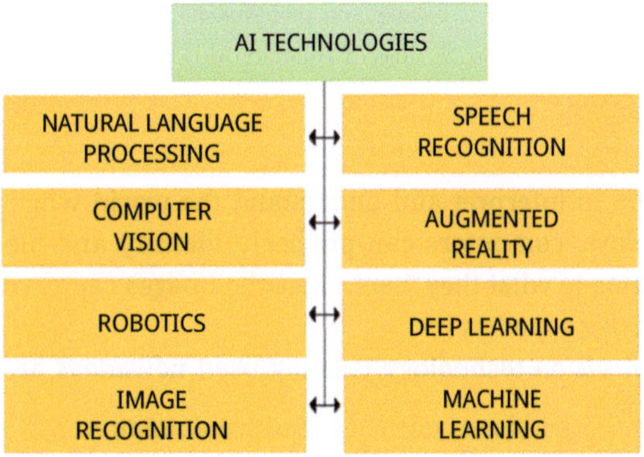

Figure 3: AI technologies.

execute. AI is enabling the vehicles to see, hear, think, and make decisions as the human drivers do [36]. AI perception cycle for autonomous vehicles can be broken down into three main components:

- Live data collection and communication systems
- Autonomous driving platform
- AI-based functions

2.2 Internet of things (IoT)

The numerous interconnected devices and sensors connected to the Internet and collecting and transferring data to the next node for processing is the Internet of things. Nowadays, almost every electronic device is being manufactured in a way to connect to the Internet and act as a smart thing. These devices are intelligent, and are able to collect data from sensors and cameras connected to them [37]. They are able to perform their desired tasks without the involvement of humans. IoT is constructing a fabric of the smart devices around us. The term "IoT" is basically used for a device which has the ability to connect to the Internet and communicate with the network without any human intervention [38].

More and more industries and businesses have been adopting IoT and smart devices technology in their daily processes to gain more efficiency and productivity.

2.2.1 How does IoT work?

All the IoT smart devices are equipped with sensors which are further connected to an IoT platform. The IoT platform further integrates data from various connected devices and applies various analytic tools to bring the most valuable information which can be used for various purposes. These platforms are designed in such a way that they are capable of extracting exactly what is required and is useful for the system, and ignore or remove any other data. This extracted data is then used to detect patterns and inferences, and recommendations are made, and it is further used to detect problems and errors before they occur [39].

For example, for a car manufacturing business, IoT can help increase the business potential in a number of ways. Figure 8 depicts the working of IoT. Sensors can be used to detect the areas in the showroom that are more popular and where the customers spend their most time. Sales data can be studied to pin point which components are most loved by the customers and are being sold fast. Sensors and actuators can be used to track the inventory which will not allow any item to go out of stock. All this information will allow the business owners to make smart decisions and make the processes more efficient and increase profits. They can be used in tasks that are dangerous and where humans cannot reach without difficulty. Smart devices also help in automating tasks and jobs that need to be performed regularly or on a daily basis.

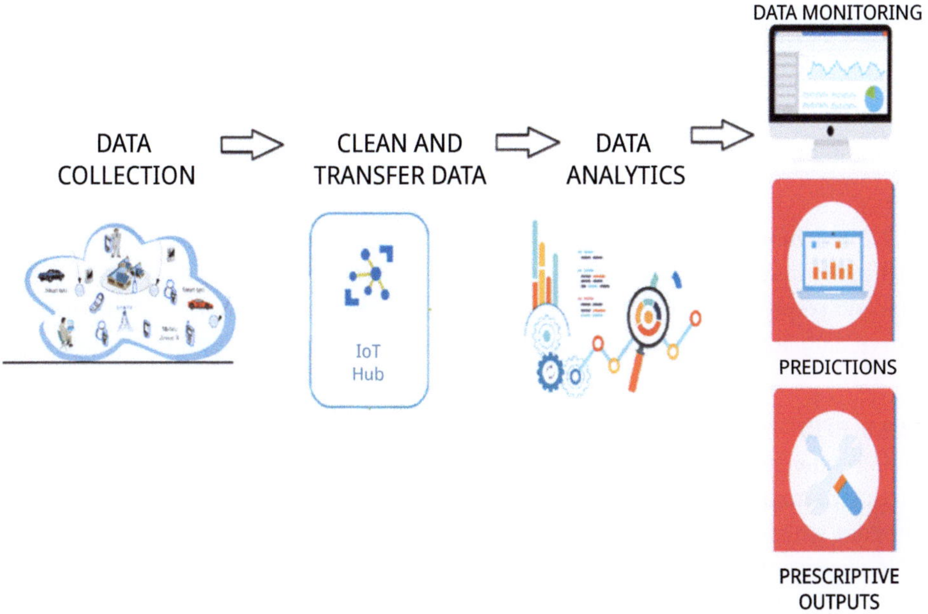

Figure 8: Working of IoT.

2.2.2 IoT technologies

A number of technologies are involved in implementing the concept of IoT in real life. Some of them are listed below [37]. Figure 9 lists some IoT technologies.

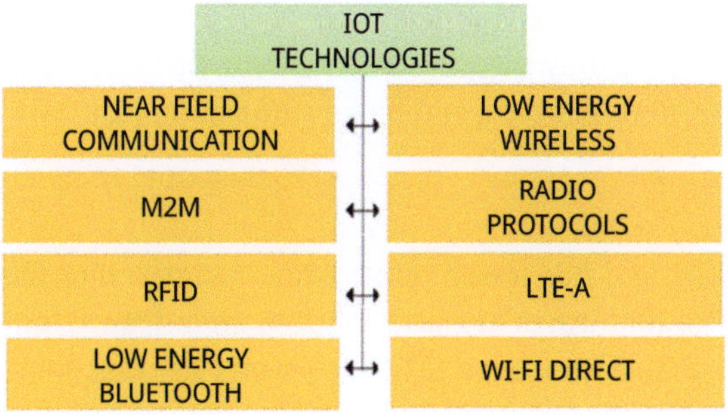

Figure 9: IoT technologies.

2.2.2.1 Near-field communication

Near-field communication (NFC) is a contactless communication protocol between portable smart devices like smartphones, tablets, speakers, and wireless earphones.

Communicating contactless enables the users to wave their smartphones or tablets over another NFC-compatible device and send data and information without touching the devices or clicking and pairing them and performing other setup steps beforehand. They contain NFC tags with unique identification information for every device. It helps in playing music, paying at NFC-enabled stores and learning easily [40].

2.2.2.2 Machine-to-machine communication

Machine-to-machine (M2M) communication is the technology that allows devices to send and receive information in an autonomous form without the need of any human intervention. It can occur using wired as well as wireless communications channel [41].

2.2.2.3 RFID

Radiofrequency identification (RFID) is a wireless communication system which comprises two main components: tags and readers. The reader consists of one or more antennas which emit radio waves and receive signals from the tags. RFID tags use the radio waves emitted by the RFID reader to communicate with them. The tags communicate their identity and other such information to the nearby readers. Tags are of two types: active and passive. Passive RFID tags do not have a battery of their own and powered by the waves emitted by the readers. Active tags are powered by their own batteries [42].

2.2.2.4 Low-energy Bluetooth

Bluetooth low energy (BLE) was first introduced by Bluetooth SIG in 4.0 specification of Bluetooth. BLE can be generalized as a Bluetooth type that uses less power and energy when compared to normal Bluetooth standard. It was developed specifically for IoT devices due to their constraint energy reserves. The low data rates of BLE make it very efficient and suitable for use situation where only the state data needs to be exchanged. BLE is used in smartwatches, fitness trackers, beacons, and home automation [43].

2.2.2.5 Low-energy wireless

Low-energy wireless uses lesser energy and has lesser range when compared to the standard wireless communication. The data rates are also reduced significantly but are perfectly suitable for low-powered and less-range IoT sensors and devices. Low-energy wireless extends the life of the devices through less use [44].

2.2.2.6 LTE-A

Long-term evolution-advanced is the latest version of LTE standard available. It supports very fast data transfer rates compared to previous versions. LTE-A provides a much wider range to the small IoT devices and sensors with very high uptime and connectivity and data rates. It provides in-built security parameters and highly scalable and robust traffic management capabilities. The data transmission and receiving over a 4G network can be achieved at a much lesser cost per bit when compared to other technologies. LTE-A integration has started in IoT devices for healthcare, automobiles, security cameras, and utility meters [45].

2.2.2.7 Wi-Fi direct

Wi-Fi direct is a wireless communication protocol which enables devices to communicate in a peer-to-peer (P2P) communication model without the use of any centralized common entity. It uses the combination of the speed to Wi-Fi and the ease of the Bluetooth technology. It is being used in IoT devices for low-cost data transmission and communication at a faster data rate. Sensitive data collected by the IoT devices can be secured with the use of this technology [46].

2.2.3 IoT standards

Some of the well-known IoT standards are listed in this section [47]. Figure 10 lists some IoT standards:

IPv6
Zigbee
LiteOS
OneM2M
DDS
AMQP
CoAP
LoraWAN

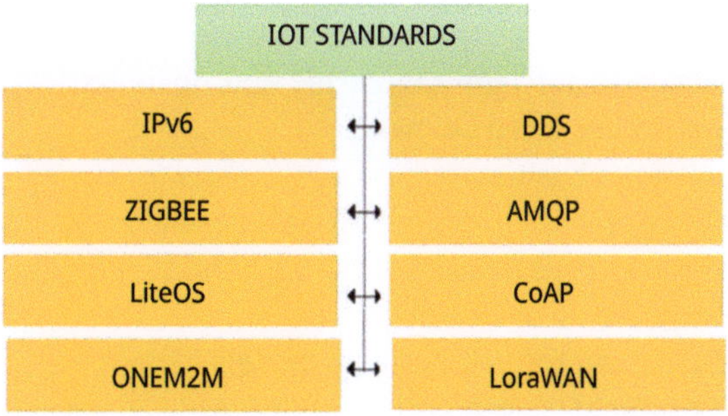

Figure 10: IoT standards.

2.2.4 IoT real-time applications

IoT is being used in almost every sphere of life nowadays [48]. Some of the most important applications of IoT are listed below. Figure 11 lists some applications of IoT:

- Wearables
- Health
- Traffic monitoring
- Fleet management
- Agriculture
- Hospitality
- Smart grid and energy saving
- Water supply

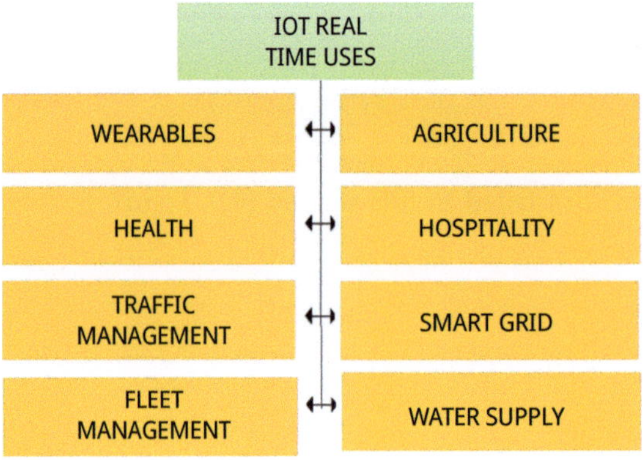

Figure 11: IoT real-time uses.

2.2.5 Advantages of IoT

IoT has proved its worth since its inception into the industries and business [49]. Some of the benefits of using an IoT system are listed below:

- Helps in monitoring all the process of the business
- Helps in improving customer experience
- Saves money and time
- Increases productivity of the employees
- Helps in adapting and integrating new and refined business models
- Helps in making future proof and profitable decisions
- Helps in increasing revenue

2.3 Internet of drones (IoD)

Unmanned aerial vehicles (UAVs) or drones are definitely going to exploit the future. Just like IoT, IoD will also help people make their life comfortable and easier. Drones are the areal devices that fly in the air and collect data in forms of images, sounds, and videos with the camera's provided in it and keep track of the happenings around them. They do not need any human to control or operate them [50]. They further transmit the data to the gateways for further processing and information extraction process. They will also be used to work as flying portable base stations for many purposes in the near future. They will be able to monitor places where humans cannot reach, or reaching to these places is risky and life threatening. They can be used in monitoring disaster-hit areas without any further loss of life and property. They will help in gathering big data for analysis and ML processes and at the same time make our cities even smarter. IoD can be treated as the subset of IoT. IoT acts as the backbone for IoD to operate and work and provides controlled and coordinated access to the airspace for UAVs [51].

2.3.1 Drones

Drones were developed recently in the twentieth century and have gained a lot of popularity since then. Huge technological advancements have been made since its first production. Size has decreased considerably; battery power has increased from a few minutes to a few hours on a single charge, area covered and control range have increased tremendously, and camera quality has improved from standard definition and high definition to full HD quality and ultra-HD as well. Inception of microphones was a big achievement in the drone industry [52]. Huge storage space has allowed to record continuously without the fear of losing or overwriting on previous videos. The integration of AI, ML, and deep learning techniques was the next big milestone achievement in the drone industry.

The main components of an UAV are controller, communication system, sensors, camera, a power source (battery), and mechanical components which help in flying [53]. Figure 12 depicts a drone and its parts.

2.3.2 Development of IoD

Four basic steps are required for development of an IoD system.

The first step is to install and discover the sensors, actuators, cameras, and other smart devices to communicate with the UAV. Deciding the covering area of a drone is also planned here.

Data generated by the devices is in analogue form, which needs to be converted into digital form before it can be used for further processing. This step is dedicated to the conversion of the data.

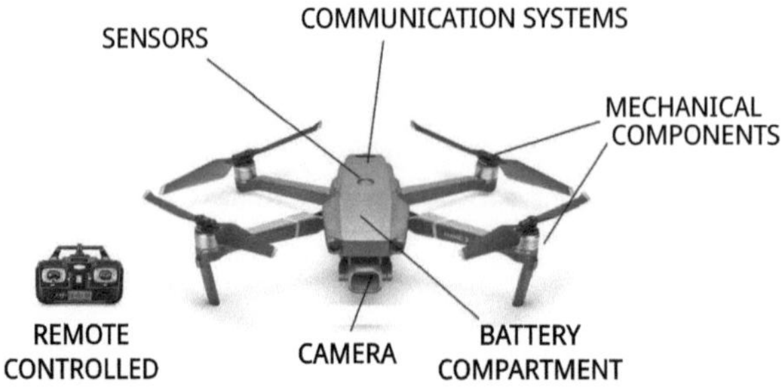

Figure 12: A drone.

Data is sent to the next node in the network. It can be the router which further connects to the drones of the sensors and devices can directly connect to the drones to make the process faster with less latency. These drones can either process the data on their own or send it forward for further processing [54].

Drones can also analyze the data and apply analytics and send a reply back to the concerned device to perform an action needed. They can also control and send commands to other devices based on the information received from adjacent or neighboring devices. They can also communicate with other drones and aircrafts nearby [55].

2.3.3 Relevant networks for UAVs

In this section, we have listed a few networks relevant to UAVs [53]:

Air traffic
Cellular networks
Internet

2.3.4 Attacks on IoD

There are a number of attacks possible on the drones in the IoD. In this section, we have listed a few attacks that can take place on the IoD network [56]. Figure 13 lists some attacks on IoD.

Integrity attacks:
These attacks attempt to corrupt or make the data unreadable. A few examples of integrity attacks are
Substitution/altercation of information
Message forgery
Man in the middle

Access control modifications
Confidentiality

The attacks that compromise the confidentiality of the data or the users are known as confidentiality attacks. A few examples of this type of attacks are
Identity spoofing
Unauthorized access
Replay attacks
Eavesdropping
Availability

The attacks that compromise the availability of the resources thereby interrupting the normal services for the users are known as availability attacks. A few examples of availability attacks are
Physical attacks
Channel jamming
Denial of service
DDoS attacks
GPS spoofing
Routing attacks
Trust

The attacks that compromise the trust of the users on the services are counted under trust attacks. A few examples of trust attacks are

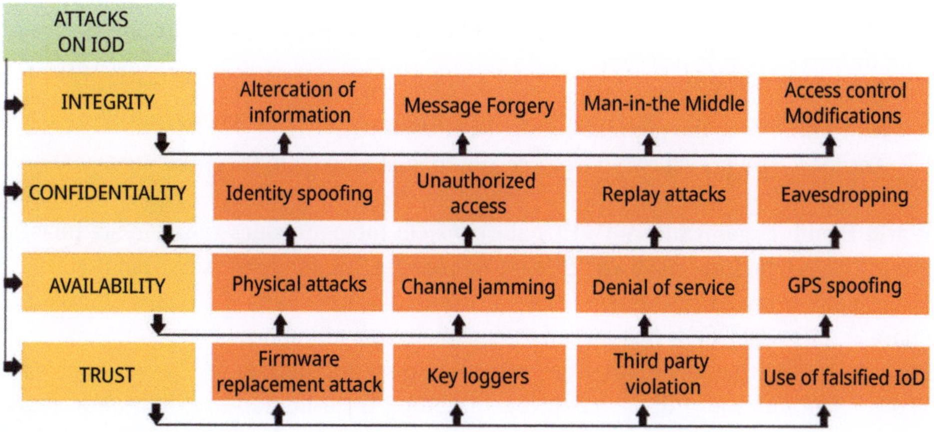

Figure 13: Attacks on IoD.

Firmware replacement attack
Key loggers
Third parties' violation
Use of falsified IoD

2.3.5 IoD real-time implementations

Nowadays, IoD has found a way into almost every possible sector of the human life. In this section, we list a few real-life uses of IoD [57]:

Construction and infrastructure
Energy/disaster relief
Smart city monitoring
Smart agriculture
Healthcare
Insurance
Weather forecasting

3 The pandemics and their effects

Pandemic is an outbreak of a disease that spreads across continents, not just countries. It has a more severe effect on the population and takes more lives than an epidemic. A disease is declared as a pandemic when it becomes severe and spreads rapidly through the countries and continents.

Death toll of a pandemic depends on a few factors listed below:
Number of people infected
How severe is the illness caused?
How vulnerable the population is to the illness?
Are there any preventive measures and how effective are they?

World Health Organization's (WHO) alert system for pandemics range in six phases. Phase 1 being the least risky and phase 6 denoting a full pandemic situation [58].

Phase 1: An animal virus known to cause disease has caused no infections in humans.
Phase 2: An animal virus has caused infections in some humans.
Phase 3: There are a few cases of the infection in scattered cases or clusters in human communities. Illness might be spreading from human to human but is not severe enough to cause and spread community-level outbreaks.
Phase 4: Outbreaks are confirmed at the community level, and human-to-human spread of the illness is also confirmed.

Phase 5: The disease is confirmed to be spreading in population of more than one country.

Phase 6: The disease is confirmed to be spreading at the community level outbreak in a country in different region than the host country.

3.1 Pandemics in the last century

Pandemics have hit us tremendously in the last as well as the current century. They have come unannounced and we have dealt with it but not before a large number of lives were lost. In this section, we have highlighted a few recent pandemics and their effects on our societies. The rapid population growth, need for more and more resources to sustain life, and other needs of the humans leading to immense changes to the global environment have led to an increase in the rate at which the pandemics and epidemics occur. In 1918, the influenza pandemic, better remembered as the Spanish flu, occurred. In 1957, the Asian flu emerged in East Asia. In 1968, the H3N2 virus caused the Hong Kong flu. In 1977, the H1N1 virus caused the Russian flu. In 2009 again, the H1N1 virus caused the swine flu, and the current coronavirus (COVID-19) is caused by the SARS-CoV-2 virus [1].

3.1.1 Spanish flu (1918)

Spanish flu was also known as the great influenza. It was an unexpectedly deadly global influenza which was caused by the H1N1 influenza virus. The index case was reported in March 1918 in Kansas City of the United States. Gradually, cases started to be reported from France, Germany, and the United Kingdom in April. Within the span of 2 years, almost one-third of the global population, which estimated to around 500 million, were reported infected [59]. Around 142 million people were estimated to be dead in four waves of the pandemic, making it the deadliest pandemic in the history of human kind. India reported its first case of the flu in May 1918. The total death was estimated to be around 12–17 million in India alone.

3.1.2 Asian flu (1957)

Asian flu was a global pandemic influenza caused by influenza A virus H2N2. The index case was reported in Guizhou in southern China in early 1957. More cases begin to be reported in the adjacent province, Yunnan, in early March. The flu spread in the whole China by the middle of March. China in 1957 was not a member of the WHO; therefore, the outbreak was not reported. The first case outside China was reported in Singapore in February 1957. On April 17, 1957, cases were reported in Hong Kong.

India reported a million cases by June. The pandemic reached the United Kingdom and the United States in late June [60]. Estimated deaths stood at 14.2 million throughout the world. India reported 1.5 million cases and 1,055 deaths.

3.1.3 Hong Kong flu (1968)

Just after 10 years of the Asian flu, another pandemic was reported which was caused by the H3N2 of the influenza A virus. The index case was reported on July 13, 1968 in Hong Kong. Within 2 weeks, the outbreak reached its peak. Outbreaks were reported in Vietnam and Singapore in July. The flu reached India, Philippines, Australia, and northern Europe by September. It was widespread in the United States by December. It reached Japan, South America, and Africa in 1969 [61]. An estimate of 1.4 million deaths were reported. No significant number of deaths were reported in India.

3.1.4 Russian flu (1977)

Within the next 10 years of the Russian flu, another pandemic was reported which was caused by the H1N1 influenza strain. The index case was reported in Northern China in May 1977. Soon after, cases were reported in Soviet Union. The flu affected the population under the age of 25–26 years. It was speculated that the virus was released to the public through a laboratory accident. Later the year, the flu was detected in China, Hong Kong, and Siberia. By the end of 1977, the virus reached the United Kingdom. It reached the United States in January 1998 [62]. A total of 0.7 million people were reported dead due to the pandemic. India did not report any deaths due to the pandemic.

3.1.5 Swine flu (2009)

Swine flu was caused by the H1N1 influenza virus. The index case was detected in the United States in April 2009. It was at its peak during mid-May and June in the United States. The estimated death was less than 0.3 million worldwide. India reported its first case in May [63]. Around 31,000 cases were reported in India with 1,841 deaths.

3.1.6 COVID-19 (2019)

The Coronavirus 2019 pandemic is an ongoing global pandemic caused by the SARS-CoV-2 virus. The index case was detected in December 2019 in the Wuhan province of China. All the attempts to contain and stop the spread of the virus failed. More than

20 countries confirmed cases in the beginning of March. By the end of March more than 40 countries confirmed more than 500 cases each. India got its first confirmed case on March 1 [64]. As of writing of this chapter, 326 million cases have been recorded with 21.5 million deaths, and India has witnessed 37.4 million cases and less than 0.5 million deaths.

In Table 1, we have tried to show the impact of the six pandemics on the human civilizations.

Table 1: Impact of pandemics.

Pandemic	Index case	Source	Most affected countries	Confirmed cases (m)	Deaths (million)
Spanish flu (1918)	USA	H1N1	USA, Spain, Serbia, Mexico, **India**	500	142
Asian flu (1957)	China	H2N2	China, Singapore, Hong Kong, USA, UK, **India**	25	14.2
Hong Kong flu (1968)	Hong Kong	H3N2	Hong Kong, Vietnam, Singapore, **India**, Philippines		1.4
Russian flu (1977)	China	H1N1	Soviet Union, China, Hong Kong, Siberia	5	<0.7
Swine flu (2009)	USA	H1N1	USA	1,400	<0.3
COVID-19 (2019)	China	SARS-CoV-2	China, USA, Italy, Iran	43	21.5

3.2 The effects of the pandemics

Pandemics and epidemics affect each and every sector of the society, education, lei sure, healthcare, construction, sports, and so on; all are adversely affected. Sometimes they have even disrupted the day-to-day lives of human beings as well. The pandemics demand emergency healthcare response on the global scale [65]. They lead to a loss of a large number of human lives throughout the world and present an unprecedented challenge to the health of the public, the food system, the medical facilities and care systems, and the work systems. It causes devastating economic and social disruptions. All large part of the population is pushed toward poverty and malnutrition and other ailments.

Below we have mentioned the effects of pandemics on some sectors worldwide.

3.2.1 Impact on GDP bringing recession

When the economy of the country increases and grows, the country makes more and more wealth and more new jobs are created. But in pandemic and epidemic conditions, the GDP of the affected country declines because all the resources and efforts are shifted toward people's health, reducing and eliminating the impacts of the pandemic and the disease. During the COVID-19 crisis, International Monetary Fund (IMF) made an estimate that the global economy reduced by 4.4% in 2020. It is the worst decline only after the great depression of the 1930s [66].

3.2.2 Impact on job seekers

Job seekers and unemployed people play a major role in the growth of the country. People lose their jobs or are terminated in pandemic and epidemic situations, simply because the business or the industry is not making enough money to pay their employees. No work is carried out which means business gets no payments which in turn makes the employees wait for their salaries. New job seekers are also left unattended as businesses do not have investments to pay them. During the current COVID-19 pandemic, unemployment increased in many countries at unimaginable rates [67]. According to the IMF, 8.9% people lost their jobs in 2020.

3.2.3 Impact on stock market

Pandemics bring the flow of cash and transactions to minimum. The banks are forced to decrease the rate of interest they provide to their customers. Since the flow of money is reduced, the investments in the form of stock markets and other trading platforms get a hit and are severely reduced. In the COVID-19 crisis, stocks like Dow Jones, FTSE, and Italy MIB experienced a decline of up to 40% in the start of 2020. As the pandemic condition eases through and the flow of money gains momentum, these stocks are also predicted to gain their stipulated ranges [68].

3.2.4 Impact on tourism

Tourism is one of the worst hit sectors in case of pandemics or epidemics, which have the ability to spread from human to human. The highly contagious diseases and human-to-human transmission of the disease force the people to stay away from infected people or even the healthy one in order to keep themselves protected and disease free. These diseases have the ability of spreading from one to another even before he/she displays symptoms themselves. This is one of the main reasons of the spread of the current COVID-19 disease. Global lockdowns, termination of the international as well as domestic flights, termination of all transportation systems, ban on people from coming out of their homes, wearing of masks, and maintaining social distancing were all implications of the coronavirus disease [1, 69].

3.2.5 Impact on agriculture

The occurrence of pandemics does not spare the agriculture sector as well. With all the resources getting diverted toward the healthcare of the people and prevention of the spread of the pandemics, the physical labor-ridden agriculture sector gets a bad hit. Transportation of raw materials, fertilizers, seeds, as well as the end products does not take place at the required strength. The end products that start to rot within a few days are not consumed or stored properly [70]. Large number of farm labors and internal migrants head back toward their home due to loss of business or work. In the current COVID-19 pandemic, more than 50 million migrants traveled back to their native places once the lockdown was implemented in India.

4 Role of AI, IoT, and IoD in pandemics

About 56.6% of the total population of the world live in the urban areas, which is estimated to increase to 68% by 2050. In 1950, only 30% of the world population was living in the cities. It was 2007 when more people lived in the urban area than the rural areas. Figure 14 depicts this population trend.

With the rapid increase in the population and limited amount of resources and land for cultivation and living, we need to come up with more sustainable development techniques. The smart city concept is a promising innovation with sustainable social, economic, and political goals. With the use of technology and computers, we have to build a city which conserves resources for the future generations, make the life comfortable for the current generation, and at the same time make the environment less polluted and safe for the human kind. Development of smart cities is currently the top priority in a number of governments nowadays. In the events of pandemics and epidemics, smart cities will be well equipped to face the diseases, and with the help of technologies like IoT, big data, AL, and IoD, cities can perform continuous monitoring, offer strict warnings, and make quick decisions. The smart cities and smart technologies can also benefit the healthcare sectors significantly in these adverse times.

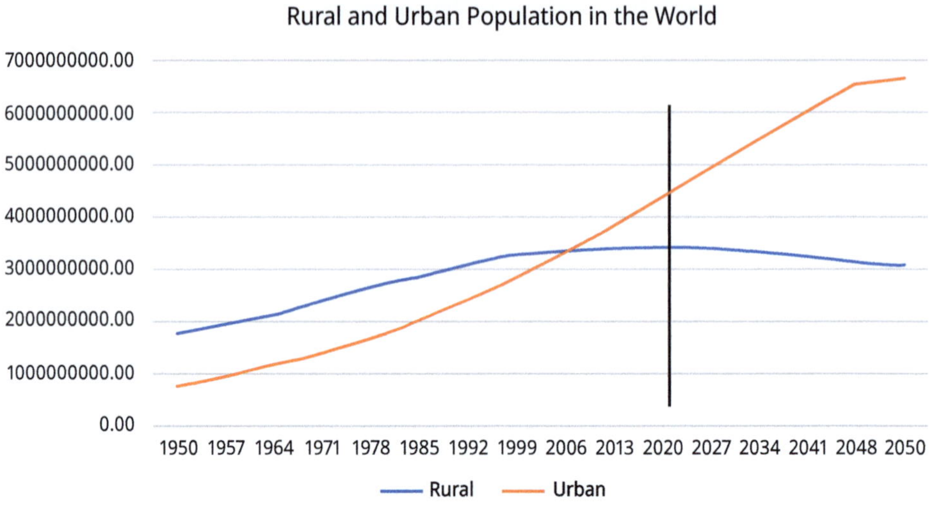

Figure 14: Year-wise rural and urban population of the world.

4.1 AI in the event of pandemics

AI that worked upon properly has the potential of avoiding or at least minimizing the effects of the pandemics, epidemics, and the onset of diseases and abnormalities. In the current COVID-19 pandemic, AI has been working tirelessly assisting the limitations of the human knowledge in the huge venture of understanding, limiting and tracking the spread of the disease. AI-powered projects using the technologies like data science, ML, and big data can be used in a number of domains to predict, explain, and manage the different scenarios caused by the global as well as local health crisis. The use of AI in the healthcare domain can lead to early detection as well as prediction of COVID-19 symptoms and hence controlling and reducing its spread. AI algorithms can be used to screen as well as track patients and predict future infections and abnormalities.

4.1.1 Prediction and tracking

Healthcare professionals can study and track the transmission rate of a disease or an abnormality by the use of AI algorithms and AI models.

Susceptible, infectious, and recovered (SIR) model can be used in conjunction with AI in order to analyze and make predictions and forecasting the growth and development of unknown viruses and variants which can become lethal if kept unmonitored and uncontrolled. AI-based Global Epidemic and Mobility (GLEaM) model is capable of making a simulation of the spread of a disease across the globe. It can help the healthcare professionals and researchers in developing case studies, test their hypothesis, if any, and justify it, in order to save the humans from the diseases, on the spread of the disease. It can help in understanding the recognized variants of the pandemic. It can also help researchers in studying the efficacy and results of various interpolation strategies, analyze threats through various model scenario techniques, and forecast any new and developing infectious diseases.

Another AI-based system, Transportation Analysis and Simulation (TRANSIMS), works on the principle of unconventional computational and analytical techniques in order to survey a region's transportation system and forecast the spread of a disease or illness based on the local interactions and habits of the people. It has the ability to mimic the patterns of transit of all the individuals of an area for a complete 24-h period on the basis of the data received from the surveys, including the data and stats on the intensity of congestion and traffic, time-dependent delays for the complete transit network and the roads, and queues at intersections. These AI-based models can accurately predict the number of cases and the rate of transmission for a new illness.

AI can be used for anomaly detection (AD). It has the ability to identify abnormal and unfamiliar patterns present in a medical image, such as MRI scan, CT scan, and X-ray imaging. AD can be used to single-dimensional as well as multidimensional data. AD-driven processes were very hectic and time-consuming for doctors and medical practitioners to analyze and provide therapy and updates for patients without the AI technology. With the data generated by AD, AI can prove its worth in identifying the most and least risky and vulnerable regions simply by tracking and tracking the figures of confirmed cases and giving suggestions and recommendations for the necessary actions to be taken in order to recommend the necessary actions to cut back the spread.

For the current COVID-19, AI is helping in identifying and forecasting COVID-19 outbreaks in various regions by using multidimensional data. Normally, AI tools work on single-dimensional data type, which sometimes may lead to inaccurate prediction of the escalation of the disease. In these cases, multidimensional data help the AI tools in making better decision with greater reliability and accuracy.

4.1.2 Vaccine discoveries and predictions based on AI

If an outbreak occurs, various approaches based on AI can be used to design vaccines or antidotes. NLP models, like language modeling techniques, can be helpful in driving a powerful, useful, and safe vaccine. The AI algorithms analyze huge amounts of data, including geographical locations and the social interactions of the patients, and come up with recommended treatments, clearing the path for the development of the vaccine. AI can be used with various other ML programs such as Vaxign ML platform, which is implemented on supervised learning model to expedite the discovery process.

Currently, AI is pushing COVID-19 research in three major areas:
Binary diagnosis: to check the presence of COVID-19
Studying lung abnormalities
Eliminating non-COVID-19 pneumonia from COVID-19

AI algorithms, if trained properly, can forecast the development of acute respiratory distress syndrome in patients. They can also notify the medical staff for the need of oxygen treatment or incubation in the patients. Different AI platforms can help the medical staff in determining and generalizing the treatments to patients from different nations and geographical locations. They can further help in integrating imaging and clinical information and analyzing the medical image data and customize the medicines being given to each and every patient. Further, with the use of NLP in clinical reports and diagnosis, ML models are learning from clinical images to foresee the need of intensive care for the patients.

4.1.3 Developing AI-driven insights for future pandemic

Hospitals and healthcare firms and institutions, today, find themselves in grave requirement of a technology with real-time and quick decision-making in order to reduce and stop the spread of the coronavirus as well as any other disease which may follow. The ability of AI to imitate the intelligence of humans in a skilled way is helping the healthcare workers to learn and recognize the nature of the causing agent and developing the vaccines and medicine and taking quick steps to reduce its spread. The technology is directing screening of the people, analysis of the data received, and making forecast and keeping a track of the current and probable future infections. It also helps in tracking the cases which are confirmed and recovered as well as the fatality cases which enable the doctors, physicians, and other healthcare workers to gain important insights on how to treat the patients and work toward ending the pandemic.

4.2 IoT in the event of pandemics

IoT devices deployed at various places can speed up the detection of anomalies and capturing information. They will make the detection process faster and efficient. The COVID-19 pandemic has highlighted the lack of reliable and robust response system we currently have in a pandemic situation. IoT can play a significant role in the future in times of crisis and emergency, provided it is used accurately and efficiently. IoT data can be used to detect patterns, make recommendations, and provide insights during outbreaks. IoT can provide valuable assistance in future pandemics in the following ways.

4.2.1 Data collection

Technology companies can provide data to analyze different parameters and streams such as movement of people and rise of different chemicals and other wastes in the environment like soil, air, and water. This data can be used to track the implementations of proper guidelines set up by the government. The geographical and healthcare data can help the policymakers and officials in introducing reliable and updated solutions and new policies to control future breakouts. The data can also serve in research and development process, in turn improving the healthcare infrastructure and methods and medical treatment procedures.

4.2.2 Healthcare solutions

Healthcare is another field where IoT technology can be very useful. IoT is integral for the digital transformation of the healthcare industry. Some of the essential applications of IoT during a pandemic can be remote monitoring of the patients, management of the inventory, telehealth and telemedicine. During the global health crisis, when hospitals are crowded with infected patients, the treatment of patients suffering from chronic diseases becomes difficult. Such cases also increase the workload of the health workers and expose them to the virus. Remote patient monitoring and medical assistance will be a game-changer as it will provide better healthcare and reduce the risk of cross-infection.

IoT can also be leveraged for inventory management in emergencies to enhance drug management and ensure the availability of critical equipment. Telehealth is the use of digital knowledge and communication technologies for receiving healthcare services. Telehealth is helpful for patients suffering from mobility issues since it allows treatment of patients without an in-person visit using telecommunication technology.

4.2.3 IoT solutions

In the current COVID-19 pandemic, as the probability of infection is immense, there is crucial necessity for patients to be monitored regularly and connected with doctors proactively in the different phases of the COVID-19 infection. IoT sensors and devices can collect the data and information from the patients and accelerate the detection process. This can be achieved by observing the body temperature at various time intervals, taking and analyzing samples from probable cases. Various IoT devices can help in monitoring the status of the patients remotely when they have been asked to be in isolation. They can also help in cleaning and disinfecting areas and rooms without any human involvement. The next vital step is to avoid reinfection for the previously healed patient. For the purpose of preventing reinfection, or even new people getting infected, social distancing needs to be practiced which can easily be achieved using IoT devices such as wearable bands and various crowd monitoring devices. IoT technology, during the hard COVID times, has proven its worth and usefulness in almost every domain of the society.

4.3 IoD in event of pandemics

IoD is still in its early days. But the COVID-19 pandemic has shown us that the uses of drones are virtually limitless with effective use in case of emergencies as well. Currently, cellular networks are providing the required startup infrastructure to the acceptance of drones, and the potential of drones only increases as the 5G networks gain momentum, expand, and become a reliable source of communication.

The implementation of IoT within drones, known as IoD, enables the drones to perform a number of tasks like searching for people or vehicles or objects, monitoring an area for unwanted activities or level of pollutants, and delivering of items to the people. Drones can be controlled and operated with the use of smartphones and/or a controller which makes them efficient for various tasks in the field like agriculture, military purposes, and healthcare. Nowadays, drones are equipped with thermal sensors that take thermal images of the people or animals, known as thermal drones. Other types of drones are the surveillance drone, medical drones, disinfectant drones, announcement drone, and so on. The multipurpose drone can be used in the healthcare domain and, particularly in the fight against any future pandemics as well as current COVID-19.

4.3.1 The 5G wave

As the 5G technology continues to gain strength in the cellular networks, people and manufacturers start switching from 4G to 5G. The drones will also evolve and start to move from large cities to rural areas strongly helping in closing the digital gap between the two and start to deliver new services and benefits to every community.

As the drone technology evolves over time, it will become a more common system. It will move from being a "nice-to-have" to a "must-have" IoT device, and at the same time an essential service for connecting and joining people from around cities in ways not perceived before.

4.3.2 Finding the red flags

IoD can be another method to accelerate the method of detecting and locating infected people and contamination zones during pandemics. Drones will reduce the human-to-human interactions significantly and can even reach the areas which are harder to access. The drones with the capability of thermal imaging can be designed in such a way that it can capture the temperature and other details of people at a crowded place and can also be helpful for the early diagnosis of the infected. These drones can be integrated with AI and other IoT devices to pin point people with higher temperature levels (fevers). This drastically decreases human-to-human interactions and at the same time consumes less time when compared to gun thermometer devices.

4.3.3 Mass disinfection and sterilization

Keeping areas with high level of abnormalities and infection reports can be sprayed with disinfectants and sterilized with the help of drones. The drones can easily enter the contaminated and toxicated zones and reduce the contamination of the virus and prevent the workers from getting infected. Disinfectants can also be sprayed in large water bodies, where the level of toxicants is high and can lead to bigger problems.

4.3.4 Medicine and essential delivery

Drones can help in transferring the kits, medicines, as well as essential items to the at-home patients as well as hospitals. They can also carry back the samples from the patients to the hospitals or testing places to eliminate the interactions with humans. These types of drones will greatly reduce the hospital visits and increase the access to medical care more convenient and easier. Using medical drones will reduce the delivery time and increase the diagnosis speed. The drones can be used for numerous other purposes such as postal and grocery services while the people are not able to do the same.

4.3.5 Surveillance drone

The surveillance drone is designed and developed in such a way that it can monitor crowds as well as various sites where the toxicity level is above normal. The drone is capable of announcing important information with the help of speakers equipped in it. This allows for quick and clear information transfer in case of emergencies and at places with low accessibility to the Internet.

5 Conclusion

AI, IoT, and IoD can help develop connected and responsive healthcare systems to deal with outbreaks. However, it still requires further innovation, investment, and research. IoT data can provide useful insights, using AI, for policymaking in dealing with outbreaks, epidemics, and pandemics. Telecom operators can further investigate and assist manufacturing industries in dealing with the pandemic crisis. Government agencies and individual organizations should invest in crisis planning and recovery strategy to prevent significant loss of life, property, and economic shocks. The governments need to allocate funds for response plans, and IoT and IoD projects that will help vastly in the prevention and minimizing the risks of the future pandemics. IoT service providers can focus on resolving data security, accuracy, overload, and privacy issues. For further adoption of IoT and IoD technologies in healthcare, IoT and IoD functions should be aligned with global healthcare regulations. IoT and AI can help in creating patterns of the spread of the contagion to predict future outbreaks well in advance.

The use of the data collected from diseases such as Ebola and Zika outbreaks has given us immense knowledge to address global health issues and led to some best practices that are now facilitating the use of IoT and IoD. The current pandemic has also given us huge amount of data to play with and learn about the outbreaks. This has triggered widespread hype and optimism about the capacity of these technologies to fight pandemics. Yet, the current trend opens up myriad questions that require further scrutiny.

References

[1] Alam, M., Parveen, R. COVID-19 and tourism. International Journal of Advanced Research, 2021, 9(4), 788–804 Available at: https://doi.org/10.21474/ijar01/12766.

[2] Shur, M. Describing and predicting COVID19 evolution using pandemic equation. In: International Conference on Big Data, 2020.

[3] Arroub, A., Zahi, B., Sabir, E., Sadik, M. A literature review on smart cities: Paradigms, opportunities and open problems. In: International Conference on Wireless Networks and Mobile Communications (WINCOM), Fez, Morocco, 2016.

[4] Mtshali, P., Khubisa, F. A smart home appliance control system for physically disabled people. In: Conference on Information Communications Technology and Society (ICTAS), Durban, South Africa, 2019.

[5] Wang, X., Li, X., Leung, V. C. M. Artificial intelligence-based techniques for emerging heterogeneous network: State of the arts, opportunities, and challenges. IEEE Access, 2015, 3, 1379–1391.

[6] Alam, M., Khan, A. H., Khan, I. R. Swarm intelligence in MANETs: A survey. International Journal of Manufacturing Technology and Management, 2016, 5(5), 141–150.

[7] Alam, M., Khan, I. R. Internet of things as key enabler for efficient business processes. SSRN Electronic Journal, 2019. Available at: https://doi.org/10.2139/ssrn.3806408.

[8] Alam, M., Khan, I. R. Application of AI in smart cities. In: Industrial Transformation, Delhi, Taylor & Francis Group, 2022, 61–86.
[9] Kar, A., Subash, A., Rao, V. U. Reactive artificial intelligence using big data in the era of precision medicine. JAMA Surgery, 2020, 155(7), 671.
[10] Schmidt, M., Berg, E., Friedlander, M., Murphy, K. Optimizing costly functions with simple constraints: A limited-memory projected quasi-newton algorithm. In: International Conference on Artificial Intelligence and Statistics (AISTATS), Florida, USA, 2009.
[11] Scassellati, B. Theory of mind for a humanoid robot. Autonomous Robots, 2002, 12(1), 13–24.
[12] Gorbenko, A., Popov, V., Sheka, A. Robot self-awareness: Exploration of internal states. Applied Mathematical Sciences, 2012, 6(14), 675–688.
[13] Andreas, K., Haenlein, M. Siri, Siri, in my hand: Who's the fairest in the land? On the interpretations, illustrations, and implications of artificial intelligence. Business Horizons, 2019, 62(1), 15–25.
[14] Lieto, A., Bhatt, M., Oltramari, A., Vernon, D. The role of cognitive architectures in general artificial intelligence. Cognitive Systems Research, 2018, 48, 1–3.
[15] Barrett, A. M., Baum, S. D. A model of pathways to artificial superintelligence catastrophe for risk and decision analysis. Journal of Experimental & Theoretical Artificial Intelligence, 2017, 29(2), 397–414.
[16] El-Najdawi, M. K., Stylianou, A. C. Expert support systems: Integrating AI technologies. Communications of the ACM, 1993, 36(12), 55–66.
[17] Rani, P. J., Bakthakumar, J., Kumaar, B. P., Kumaar, U. P., Kumar, S. Voice controlled home automation system using Natural Language Processing (NLP) and Internet of Things (IoT). In: Third International Conference on Science Technology Engineering & Management (ICONSTEM), Chennai, India, 2017.
[18] Mihalcea, R., Liu, H., Lieberman, H. NLP (Natural Language Processing) for NLP (Natural Language Programming). In Computational Linguistics and Intelligent Text Processing. CICLing 2006, Springer, Berlin, Heidelberg, Springer, 2006.
[19] Forsyth, D., Ponce, J. Computer Vision: A Modern Approach, 2nd edition), Prentice Hall, Boston, Massachusetts 2011.
[20] Baumgart, B. G. A polyhedron representation for computer vision. In: National Computer Conference and Exposition, 1975.
[21] Torresen, J. A review of future and ethical perspectives of robotics and AI. Frontiers in Robotics and AI, 2018, 4. Available at: 10.3389/frobt.2017.00075
[22] Rosenschein, S. J. Formal theories of knowledge in AI and robotics. New Generation Computing, 1985, 3(4), 345–357.
[23] He, K., Zhang, X., Ren, S., Sun, J. Deep residual learning for image recognition. In: IEEE Conference on Computer Vision and Pattern Recognition (CVPR), Las Vegas, NV, USA, 2016.
[24] Sun, Q.-S., Zeng, S.-G., Liu, Y., Heng, P.-A., Xia, D.-S. A new method of feature fusion and its application in image recognition. Pattern Recognition, 2005, 38(12), 2437–2448.
[25] Khotanzad, A., Hong, Y. H. Invariant image recognition by Zernike moments. IEEE Transactions on Pattern Analysis and Machine Intelligence, 1990, 12(5), 489–497.
[26] Halle, M., Stevens, K. Speech recognition: A model and a program for research. IRE Transactions on Information Theory, 1962, 8(2), 155–159.
[27] Khan, I. R., Goyal, A., Alam, M. Augmented reality application for newspapers. SSRN Electronic Journal, 2021, 252–258. Available at: 10.2139/ssrn.3927827
[28] LeCun, Y., Bengio, Y., Hinton, G. Deep learning. Nature, 2015, 521(7553), 436–444.
[29] Jordan, M. I., Mitchell, T. M., Machine learning: Trends, perspectives, and prospects, Science, 349, 6245, 255–260, 2015.
[30] Wu, F., Yen, Z., Yunhe, H., Ni, Y. Applications of AI techniques to generation planning and investment. Power Engineering Society General Meeting, 2004, 1, 936–940.

[31] Vincent, D. R., Deepa, N., Elavarasan, D., Srinivasan, K., Shauhdary, S. H., Iwendi, C. Sensors driven AI-based agriculture recommendation model for assessing land suitability. Sensors, 2019, 19(17), 3667.

[32] Bartoletti, I. AI in Healthcare: Ethical and Privacy Challenges, Springer International Publishing, London, UK, 2019, 7–10.

[33] O'Leary, D. E. AI in accounting, finance and management. Intelligent Systems in Accounting, Finance and Management, 1995, 4(3), 149–153.

[34] Carron, M. S. The transformative effect of AI on the banking industry. Banking & Finance Law Review, 2019, 34(2), 169–214.

[35] Adam, M., Wessei, M., Benlian, A. AI-based chatbots in customer service and their effects on user compliance. Electron Markets, 2021, 31, 427–445.

[36] Ma, Y., Wang, Z., Yang, H., Yang, L. Artificial intelligence applications in the development of autonomous vehicles: A survey. IEEE/CAA Journal of Automatica Sinica, 2020, 7(2), 315–329.

[37] Alam, M., Khan, I. R., Tanweer, S. IOT in smart cities: A survey. Juni Khyat, 9 May 2020, 10(5), 89–101.

[38] Alam, M., Khan, I. R., Siddique, S. A., Wiquar, R., Anwar, H. IoT and AI as key enabler of growth of smart cities. In: 2nd International Conference on ICT for Digital, Smart and Sustainable Development, New Delhi, 2020.

[39] Reggio, G., Leotta, M., Cerioli, M., Spalazzese, R., Alkhabbas, F. What are IoT systems for real? An experts' survey on software engineering aspects. Internet of Things, 2020, 12, 100313.

[40] Lazaro, A., Villarino, R., Girbau, D. A survey of NFC sensors based on energy harvesting for IoT applications. Sensors, 2018, 18(11), 3746.

[41] Alam, M., Nielsen, R. H., Prasad, N. R. The evolution of M2M into IoT. In: First International Black Sea Conference on Communications and Networking (BlackSeaCom), Batumi, Georgia, 2013.

[42] Jia, X., Feng, Q., Fan, T., Lei, Q. RFID technology and its applications in Internet of Things (IoT). In: 2nd International Conference on Consumer Electronics, Communications and Networks (CECNet), Yichang, China, 2012.

[43] Pallavi, S., Narayanan, A. V. An overview of practical attacks on BLE based IOT devices and their security. In: 5th International Conference on Advanced Computing & Communication Systems (ICACCS), Coimbatore, India, 2019.

[44] Nair, K., Kulkarni, J., Warde, M., Dave, Z., Rawalgaonkar, V., Gore, G., Joshi, J. Optimizing power consumption in IoT based wireless sensor networks using Bluetooth Low Energy. In: International Conference on Green Computing and Internet of Things (ICGCIoT), Greater Noida, India, 2015.

[45] Gao, Y., Qin, Z., Feng, Z., Zhang, Q., Holland, O., Dohler, M. Scalable and reliable IoT enabled by dynamic spectrum management for M2M in LTE-A. IEEE Internet of Things Journal, 2016, 3(6), 1135–1145.

[46] Belghazi, Z., Benamar, N., Addaim, A., Kerrache, C. A. Secure WiFi-direct using key exchange for IoT device-to-device communications in a smart environment. Future Internet, 2019, 11(12), 251.

[47] Porkodi, R., Bhuvaneswari, V. The Internet of Things (IoT) applications and communication enabling technology standards: An overview. In: International Conference on Intelligent Computing Applications, Coimbatore, India, 2014.

[48] Chen, S., Xu, H., Hu, L. D. B., Wang, H. A vision of IoT: Applications, challenges, and opportunities with China perspective. Internet of Things Journal, 2014, 1(4), 349–359.

[49] Formisano, C., Pavia, D., Gurgen, L., Yonezawa, T., Galache, J. A., Doguchi, K., Matranga, I. The advantages of IoT and cloud applied to smart cities. In: 3rd International Conference on Future Internet of Things and Cloud, Rome, Italy, 2015.

[50] Lee, C.-Y. Cooperative drone positioning measuring in internet-of-drones. In: 17th Annual Consumer Communications & Networking Conference (CCNC), Las Vegas, NV, USA, 2020.

[51] Cavoukian, A. Privacy and drones: Unmanned aerial vehicles. In: Information and Privacy Commissioner of Ontario, Ontario, Canada, 2012, pp. 1–30.

[52] Gharibi, M., Boutaba, R., Waslander, S. L. Internet of drones. IEEE Access, 2016, 4, 1148–1162.

[53] Alam, M., Chamoli, A., Hasan, N. Smart Cities and Internet of Drones, 2022.

[54] Guillen-Perez, A., Sanchez-Iborra, R., Cano, M.-C., Sanchez-Aarnoutse, J. C., Garcia-Haro, J. WiFi networks on drones. ITU Kaleidoscope: ICTs for a Sustainable World (ITU WT), Bangkok, Thailand, 2016, pp. 1–8, doi: 10.1109/ITU-WT.2016.7805730.

[55] Shan, L., Miura, R., Kagawa, T., Ono, F., Li, H.-B., Kojima, F. Machine learning-based field data analysis and modeling for drone communications. IEEE Access, 2019, 7, 79127–79135.

[56] Lin, C., He, D., Kumar, N., Choo, -K.-K. R., Vinel, A., Huang, X. Security and privacy for the internet of drones: Challenges and solutions. IEEE Communications Magazine, 2018, 56(1), 64–69.

[57] Hall, R. J. An internet of drones. IEEE Internet Computing, 2016, 20(3), 68–73.

[58] Phases, T. W. P. Pandemic Influenza Preparedness and Response: A WHO Guidance Document, Geneva, World Health Organization, 2009.

[59] Aassve, A., Alfani, G., Gandolfi, F., Moglie, M. L. Epidemics and trust: The case of the Spanish Flu. Health Economics, 2021, 30(4), 840–857.

[60] Jackson, C. History lessons: The Asian Flu pandemic. British Journal of General Practice, 2009, 59(565), 622–623.

[61] Joffe, H., Lee, N. Y. L. Social representation of a food risk: The Hong Kong Avian Bird Flu epidemic. Journal of Health Psychology, 2004, 9(4), 517–533.

[62] Gregg, M. B. The Russian Flu. JAMA, 1978, 240(21), 2260.

[63] Myers, L. B., Goodwin, R. Determinants of adults' intention to vaccinate against pandemic swine flu. BMC Public Health, 2011, 11(no), 1.

[64] Alam, M., Parveen, R., Khan, I. R. Role of information technology in Covid-19 prevention. International Journal of Business Education and Management Studies, 2020, 5(1), 65–75.

[65] Jorda, O., Singh, S. R., Taylor, A. M. Longer-run economic consequences of pandemics. The Review of Economics and Statistics, 2022, 104(1), 166–175.

[66] Maliszewska, M., Mattoo, A., Mensburgghe, C. V. D. The potential impact of COVID-19 on GDP and trade: A preliminary assessment. World Bank Policy Research Working Paper 9211, 2020.

[67] Crayne, M. P. The traumatic impact of job loss and job search in the aftermath of COVID-19. Psychological Trauma: Theory, Research, Practice, and Policy, 2020, 12(S1), 180–182.

[68] Zhang, D., Hu, M., Ji, Q. Financial markets under the global pandemic of COVID-19. Finance Research Letters, 2020, 36, 101528.

[69] Zenker, S., Kock, F. The coronavirus pandemic – A critical discussion of a tourism research agenda. Tourism Management, 2020, 81, 104164.

[70] Siche, R. What is the impact of COVID-19 disease on agriculture? Scientia Agropecuaria, 2020, 11(1), 3–6.

Shishupal Kumar, Kumari Nidhi Lal*

A prediction approach of coronavirus disease 2019 cases in India using regression analysis modeling of machine learning

Abstract: A significant international epidemic and serious public health concern have been brought on by the arrival of the severe acute respiratory syndrome coronavirus 2 (SARS-CoV-2; also known as the coronavirus virus or 2019-nCoV) illness (COVID-19) in China at the end of 2019. As of February 20, 2021, India had been home to more than 10,977,387 confirmed cases and 156,240 fatalities, according to the data from the World Health Organization (WHO). The WHO designated COVID-19 as the sixth public health emergency of global concern on January 30, 2020. On May 15, 2020, 81,990 cases have been verified in India. In this regard, the Indian Council of Medical Research takes action to fulfill the wishes of coronavirus patients by offering them intensive treatment. Between April 1 and May 14, 2020, the daily COVID-19 infection rate in India was regularly between 20.64% and 30.81% of patients who are actually sick. India is now coping with the epidemic issue. In India, the number of patients who have become infected since May 14 has roughly followed an exponential trajectory. If this pattern continues for another week, there will be between 1 lakh and 13 lakh infected persons by the middle of March, and India will face a grave situation. By mid-March 2020, there will be a demand for up to 710,761 hospital isolation beds since intensive care units will then be at capacity. In this chapter, we covered the COVID-19 preparations and their effects on the world's second-most populous nation. A prognostication model is suggested as a contribution to accurately predict COVID-19 corroborated instances. Our study could help political leading lights and health-conscious organizations to allocate the necessary employees, beds, and intensive care facilities in handling the issue over the coming days and weeks.

1 Introduction

At the end of December 2019, when all countries of the world were engaged to celebrate the new year 2020, the residents of a city named Wuhan in China started to suffer from a novel COVID-19 disease. The common symptoms of COVID-19 are dry cough, throat

***Corresponding author: Kumari Nidhi Lal**, Department of Computer Science and Engineering, Visvesvaraya National Institute of Technology, Nagpur, India
Shishupal Kumar, Department of Computer Science and Engineering, Indian Institute of Information Technology, Nagpur, India

https://doi.org/10.1515/9783110767681-011

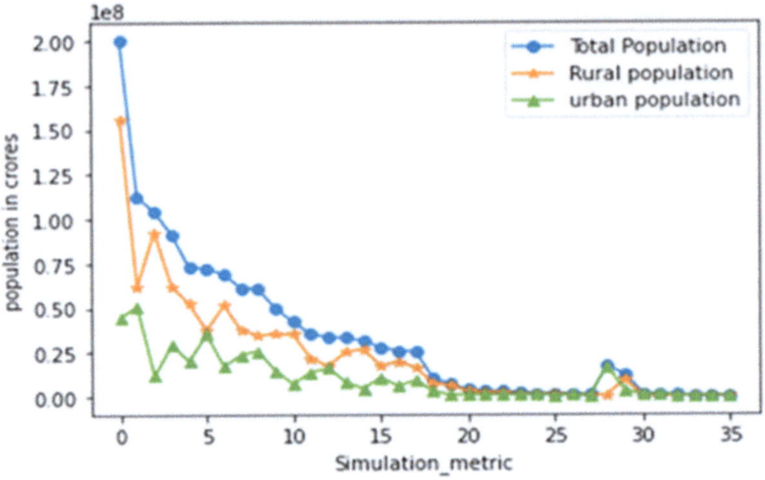

Figure 2: Population in India.

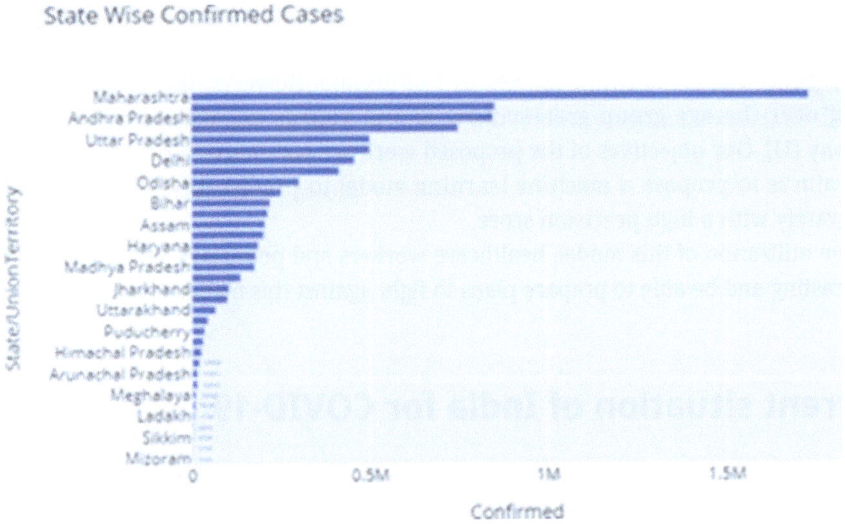

Figure 3: Confirmed COVID-19 cases in all the states of India.

condition remains the same, then the counting of confirmed cases will get higher in comparison to Italy, Spain, and the USA.

Fang et al. [5] mentioned that humans having some autoimmune diseases like cancer, HIV-AIDS, and diabetes are more prone to be a victim of COVID-19. In India, out of a total of 118 deaths, more than 80% of persons have some disorders of autoimmune diseases. In this regard, one assumption is to eat particular foods that are used to boost the immune system. In this way, India can win the battlefield against COVID-19 [13].

However, if this is a true case, then what about other developed countries like Italy and Spain? What is the reason for the high death toll rate in Italy and Spain compared to India? Do the residents of Italy and the USA not include immune booster-related foods? Along with food, another important term that plays a vital role in spreading COVID-19 is temperature. In India, there are mainly three weather seasons: summer, rainy, and winter. The summer season is from April to June with a maximum temperature of 45 °C. Therefore, another discussion point is the impact of temperature on COVID-19. Viruses can indeed be active for more hours in cold places rather than in hot environments. However, there is no research-related proof over it, which can assure that COVID-19 does not show its full progression inside hot countries [8].

Along with this, there are various factors that can play a huge role in increasing COVID-19 patient count in India. Lack of support from the community upon the lockdown decision taken by the government provides a great impact on this situation. If the population is high, then there will be numerous problems that occur in the management. In India, people are not following the restrictions of public gatherings due to their spiritual thinking. People are not able to understand the seriousness and caution regarding this disease. The outcome will be just because of a few humans, hundreds/thousands/lakhs may be infected and get suffered. However, the government has done many advertisements and online programs to distribute awareness of COVID-19. Another factor that plays a role in spreading COVID-19 is that some people hide after being suspected or confirmed of COVID-19 after testing. They are not following the quarantine or isolation procedures. Also, some of them tried to hide their travel history or listing of visited places and persons. In this regard, the government of India is taking strict actions in favor of fines or imprisonment against these people. In these stated measures, the only panic concern is: how can we prevent or stop the infection of COVID-19?

Along with these conditions, the growth of confirmed cases in India is lower than in other countries like the USA, Italy, France, and Spain. In this regard, the WHO admires the prime minister of India for taking preventive steps like lockdown, use of sanitizers, wearing of a mask, and suspending local gatherings at the start of the COVID-19 cases. However, some aspects arise over it like random testing of samples, and few testing processes are done by medical authorities [16]. For more accurate identification, private labs are involved in the testing process of COVID-19 as instructed by the government [10].

Currently, Indian Council of Medical Research describes four stages of COVID-19 spreading in India. In stage 1, only the first starting cases having a travel history in one of the infected countries are diagnosed. In stage 2, after the virus reaches the destination country through the body of the victim, it spreads over his/her close relatives and friends. In stage 3, the local transmission of the virus begins, and sometimes it is called community transmission. In this stage, the history of the origination of the virus could not be traced. In stage 4, the condition of spreading the virus becomes uncontrollable. In the current situation, India lies in stage 3 and the origin of virus spreading is not

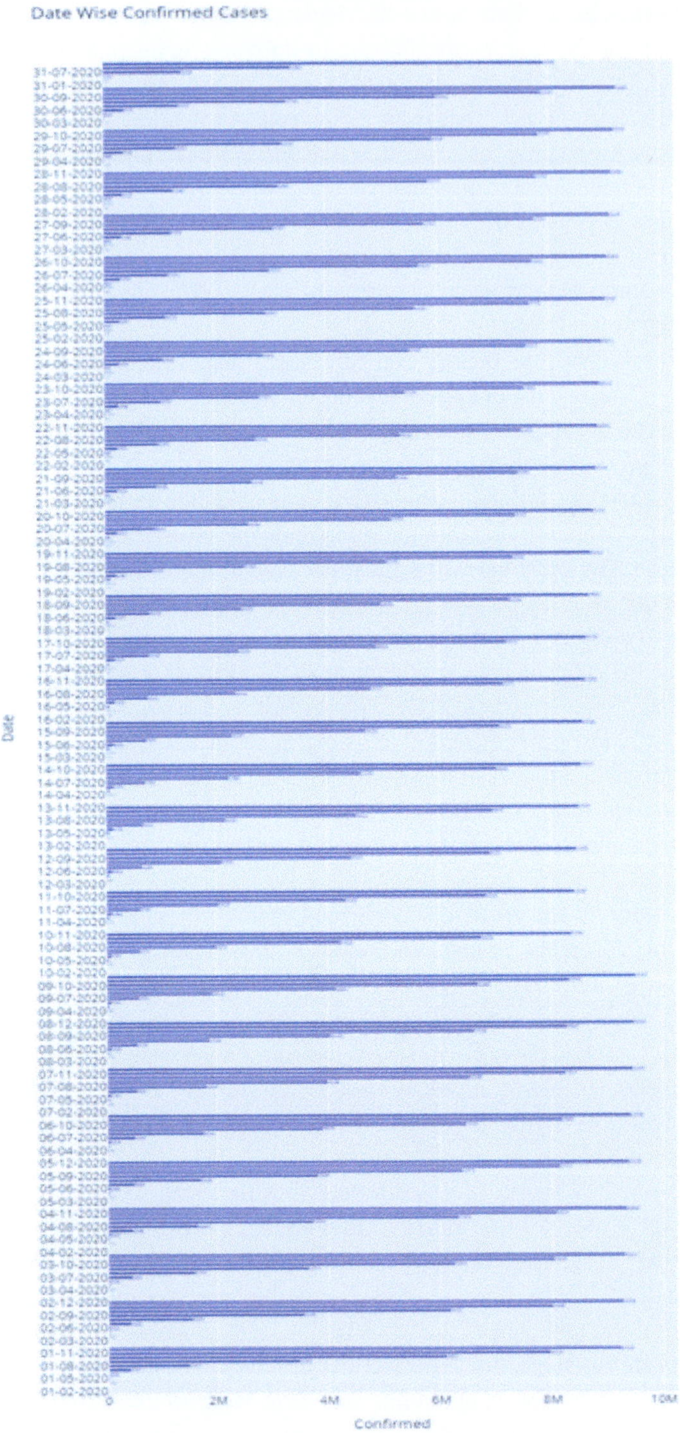

Figure 4: Confirmed cases of growth of COVID-19 in India.

easily accessible. Regarding this, the government of India needs the preparation of medical facilities to be sustained into stage 3. The interventions implemented throughout India include complete lockdown of cities, active case surveillance, rapid investments in increased testing capacity, isolation of cases, ventilators, treatment of severe cases, quarantine of cases and high-risk groups, and behavioral risk-reduction strategies, such as the compulsory use of masks in the general population [18, 20].

India is a developing country with the highest population in which the facilities are not up to a remarkable way. The government hospitals will have to increase the number of beds and isolation wards to treat COVID-19 patients. A dataset that comprises the data of COVID-19 cases in India up to May 14, 2020, is collected [26]. The collective measures of the dataset are presented in Figures 4–6. The government of India provides free testing services and treatment to infected COVID-19 patients through public sector hospitals [14]. However, the facilities regarding isolation wards and cleaning of washrooms are not up to the level. There are some cases in which the patients have attempted to run away from hospitals without informing medical authorities. Moreover, the treatment facility is provided by private hospitals with high charges. This high cost cannot be borne by the common middle- or low-class people of India. Currently, India has 29,899 total hospitals with a capacity of 739,024 beds. Out of the total beds, only 279,588 reside in the rural area and 431,173 beds reside in an urban area. Besides these, to cope with the lakhs of COVID-19 cases, the government of India has prepared railway coaches to act as isolation wards by having thousands

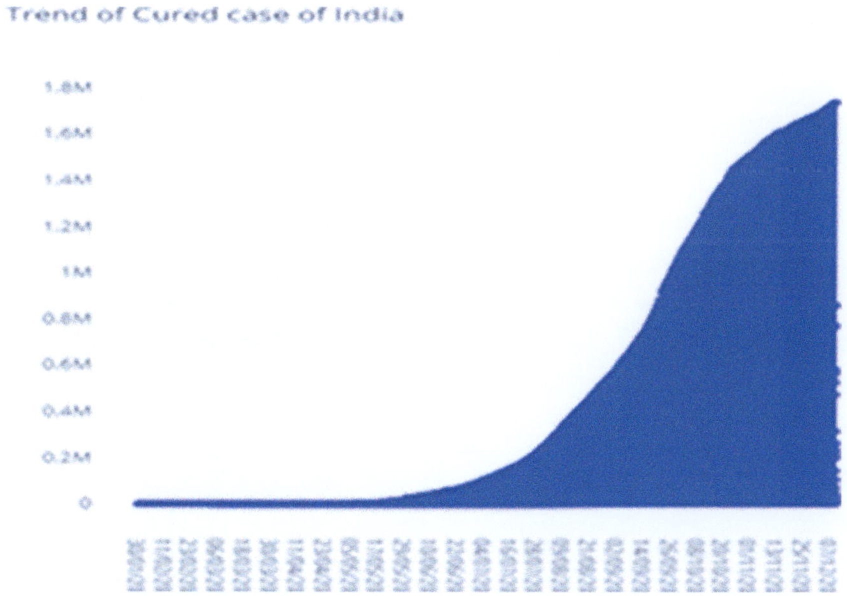

Figure 5: Cured cases of COVID-19 in India.

of capacity per train. Besides, the government also provides extensive care and protection to the working team and their family including doctors and medical staff. The prime minister of India provided an emergency relief fund where people can contribute and help in the government's fight against coronavirus [19]. A Reuters report has now said that the Indian government may bring an INR 2.3 Tn relief fund for the poor sections of the population and businesses [17].

3 Our contributions

In this chapter, the aim is to build a machine learning-based prediction model to forecast the confirmed cases of COVID-19 in India. In this way, the model can be utilized by the politicians and health service providers to take some necessary and preventive steps against COVID-19-related situation of India as indicated in Figure 7. Therefore, we proposed a model that predicts the confirmed cases of COVID-19 with 96% accuracy. To build the model, we utilized a dataset provided by Kaggle [21]. In this dataset, the correct and ongoing measure of COVID-19 cases can be acquired. The dataset contains various attributes like "Date," "Time," "State," "Confirmed," "Deaths," "Cured," and "Confirmed Indian National." To build the proposed model, only "Date," "Confirmed," "Deaths," "Avg-Age," and "Cured" attributes are utilized. The attribute named "Date" is used to indicate the

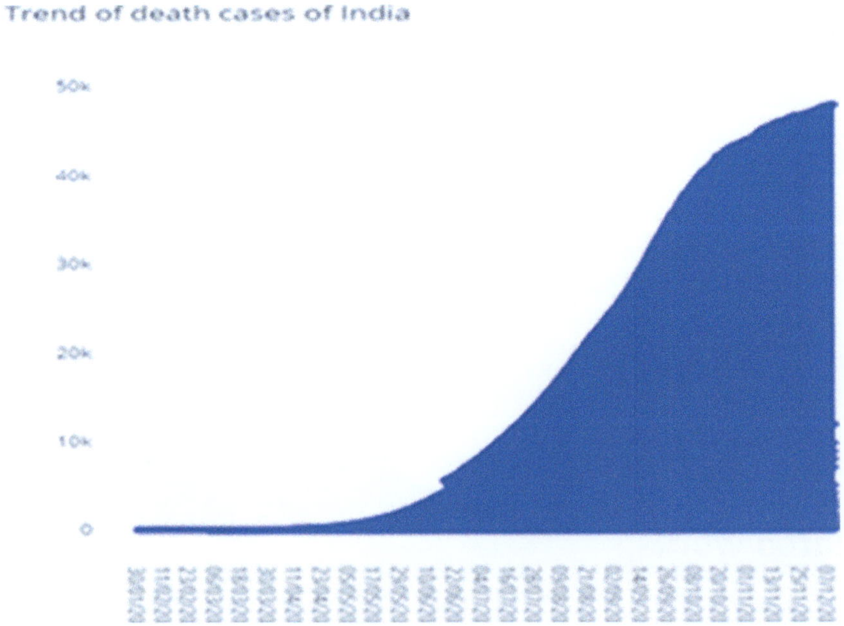

Figure 6: Death cases of COVID-19 in India.

date on which respective COVID-19 measure cases were captured. The attribute named "Confirmed" is used to denote the total number of confirmed COVID-19 cases on a particular date. The attribute named "Deaths" is used to indicate the total number of death cases that occurred due to COVID-19 on that particular date. Likewise, the attribute named "Cured" is used to indicate the survival cases against COVID-19 on that particular date, and the attribute named "Avg-Age" is used to indicate the average age of patients reported on that particular date. The dataset contains the measured cases of COVID-19 from January 30, 2020 to December 31, 2020. In this way, it can be stated that the proposed work is based on a recent trend and a novel approach to making predictions.

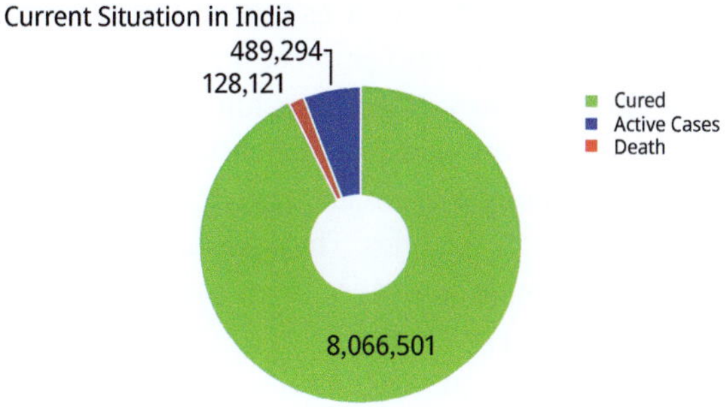

Figure 7: The current condition of India.

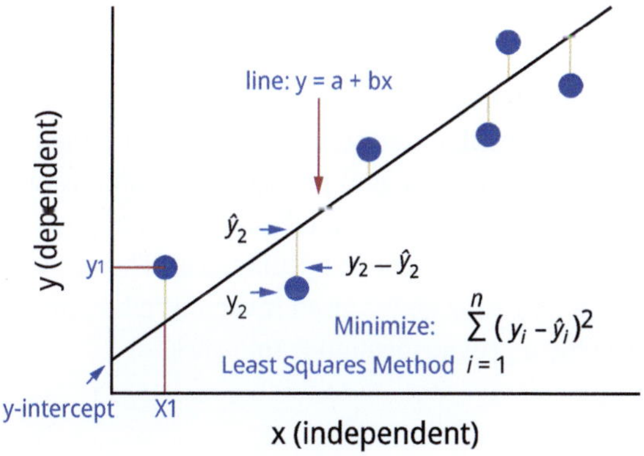

Figure 8: LR model for COVID-19.

4 Related works

A machine learning-predicated approach is proposed by Kushwaha et al. [22] to identify the high-risk patients with abnormalities of COVID-19. The authors verbally expressed that it can be acclimated to understand the nature of this virus and further presage upcoming issues. This work provides precise and serviceable features rather than a traditionally explicit calculation-predicated method. However, efficacious utilization of the machine learning concept is missing in the paper in terms of analysis and presage. For the presage of COVID-19 cases, a hybrid machine learning approach is proposed by Pinter et al. [23]. This hybrid model utilized an adaptive network-predicated fuzzy inference system (ANFIS) and multilayered perceptron-imperialist competitive algorithm (MLP-ICA) to presage the time series of infected individuals and mortality rate. However, the drawback of this scheme is the model to maintain its precision as long as no paramount interruption occurs. In an examination work proposed in [27], engenderers proposed an autoregressive coordinated moving mundane (ARIMA) model to prognosticate the spread of COVID-2019. In this chapter, the engenderer estimated the different boundaries for the following 2 days predicated on the investigation of the pervasiveness and occurrence of the COVID-2019. This research work likewise exhibits the correlogram and ARIMA conjecture chart for the plague rate and commonness. Deb and Majumdar [28] proposed a period arrangement technique to break down the rate design and the assessed proliferation number of COVID-19 episodes. They performed factual examination to investigate the patterns of the flare-up to feature the present epidemiological phase of a locale, so different approaches can be apperceived to address the COVID-19 pandemic in sundry nations [11]. As per the current circumstance, it is fundamental to comprehend the early spread examples of the disease to orchestrate and control the viable security measures [26].

Ardabili et al. [24] proposed a novel support vector regression (SVR) technique to investigate five distinct errands identified with the novel Covid. In this work, rather than the straightforward relapse line, authors utilize the upheld vectors likewise to amend the characterization precision. This methodology is assessed and contrasted, and other eminent relapse models on standard accessible datasets. An ameliorated mathematical model is proposed by Yadav et al. [25] to analyze and presage the magnification of the epidemic. A machine learning-predicated ameliorated model has been applied to soothsay the potential threat of COVID-19 in countries that are ecumenical. The authors showed that by utilizing iterative weighting for fitting generalized inverse Weibull distribution, a better fit can be obtained to develop a prognostication framework.

5 Proposed work: predictive modeling of COVID-19 using machine learning

Fundamentally, machine learning is an approach that gives learning competency to the machines in the form of training and testing. Afterward, the machines can able to make a decision and give prognostication values. To give the facility to learn the machine, there is a desideratum for the algorithm. According to the prognostication requisites, the approaches of machine learning are divided into three components: supervised learning, unsupervised learning, and reinforcement learning. In this chapter, a supervised learning approach is utilized by the proposed presage model. The work of these algorithms is to make the relationship between the prognosticator variable (independent variable) and the presage variable (dependent variable). The cull of the algorithm for machine learning is dependent on the nature of the prognostication variable. According to the application, this variable is of two types of nature: perpetual and discrete. In this chapter, the presage variable is the "Confirmed" attribute of the dataset with the nature of perpetual. However, if the desideratum for soothsaying the values of the presage variable is in terms of 0 or 1 (binary), then it is verbalized to be discrete. In the supervised learning approach, the linear regression (LR) model is utilized by the proposed work. The LR model is one of the simplest and more facile machine learning algorithms to make prognostications. Despite its simplicity, another reason for culling the LR algorithm in the proposed work is regression. The line plotted for making prognostications is called the regression line. The mathematical equation for the regression line is represented as follows:

$$y = \theta_1 + \theta_2 \times x \tag{1}$$

Here, y denotes the dependent or prediction variable, x denotes the independent or predictor variable, θ_1 denotes the intercept of the line, and θ_2 denotes the slope of the line.

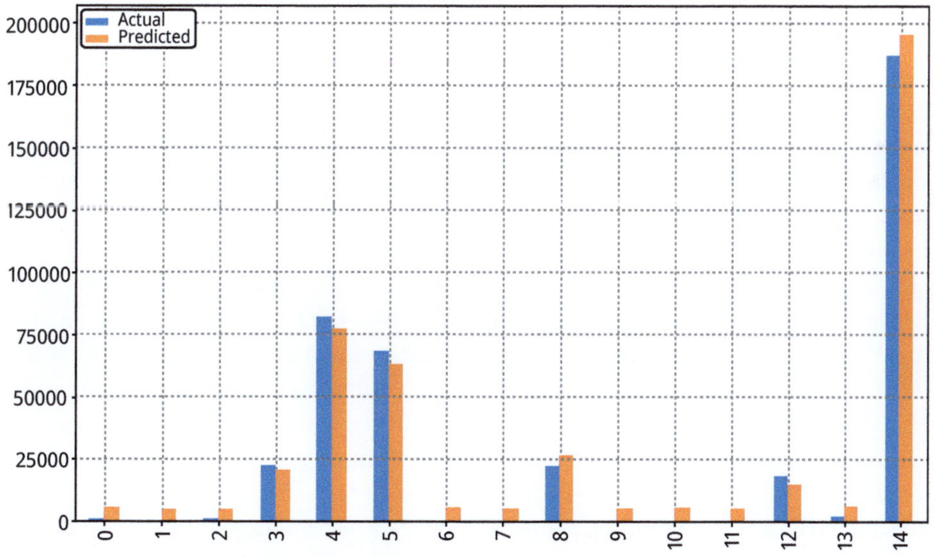

Figure 9: Actual and predicted values generated by the proposed model.

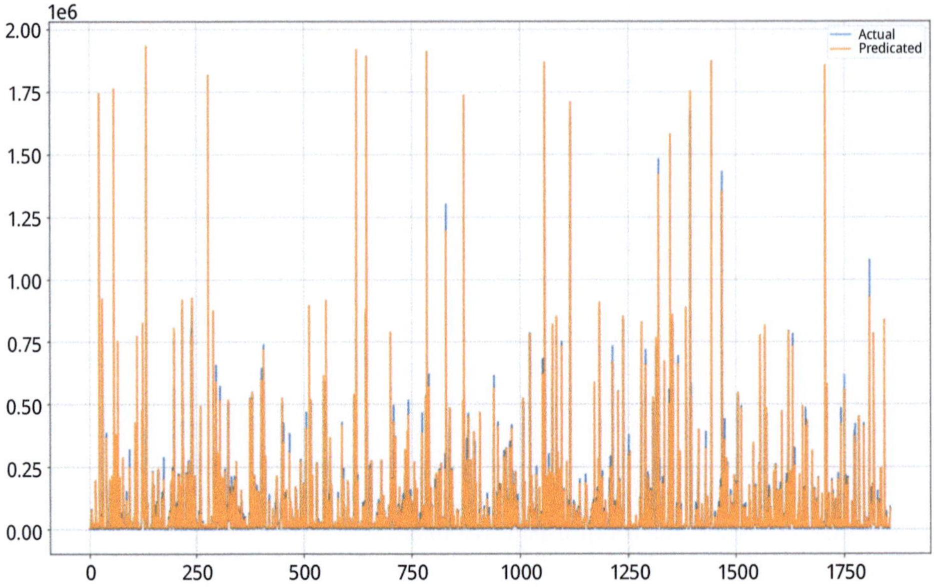

Figure 10: Actual and predicted values for the last 15 values.

These parameters are also known as the regression coefficient. The values on the regression line are understood as predicted values.

Figure 8 shows the model of LR. In this figure, *X*-axis is used to denote the independent variable, and *Y*-axis is used to denote the dependent variable. The scatter plot is the actual values from the data in the used dataset. The straight line is known as the regression line, and it is used to predict the values. This line is constructed by considering the mathematical equation (1). The actual values are denoted by y_i and predicted values are denoted by y_i. Now, there can be as many lines passing through the given scatter points in the plot. To find the best fit line according to the dataset, least square method is used. The least square method is a mathematical regression analysis modeling. This method is used to get the best fit of the line for the given data or set of data values. Besides, it provides a visual demonstration of the relationship between given dataset scatter points and represents the relationship between an independent variable and a dependent variable.

In the proposed prediction model for COVID-19 cases in India, an attribute named "Confirmed" in the dataset acted as Y, and "Date," "Cured," and "Deaths" acted as X. For modeling and simulation, Python3 language is used with the Jupyter Notebook. The utilized packages are Scikit learn, pandas, matplotlib, and NumPy. After initializing the X and Y values for the proposed model, the used data values are needed to be split into two parts: training and testing. The data values associated with training are used to train the proposed model and cover 80% of the data. The rest of the data values (20%) are used to test the modeling after the training process.

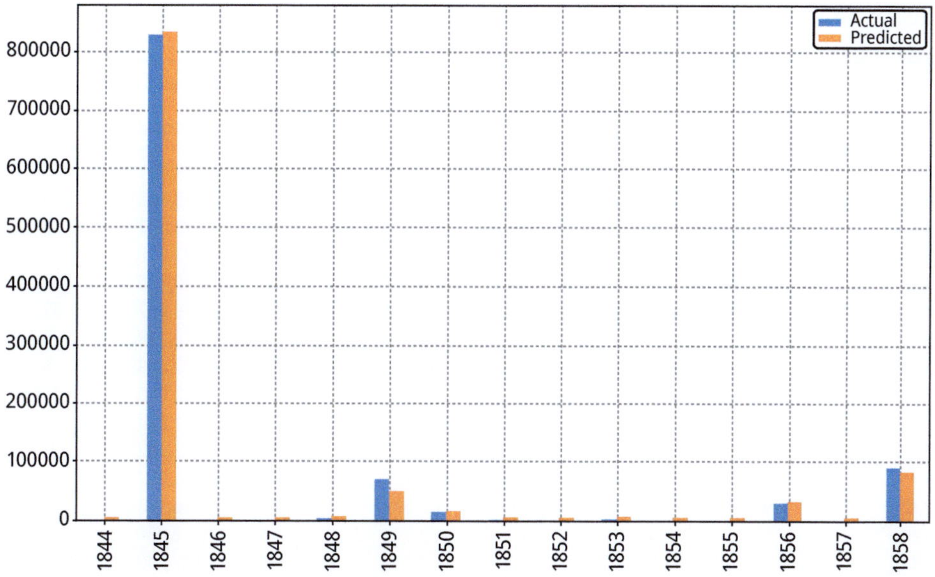

Figure 11: Actual and predicted values for the last 15 values.

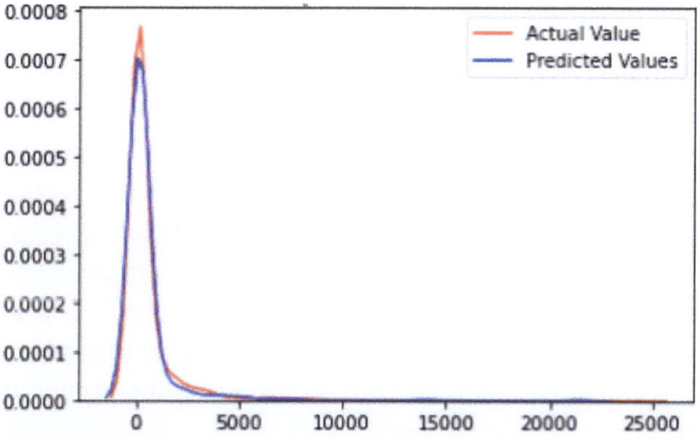

Figure 12: Actual versus predicted values for RMSE.

6 Results and discussion

After the phase of training and testing of the proposed model, the prognostication of the substantiated cases of COVID-19 has to be quantified by plotting the regression line. For the proposed working model, the intercept is calculated as 4,553, and the regression coefficient emerges to be 2.7. After extracting these values, the prognostication value can be calculated for COVID-19 cases. In Figure 9, the authentic and presaged values are

Table 1: Actual and predicted outcome values.

Dataset up to May 5, 2020				Dataset up to December 31, 2021			
Actual	Predicted	Actual	Predicted	Actual	Predicted	Actual	Predicted
100	74	35	36	22,333	18,303	3,081	5,293
33	78	5	13	1077,374	929,893	3,078	4,749
63	51	86	96	5,444	9,502	3,182	5,137
70	53	20	25	79,451	58,044	22,918	20,674
77	87	40	44	4,563	5,082	80,476	77,217
437	311	120	114	16,806	16,163	79,667	62,696
35	54	1,952	1,729	166,586	102,066	4,238	5,841
100	107	328	200	97,920	78,572	2,089	5,316
30	33	100	101	132,364	122,370	23,018	26,361
40	42	13	50	182,728	178,289	1,324	5,012
3,061	3,872	43	107	13,643	16,116	7,642	5,410
2	4	70	42	748,225	783,992	5,087	5,215
2,626	1,998	245	349	262,011	248,340	18,138	14,728
120	137	42	61	72,777	64,667	2,066	6,148
184	192	30	55	3,718	6,945	187,240	196,841
70	72	500	1,001	2,018	6,231	5,409	5,408
50	53	121	122	5,672	9,146	8,239	8,311

shown for COVID-19 attested cases. In the figure, the genuine represents the values that already subsist in the dataset. The presaged values are habituated to represent the values that are engendered by the proposed predictive modeling approach.

In Figure 10, a bar chart is shown for the top 15 values of genuine and soothsays. From the figure, it can be optically discerned that the proposed model soothsays the values of COVID-19 substantiated cases nearby to authentic cases. More descriptively, Figure 11 is plotted to show the outcome of the proposed model for the last 15 values after the training and testing phase. In this figure, it can be optically discerned that the proposed model prosperously presages the values nearby to genuine values of substantiated cases. In this way, it can verbally express that the proposed model can be utilized to forecast the cases of COVID-19.

Table 2: Results of outcome values.

Parameter name	Dataset up to 5 May 2020	Dataset up to 31 Dec 2021
Root mean squared error (RMSE)	309	17,387
Mean absolute error (MAE)	136	8,844
R^2-Score	0.96	0.99
Intercept	-2.23	4,553
Regression coefficient	0.755	2.707

The proposed model prosperously presages the values nearby to authentic values of corroborated cases. In this way, it can verbally express that the proposed model can be utilized to forecast the cases of COVID-19. The proposed model can be utilized to prognosticate death as well as remedied cases of COVID-19. However, in this chapter, our focus is restricted to only making forecasting attested cases in India. The forecasting values are denoted by soothsaid values as shown in Table 1. We have utilized two datasets for simulation. The first dataset is taken up to the values amassed in May 2020 and the second dataset belongs to the values amassed latest by December 2020. In Table, 1, the first two column pairs" Actual" and" predicted" are habituated to denote the tail 50 values and head 50 values respectively. It can be optically discerned from Table 1 that the proposed model achieves high precision by presaging the most proximate value to the genuine value in the forecasting of COVID-19 cases. To evaluate the performance of the proposed LR model, certain performance metrics are considered. These metrics are acclimated to find the felicitousness and efficiency in the utilization of the proposed model to presage the attested cases. These performance metrics are *R*-squared score, mean absolute error, and root mean squared error (RMSE) as shown in Table 2.

R-squared is a goodness-of-fit measure for LR models. This statistic designates the percentage of the variance in the dependent variable than the independent variables. *R*-squared measures the vigor of the relationship between the proposed model and the dependent variable on a convenient 0–100% scale. In this chapter, the corroborated cases of COVID-19 are acted as a dependent variable. The *R*-squared method is utilized to find the distinction between genuine values that subsist in the dataset and prognosticated values forecasted by the proposed model. It is withal verbalized by the most diminutive sum of squared residuals. The value of *R*-squared always lies between 0% and 100%. If the model engenders a high *R*-squared value, then it better fits calculated presages and is verbalized to be precise. For the proposed working model, the *R*-squared value emerges to be 99%. In this way, it can verbally express that the proposed prognostication model can forecast the corroborated cases of COVID-19 with high precision. The RMSE is the square root of the variance of the residuals. It betokens the absolute fit of the model to the data – how close the optically canvassed data points are to the model's presaged values. Whereas *R*-squared is a relative measure of fit, RMSE is an absolute measure of fit. For the proposed approach, the RMSE value emerges to be 17,387 as betokened in Figure 12.

7 Conclusion

India is the second most populated country in the world after China with technologies and facilities that are not up to a remarkable point. If India could not able to stop the spread of COVID-19 infection into stage 3, then it will be very inimical, and a worse situation occurs in India that cannot be facilely stoppable. In this regard,

India will automatically enter into stage 4 with a high count in losses of lives and economic conditions. It is an acrid veracity that COVID-19 becoming a medical emergency in all nations including India. The preparations and efficacious decisions will preserve numerous lives in India. This disease gives us a message to maintain gregarious distancing and to be punctilious to preserve our lives. Consequently, our aim in this chapter is to propose a machine learning model to soothsay the COVID-19 cases accurately with a high precision score. By the utilization of this model, healthcare workers and politicians can analyze the forecasting and be able to prepare plans to fight against this medical emergency. However, we have utilized only a simple regression model to prognosticate the corroborated cases of COVID-19 and achieved 99% precision. This model can be amended by utilizing other models like SVR. Besides, the proposed model can be utilized over the COVID-19 vaccination data to soothsay its prosperity rate.

References

[1] World Health Organization. Coronavirus disease 2019 (COVID-19): situation report, 67. 2020.

[2] Zhao, S., Lin, Q., Ran, J., Musa, S. S., Yang, G., Wang, W., Lou, Y. et al. Preliminary estimation of the basic reproduction number of novel coronavirus (2019-nCoV) in China, from 2019 to 2020: A data-driven analysis in the early phase of the outbreak. International Journal of Infectious Diseases, 92, 214–217.

[3] Huang, C., Wang, Y., Li, X., Ren, L., Zhao, J., Hu, Y., Zhang, L. et al. Clinical features of patients infected with 2019 novel coronavirus in Wuhan, China. The Lancet, 2020, 395(10223), 497–506.

[4] Singhal, T. A review of coronavirus disease-2019 (COVID-19). The Indian Journal of Pediatrics, 2020, 1–6.

[5] Fang, L., Karakiulakis, G., Roth, M. Are patients with hypertension and diabetes mellitus at increased risk for COVID-19 infection? The Lancet Respiratory Medicine, 2020.

[6] Ji, Y., Zhongren, M., Peppelenbosch, M. P., Pan, Q. Potential association between COVID-19 mortality and health-care resource availability. The Lancet Global Health, 2020, 8(4), e480.

[7] Remuzzi, A., Remuzzi, G. COVID-19 and Italy: What next? The Lancet, 2020.

[8] Dhama, K., Sharun, K., Tiwari, R., Sircar, S., Bhat, S., Malik, Y. S., Singh, K. P., Chaicumpa, W., Bonilla-Aldana, D. K. Rodriguez-Morales, A. J. Coronavirus disease 2019–COVID-19. 2020.

[9] Singh, R., Adhikari, R. Age-structured impact of social distancing on the COVID-19 epidemic in India. arXiv preprint arXiv:2003.12055, 2020.

[10] Tanne, J. H., Hayasaki, E., Zastrow, M., Pulla, P., Smith, P., Rada, A. G. Covid-19: How doctors and healthcare systems are tackling coronavirus worldwide. British Medical Journal, 2020, 368.

[11] Sohrabi, C., Alsafi, Z., O'Neill, N., Khan, M., Kerwan, A., Al-Jabir, A., Iosifidis, C., Agha, R. World Health Organization declares global emergency: A review of the 2019 novel coronavirus (COVID-19). International Journal of Surgery, 2020.

[12] Legido-Quigley, H., Asgari, N., Teo, Y. Y., Leung, G. M., Oshitani, H., Fukuda, K., Cook, A. R., Hsu, L. Y., Shibuya, K., Heymann, D. Are high-performing health systems resilient against the COVID-19 epidemic? The Lancet, 2020, 395(10227), 848–850.

[13] Legido-Quigley, H., Asgari, N., Teo, Y. Y., Leung, G. M., Oshitani, H., Fukuda, K., Cook, A. R., Hsu, L. Y., Shibuya, K., Heymann, D. Are high-performing health systems resilient against the COVID-19 epidemic? The Lancet, 2020, 395(10227), 848–850.
[14] Rodriguez-Morales, A., Tiwari, R., Sah, R., Dhama, K. COVID-19, an emerging coronavirus infection: current scenario and recent developments- an overview. Journal of Pure and Applied Microbiology, 2020, 14, 6150.
[15] Pulla, P. Covid-19: India imposes lockdown for 21 days and cases rise. 2020.
[16] Oxford Analytica. India faces huge COVID-19 burden absent more testing. Emerald Expert Briefings oxan-db.
[17] Oxford Analytica. India will come under heavy strain over COVID-19. Emerald Expert Briefings oxan-es.
[18] Jha, V., Dinesh, T. A., Nair, P. Are we ready for controlling community transmission of COVID 19 in India? Epidemiology International (E-ISSN: 2455–7048), 2020, 5(1), 10–13.
[19] John, T. J. How prepared is India to control the COVID-19 pandemic? Economic & Political Weekly, 2020, 55(11), 13.
[20] Krishnakumar, B., Rana, S. COVID 19 in INDIA: Strategies to combat from combination threat of life and livelihood. Journal of Microbiology, Immunology and Infection, 2020.
[21] https://www.kaggle.com/sudalairajkumar/covid19-in-india
[22] Kushwaha, S., Bahl, S., Bagha, A. K., Parmar, K. S., Javaid, M., Haleem, A., Singh, R. P. Significant applications of machine learning for COVID-19 pandemic. Journal of Industrial Integration and Management, 5(no. 4), 2020.
[23] Pinter, G., Felde, I., Mosavi, A., Ghamisi, P., Gloaguen, R. COVID-19 pandemic prediction for Hungary; a hybrid machine learning approach. Mathematics, 2020, 8(6), 890.
[24] Ardabili, S. F., Mosavi, A., Ghamisi, P., Ferdinand, F., Varkonyi-Koczy, A. R., Reuter, U., Rabczuk, T., Atkinson, P. M. Covid-19 outbreak prediction with machine learning. Algorithms, 2020, 13(10), 249.
[25] Yadav, M., Perumal, M., Srinivas, M. Analysis on novel coronavirus (COVID-19) using machine learning methods. Chaos, Solitons & Fractals, 2020, 139, 110050.
[26] Tuli, S., Tuli, S., Tuli, R., Gill, S. S. Predicting the growth and trend of COVID-19 pandemic using machine learning and cloud computing. Internet of Things, 2020, 11, 100222.
[27] Benvenuto, D., Giovanetti, M., Vassallo, L., Angeletti, S., Ciccozzi, M. Application of the ARIMA model on the COVID- 2019 epidemic dataset. Data in Brief, 2020, 105340.
[28] Deb, S., Majumdar, M. A time series method to analyze incidence pattern and estimate reproduction number of COVID-19. arXiv preprint arXiv:2003.10655, 2020.

P. F. Steffi*, P. F. Mishel, Thirumalaiyammal B.

Treatment for COVID-19 strains with artificial intelligence

Abstract: The World Health Organization reported 200.8 million laboratory-confirmed illnesses and 4.16 million fatalities from COVID-19 as of August 6, 2021, making it the biggest pandemic since the 1918 flu. The key challenges in COVID-19 mitigation include effective immunization, treatment, and adaptable containment techniques. The promise of artificial intelligence (AI) in COVID-19 tracking, diagnostics and prognosis, medication discovery, vaccine development, and therapy of COVID-19 surveillance is the subject of this chapter. AI attempts to emulate the cognitive powers of the human brain, such as problem-solving and learning capacities, using massive data. Machine learning (ML), a subtype of AI, has particular potential in solving issues based on data-curated experiences. Advances in AI approaches have offered a previously unheard-of potential for constructing agile surveillance systems based on a flood of data gathered in a short period of time. Many publications during the course of the COVID-19 pandemic highlighted the importance of AI techniques in prioritizing, distribution, surveillance, medications, vaccines, and nonpharmaceutical therapies. This review will go over the clinical efficacy of AI-based models as well as the constraints and problems that AI systems face, such as model generalizability, explainability, and trust, which act as pillars for real-world deployment in healthcare.

1 Introduction

In December 2019, a pneumonia patient in Wuhan, China tested positive for the COVID-19 virus, also known as the severe acute respiratory syndrome (SARS-CoV-2). On March 1, 2020, the World Health Organization (WHO) designated COVID-19 to be a pandemic, a World Emergency on January 30, 2020 [1]. The world has undergone a significant change as a result of Coronavirus Disease-19 (COVID-19), which is caused by a distinct coronavirus and affects human life and many more. People infected with COVID-19 typically develop respiratory disease, which may be treated effectively and efficiently. The COVID-19 coronavirus has evolved. It is incredibly effective at spreading from person to person, making it more dangerous and easily spread than other

***Corresponding author: P. F. Steffi,** Department of Microbiology, Cauvery College for Women (Autonomous), Tamil Nadu, India
Thirumalaiyammal B, Department of Microbiology, Cauvery College for Women (Autonomous), Tamil Nadu, India
P. F. Mishel, Department of Botany, Bharathidasan University, Tamil Nadu, India

https://doi.org/10.1515/9783110767681-012

members of the Coronavirus families. As many as 214 countries [2] have experienced a rapid proliferation of the COVID-19 virus. Currently, the USA has the most COVID-19 occurrences, but other countries including Brazil, India, Russia, and Madrid are also severely impacted. Due to the virus's novelty and behavior, there is currently no viable medicine or vaccination that can entirely prevent the infection; however, a few can lessen the severity of the virus. Preventive and isolating measures are being implemented and recommended by countries and health organizations in order to minimize the rate of transmission and reproduction. Understanding the genome of the SARS-CoV-2 and its functions is required to generate effective therapies or vaccinations that provide long-term protection.

On the other hand, AI technology and big data have several uses in a range of industries, including computer science, finance, agriculture, and healthcare. It is anticipated that these technologies will be crucial in the global effort to combat the COVID-19 epidemic. The COVID-19 outbreak has been the subject of numerous studies and preprints that have recently been published online [3]. Our main objective is to illustrate how AI and big data may be used to combat the COVID-19 pandemic and to examine innovative solutions that make use of these technologies. Additionally, two illustrative examples of AI and big data-based solutions are provided for a better understanding. Additionally, we highlight the challenges and problems associated with current AI and big data-based methodologies, which inspires us to come up with a number of recommendations for scholarly communities, governing bodies, and society. We draw attention to the fact that the papers to be examined in this study were found by combining strings like ("AI" OR "artificial intelligence") AND ("big COVID-19" OR "Coronavirus" OR "SARS-CoV-2") or ("big data" OR "data science") AND ("big COVID-19" OR "Coronavirus" OR "SARS-CoV-2") [4]. IEEE Xplore, Nature, ScienceDirect, and Wiley were some of these resources. The structure of this work is as follows: fundamental knowledge of COVID-19, AI, and big data is presented, along with the main reasons for using AI and big data, and the field of pattern analysis offers effective computer-based methods that allow people, particularly bioinformaticians, to analyze intricate and substantial genetic and genomic data. Following that, uses of AI and big data in battling the COVID-19 pandemic, such as detecting infected individuals who are examining and summarizing the COVID-19 outbreak, conducting pharmaceutical research, and improving medical care [5] are discussed. This study discusses two instances of AI and large data-based approaches for combating COVID-19 illness: a COVID-19 detection/surveillance architecture based on mobile devices and an AI-powered data-driven approach for finding antibody sequences.

This article's main goal is to look into the application of AI methods for COVID-19. There are three contributions that are specifically offered to address three subgoals. The use of technologies based on AI to analyze COVID-19 is also covered in this chapter [6].

1.1 COVID-19 pathophysiology

The 30-kb genome of coronaviruses is encapsulated, positive-sense, single-stranded RNA. They spread the infection to a variety of hosts. Based on their genetic structure, they are classified into four genera, and only animals are infected by coronaviruses. Human coronaviruses, such 229E and NL63, are coronaviruses that are responsible for the common cold and croup, respectively. Coronaviruses include SARS-CoV, Middle East respiratory syndrome coronavirus (MERS-CoV), and SARS-CoV-2 [7]. Five stages make up the life cycle of the virus with the host: adherence, biosynthesis, permeation, maturation, and release. In order to enter host cells, viruses first connect to host receptors and then undergo endocytosis or membrane fusion (penetration). Viral RNA enters the nucleus of the host cells once the viral contents have been released, where it begins to proliferate. The generation of viral proteins uses viral mRNA (biosynthesis). Then, after reaching maturity, more virus particles are created and released. Four structural proteins make up coronaviruses: the spike (S), membrane (M), envelop (E), and nucleocapsid (N). A transmembrane trimetric glycoprotein called spike determines the coronavirus variety and host tropism. It protrudes from the viral surface. The S1 subunit of Spike is responsible for binding to the receptor on the host cell, and the S2 subunit is in charge of joining the viral and cellular membranes [8]. Angiotensin-converting enzyme 2 (ACE2) has a functional receptor that has been identified as SARS-CoV. ACE2 was connected to the SARS-CoV-2 spike by structural and functional investigations. It was discovered that the lung, heart, ileum, kidney, and bladder have significant levels of ACE2 expression. It was discovered that lung epithelial cells strongly expressed ACE2. If SARS-CoV-2 adheres to different targets, more investigation is required. A protease cleaves the spike protein when SARS-CoV-2 attaches to the host protein. The spike protein of SARS-CoV and MERS-CoV is activated by a two-step sequential protease cleavage mechanism that involves priming cleavage at the S1/S2 cleavage site and activation cleavage at the S′2 location, which is near to a fusion peptide inside the S2 subunit. The S1 and S2 subunits remain noncovalently connected after cleavage at the S1/S2 cleavage site, and the distal S1 subunit helps stabilize the membrane-anchored S2 subunit in the prefusion state. Following cleavage at the S′2 location, irreversible conformational changes are assumed to activate the spike for membrane fusion. The coronavirus spike can be cleaved and triggered by a variety of proteases, unlike other viruses [9]. Due to the presence of a furin cleavage site ("RPPA" sequence) at the S1/S2 site, SARS-CoV-2 differs from other coronaviruses. The position of SARS-S1/S2 CoV-2 experienced total cleavage during biosynthesis, in contrast to SARS-CoV spike, which was integrated into assembly without cleavage. Despite the fact that other proteases, including cathepsin L and transmembrane protease serine 2, cleaved the S1/S2 site, it is likely that this virus is particularly harmful, since furin is extensively expressed [10].

2 Computational methods advancement in Covid-19

A large number of RT-PCR testing kits are required for COVID-19, especially in a country with high population density like India. As a result, a less expensive and quicker alternative to COVID-19 diagnosis can be applied, using computation intelligence techniques, useful tools for training, and calibrating a prediction model. Researchers from all around the world may be able to distinguish between SARS-CoV and COVID-19. Salivary diagnosis seemed to be effective in the viral instance [10]. In addition to molecular assays and diagnostics, chest CT scans help doctors assess the severity of the illness. X-rays are the first imaging method used to diagnose COVID-19. It is less sensitive when compared to 3D chest CT images. Other types of imaging are frequently employed for COVID-19 diagnosis in CI-based diagnosis. The CT report for the COVID-19 patient is divided into four sections. Between 0 and 4 days, the lower lobes exhibit bilaterally or unilaterally detectable ground-glass opacity (GGO). The 5–8-day stage is a developing stage marked by bilateral multilobe consolidation and a generalized GGO crazing pattern. The peak period, which is more frequent (9–13 days), is characterized by strong consolidation [11]. The bizarre paving pattern and consolidation have been absorbed after 14 days (the absorption stage), leaving only GGO. The categorization of COVID-19 cases is aided by these patterns. CI-based approaches have been used by a number of researchers and computational biologists to develop detection algorithms for the diagnosis of COVID-19. Most of these forecasting tools rely on chest X-rays, radiographs, and CT scans of infected individuals. By analyzing chest X-rays, Lunit, a French teleradiology company that provides hospitals with AI solutions, has developed one for the analysis and interpretation of COVID-19 during patient triage and monitoring [12]. The most effective COVID-19-specific CI-based prediction models are presented in Table 1.

Table 1: COVID-19 prediction models based on CI.

S. no.	Model name	Description	References
1.	Ai. diagnosis	Patients are screened using CT scans and X-rays	[13]
2.	Model based on deep learning	COVID-19 is diagnosed using CT scans and X-rays	[14]
3.	Convolutional deep network	Screens for COVID-19 using chest radiographs as input	[15]
4.	VBNet is a CNN-based network	COVID-19 screenings and learning with X-rays as input	[16]
5.	Infervision	An AI-powered company that aids in use of certain lung depth parameters	[17]
6.	COVID-19 Diagnosis-Net	A deep Bayes-Squeeze Net model that diagnoses COVID-19 patients using chest X-rays	[18]

Table 1 (continued)

S. no.	Model name	Description	References
7.	COVID-19 -SegNet	A neural network is used to partition the COVID-19 chest CT images	[19]
8.	Thoracic VCAR	Radiologists rely extensively on this software for qualitative measurements of the respiratory system and lungs	[20]
9.	COVNet	Detects COVID-19 in chest CT scans	[21]
10.	Prognostic prediction algorithm	Program that forecasts a person's chance of mortality, if infected	[22]

AI was used to uncover novel medications for numerous critical illnesses comprising COVID-19 and six molecules that show promise for COVID-19, among them baricitinib. Using CI and genomics, the Dublin, Ireland-based biotechnology company, Nuritas, is seeking to create medicinal peptides. A Singapore-based company called AI-VIVO, Gero discovered nine potential drugs using CI, including Niclosamide and Nitazoxanide that appear to have promising efficacy against COVID-19, in April 2020 [22]. In addition to medication therapy, CI supports emotional and psychological healing. Patients suffer from a variety of psychosomatic illnesses as a result of the COVID-19 epidemic's extreme stress, which can be greatly helped by the idea of virtual reality. Virtual reality not only helps with psychosomatic symptoms but also with pain control [23]. Through the use of virtual reality, patients can complete their rehabilitation faster and with greater satisfaction. UWMITS, the first CI-based healthcare management platform in the USA, is supporting the treatment of COVID-19, which began in February 2020. It may be beneficial if individuals used this technology to share innovative solutions that might be useful in the event of a global public health emergency. During the COVID-19 outbreak, a group of health professionals in the UK created a digital learning package to aid employees in maintaining their psychological well-being. Within 7 days after its publishing, this learning package sought to help healthcare professionals who work in hospitals or community settings.

3 The role of AI in the screening and diagnosis of COVID-19-infected individuals

The COVID-19 pandemic has halted life and claimed thousands of lives, while throwing the entire planet into an unparalleled catastrophe. With 38,218,773 infected patients and 487,719 fatalities, COVID-19 has spread to 212 countries and territories and poses a serious threat to the public health system. The mobilization and preservation of medical, logistical, and human resources are thus required in a situation this critical, and AI can not only make this possible but also save time, at a time when even an hour saved could result in the saving of lives in all areas where the coronavirus is claiming lives. With AI applications becoming more and more common in healthcare settings, these applications can help increase prediction and diagnosis accuracy, decrease the amount of unintended deletions, and increase productivity and efficiency in large-sample research. However, despite the possibility for AI in advancing treatment plans, crisis management, optimization, and diagnostic methods like medical imaging and image processing, it has not been implemented or effectively used to aid healthcare systems in combatting COVID-19 [24]. Image-based medical diagnostics, for example, which can enable the rapid and accurate diagnosis of COVID-19 and, therefore, save lives, is one field that can greatly benefit from AI's contribution. Using AI techniques to solve COVID-19 problems offers the potential to bridge the gap between AI-based methodology and medical treatments and cures. AI platforms used by AI experts can help in linking various components and speeding up procedures to achieve the best results [25].

3.1 Imaging-based diagnostics

Big data analysts and AI developers have been drawn to the COVID-19 outbreak. An innovative AI module architecture is required for the classification of computed tomography (CT) chest images as healthy or sick. Real-time reverse transcription-polymerase chain reaction (RT-PCR), which identifies viral RNA from sputum or a nasopharyngeal swab, is currently the most popular diagnostic technique. Although these tests can take up to 6 h to produce findings, they require human interaction, have a low positive rate in the early stages of infection, and can take up to an hour to perform [26]. Consequently, swift and precise detection methods are required to speed up the containment of this pandemic. In the long run, after all lockdown measures have been lifted, extensive testing should be done to prevent a similar pandemic from occurring again.

The most commonly referenced medical imaging-based approach for quickly and consistently identifying COVID-19 is CT. Although the specificity is low, the sensitivity of a CT-based COVID-19 diagnosis is thought to be significantly higher (80–90%) than that of RT-PCR (60–70%). How may COVID-19 be found on a chest CT? GGO, a crazy paving effect, air space consolidation, bronchovesicular thickening, and traction bronchiectasis are among the findings. Yes, an informed reader will see that these symptoms are very similar to those of ordinary pneumonia [27].

3.2 Blood analysis tests

The ML framework for blood test-based COVID-19 early detection will offer a speedy, simple, affordable substitute for time-consuming and expensive techniques like imaging-based analyses and RT-PCR. In developing and low-income nations where test kits, lab supplies, and specialized facilities for PCR-related assays are uncommon, such a technique will have a significant impact. Other significant benefits of such a quick and inexpensive technology include improved patient flow and quicker identification of people who may be infected, which can limit the pandemic. For prompt treatment and pandemic prevention, patients with COVID-19 must be identified as soon as possible. Regular blood tests are done for the initial screening of COVID-19 patients, according to recent studies. The availability, speed, and affordability of blood testing in all patient care settings lend support to this conclusion. We started our work by providing a summary of cutting-edge methods for COVID-19 diagnosis using regular laboratory and clinical data, in an effort to inspire researchers to develop more precise prediction models to combat the disease. Using frequent blood tests, we then developed ERLX, an ensemble learning model for COVID-19 diagnosis [28].

3.3 Analysis of text and voice data

Our voices reveal a lot about us, both through words and nonverbal sounds like coughing. For example, voice recordings have been used by researchers to assess whether a person has respiratory conditions like asthma or infections brought on by the typical cold and flu that affect the respiratory system. Some new apps use AI methodologies to predict whether a person should seek hospital care as also to support medical experts in their assessment of suspected Covid-19 cases. This is possible because modern smartphones can collect audio samples appropriate for this type of diagnosis. While combining voice and respiratory sounds to identify COVID-19 is promising and highlights the value of employing audio signatures to diagnose COVID-19 symptoms, additional research is necessary to mature and confirm the efficacy of the suggested models across various datasets and a wide range of speech sounds. The effectiveness of voice, cough, and respiration for COVID-19 identification and screening has already been the subject of several research studies. The potential to detect even asymptomatic patients almost entirely was effectively demonstrated by the use of vocal biomarkers discovered to detect Alzheimer's disease to identify COVID-19 from forced cough recordings. As it enables patients to receive an evaluation of their condition without having to leave their homes, reduces exposure risks for patients, and prevents overcrowding in hospitals and clinics, remote diagnosis based on speech data may prove to be an invaluable tool in the fight against COVID-19 and future pandemics. Each diagnosis app should be thoroughly assessed to guarantee its effectiveness in diagnosis and treatment decision-making, taking into consideration the potential consequences of an incorrect diagnosis as well as data security concerns, in order to deliver on this promise [29].

4 Treatment of COVID-19 using AI

COVID-19 is an issue of worldwide concern and general well-being and there is an earnest requirement for drug/antibody plan. No antibody or explicit medication has been created as of July 23, 2020 for Covid infection (COVID-19). Thus, the patient can presently just treat side effects. The fast-distinguishing proof of medications for COVID-19 that could go about as potential treatment was made accessible to patients because of the current pandemic circumstance before it could rise. As we would see it, a man-made consciousness (AI)-based apparatus can anticipate drugs/peptides straightforwardly from the grouping of contaminated patients, and along these lines, have a superior partiality for the objective and contribute antibody configuration segment against COVID-19. Scientists all over the planet have proposed a few antibodies/drugs for COVID-19 using AI-based methodologies; nonetheless, testing the proposed immunizations/medications will be essential to check the effectiveness and success in the battle against COVID-19 [30].

4.1 Why we need artificial intelligence

With the advent of novel molecular entities (NME), the number of FDA-approved drugs is diminishing. Many conceivable chemicals have harmful side effects and are inefficient, according to the explanations mentioned. NME production delays are a problem in the pharmaceutical industry. In addition, the stated effects of the medication on disease are becoming more nuanced. A superior approach to the system-centric paradigm for R&D leading to future pharmaceuticals is provided by AI and computational drug design, which starts with defining the scope of a new drug [31].

4.2 AI's place in vaccine development

The Human Immunome's Initiative was founded as a joint initiative of the Human Vaccines Project and the Harvard T.H. Chan School of Public Health to hasten the development of vaccines using AI models. Explaining effective immunity in the elderly and highlighting the benefits of vaccines and medications, this program employs cutting-edge technologies in epidemiology, immunosurveillance, network biology, AI, and ML. The purpose is to accelerate legal evolution [32].

4.3 The search for a COVID-19 remedy has already begun

Several companies are now employing AI to locate and assess existing medications that could be used to treat COVID-19, as well as to improve clinical validation and examine patient electronic medical records (EMRs) and trial data. In India's TCSO Innovation Lab,

31 possible COVID-19 inhibitors were discovered by a team of TCS scientists. The innovative syntheses planning tool has been made available to the scientific community by the European AI-based start-up Molecule.one to help researchers quickly synthesize and analyze potential candidate chemicals for COVID-19. IBM's AI generative frameworks were also applied to three COVID-19 pharmaceutical targets, providing an additional 3,000 possible hits or compounds [33].

4.4 Viability and expansion of AI-based drug discovery strategies

Several important criteria must be met in order to create a successful public health response to a new disease outbreak, including epidemiological modelling and identifying the causative organism and fatality rate. This data used to train and prepare the AI application for its particular role, may also work well for COVID-19. It did for SARS. AI can help with predictive maintenance, improved resource allocation, quality assurance, cost reduction, and increased effectiveness. Machines can already solve issues in the same way that people do, thanks to AI technologies. Computer programs have been manually developed for many years to produce a certain outcome from a specific input. Computers can analyze vast volumes of data using AI techniques to find important trends that may be applied to create insightful forecasts. While certain specialized software with restricted applications can be easily plugged into an organization, by customizing, choosing, or developing the proper algorithms and tool calculations for the particular action, AI should be engaged [34].

5 The use of AI in predicting COVID-19 outcomes

According to current research, technologies-based AI and ML have the potential to significantly lessen the effects of viral spread. Numerous fields are researching the use of ML technologies on patient data. Two of the most important study areas are developing a model to categorize patients based on clinical outcomes and predicting infection and death rates. These research studies are crucial and will help those in the healthcare industry be well-prepared and take all required safeguards to stop the spread of the pandemic. A method for predicting sickness severity and risk markers are used in COVID-19 patients, who can be followed remotely while at home. The study also looks at how vital signs, chronic illnesses, early clinical investigations, and demographic factors affect COVID-19 patient survival and mortality. The researchers used clinical data and demographic information from COVID-19 patients at King Fahad University Hospital to test the model's functionality and effectiveness. All risk factors or vital signs that can be tracked using low-cost sensors, such as blood oxygen levels, temperature, heart rate, and blood pressure, were taken into account in the study. As problems arise, the model will act as an early warning system [35].

5.1 AI-based insights for forecasting the COVID-19 transmission

The dynamics of numerous infectious diseases can be illustrated and predicted using a variety of mathematical models. These infectious disease dynamics prediction models might take a statistical, mathematical, empirical, or AI approach. The first attempts to use AI in medicine were made in the 1970s. Initially, AI was used to develop algorithms to aid clinical decision-making, but it is increasingly being used in biological sciences, now. The influenza outbreak was previously predicted and anticipated using recurrent neural networks (RNNs) with long short-term memory (LSTM), a type of artificial neural network, with substantial competitiveness and trustworthy results. According to many simulation studies, several AI-based technologies were used to estimate COVID-19 projections during the COVID-19 pandemic. In order to predict new COVID-19 cases in various European countries in 2020, three techniques such as autoregressive integrated moving average (ARIMA), nonlinear autoregression neural network (NARNN), and LSTM will be applied [36].

The spread of COVID-19 in several countries in 2021 will be predicted using an LSTM algorithm with ten hidden units based on confirmed cases and fatalities. In India, an LSTM-based data-driven model was used to estimate cases and recoveries, while taking into account the statutory preventive measures that the government must take, such as lockdown and isolation [37].

5.2 Model prediction with AI

Based on age, gender, number of therapy days, and number of prior illnesses, ML and AI algorithms were used to predict the expected chances of life for 1,533 isolated patients in South Korea. AI-based models were developed and evaluated on 5,165 coronavirus incidences before being verified on 1,533 quarantined patients [38].

5.2.1 Hyperparameter tuning

Hyperparameter tuning is one of the most important steps in creating a successful learning model. Based on the features of the dataset and the capability of the AI-based technique, it refers to the presetting of some of the higher-level parameters, prior to model training. C-regularization, gamma, kernel, and degree parameter are some of the hyperparameters that were trained into our model. The value of C represents a trade-off between the precision of model learning and the breadth of the hyperplane margin. Since a sharp decline in the value of C could have an impact on training accuracy, we will set it to 1.0, in this case. This parameter determines the impact of the training dataset [39].

5.2.2 COVID-19 machine learning model

To begin with, a model for estimating survival probabilities was created using ML methods, including logistic regression (LR) and Support Vector Machine (SVM). LR is used with 4,000 iterations to make the prediction. The LR model had a macro accuracy of 91% on average. To compute macro-average accuracy, the model's average recall and precision were used. The macro-average handles all data classes equally, because it calculates model accuracy separately for each data class. Furthermore, SVM is applied with parameter optimization using the grid search cross-validation method, and accuracy increases to 97% [40].

5.2.3 Deep learning prediction model

A deep learning (DL)-based prediction method based on the best technique for identifying COVID-19 and comorbidities like pneumonia is the convolutional neural network and the data augmentation of radiographic images (DARI) algorithm. To create synthetic radiography data, the DARI strategy combines a generative adversarial network (GAN) model with general augmentation methods. This synthesized data assists in the detection and monitoring of COVID-19 features on radiographs by scanning CT scans. DL-based algorithms can find hidden patterns in patient radiographs that are essential to diagnosis. Anterior–posterior radiographs of the patient are correctly evaluated by DL models in 96.3% of cases, which lowers the possibility of false-positive and false-negative results. When clinicians are unable to tell the difference between COVID-19 symptoms and flu symptoms, DL platforms can help. This is especially useful in developing nations with low incomes, where large-scale RT-PCR may be unaffordable. For distinguishing COVID-19 from community-acquired pneumonia, it has a sensitivity of 87% and a specificity of 95%. As a result, it is claimed that AI-based COVID-19 diagnosis performed under a doctor's supervision is cost-effective, time-saving, and has been shown to lighten the workload of healthcare professionals, while also resolving the issue of a finite supply of RT-PCR test kits [41].

In the second stage, an Artificial Neural Network (ANN) is developed using a DL methodology to identify the population segment that has a higher chance of survival, based on factors like the typical length of hospitalization, age group, gender, region of belongingness, contacts, and comorbidities. Among other AI-based model projections, the survival probability predicted by the ANN model with Adam optimizer is found to be fairly high and highly accurate [41].

6 Artificial intelligence in drug discovery

Understanding viral manipulation is required for therapeutic development. Viral manipulation entails creating medications that take use of the virus's signaling or host cell recognition properties. Any impediment produced by either of these two can lessen the likelihood of infection. One can also investigate the suppression of signal induction. However, before vaccines can be made accessible to the general population, vaccine research requires personnel, time, and clinical trials. Therefore, immunizations cannot serve as the only effective form of treatment. We can examine existing antivirals and vaccines in order to develop treatments and immunizations against the virus. In order to create therapies and vaccines against the virus, we can evaluate the properties of current antiviral and antibiotic medications, such as high specificity, mode of action, side effects, and so on. It is important to assess the capacity of antivirals used to treat SARS, MERS, HIV, Ebola, and other viral illnesses to treat infected individuals. ML might potentially help with drug development. Researchers used Bayesian ML models with viral pseudo-type entry tests during earlier epidemics like the Ebola virus, and data from the replication assay of the Ebola virus aided in the scoring process, indicating the molecule's ability to be used in treatment. The use of the random forest method in ML-assisted medicine development study for H7N9 yielded amazing results. The adoption of such technologies is essential in pandemics that spread quickly, like COVID-19. Traditional methods of researching the properties of these drugs will take a lot of time, and the results might not be reliable either. ML can be used to repurpose medications by analyzing knowledge graphs and forecasting interactions between host and medication molecules. ML was used to build a similar knowledge network to investigate the response of the virus to baricinitib. Neural networks can be used to research the medications listed below, and clinical trials can be used to test potential new medications. Using neural networks, a method for swiftly producing extra comparable graphs was developed. Understanding the characteristics and straightforward attack areas of SARS-CoV-2 is essential before creating a medication or vaccine against it. Since they imitate the human immune system, epitope-based immunizations are safer and more effective at preventing disease. To find epitopes and create successful vaccinations, ANN (especially DL), hidden Markov models, and SVM might be used. AI could be used to develop novel medications and vaccines. For instance, the antiviral drug, barcinitib, and six other innovative medications have been found. Thus, AI has, in many ways, facilitated the development of a drug [42].

7 Artificial intelligence challenges and limitations

Current system's limitations and future challenges that AI has shown great possibilities with the Digital Mammography DREAM challenge, which examined about 640,000 digital mammograms and was based on CI-based algorithms. There are a few CI limitations that must be resolved. The current COVID-19 pandemic is also being analyzed, verified, maintained, and managed using CI-based solutions.

7.1 Requirement for huge datasets

AI algorithms are often less reliable in the absence of large datasets. As a result, substantial datasets to train and monitor, avoid, foresee, and analyze, models need to be calibrated [43].

7.2 Black-box nature

Most AI-based approaches, including ANN and DL lack insight into how outcomes are derived, and this is referred to as the "Black box model" [44].

7.3 Issues

People have trust issues with the emerging technology in AI systems implemented for medical healthcare. They are concerned that their personal information may be abused by academics for personal gain. Yet, it is vital to increase awareness of the advantages and disadvantages of AI systems and to win over the public's faith in them. Health insurers and medical researchers are accountable. These organizations should raise public awareness about the benefits of AI systems. AI has significantly impacted many industries, in addition to improving the quality of illness diagnostics, care, and control. Additionally, it has enhanced the curriculum and medical education. AI also advances our knowledge of human biology. Robots with human intelligence may eventually replace doctors to cure illnesses more effectively. This would save money and be good for the medical sector.

8 Conclusion

COVID-19 is a worldwide concern. It affects not only human lives but also the global economy. AI is a new discipline, a great tool for predictive analytics, and it played an important part in battling the lethal COVID-19. We addressed the role of AI in four major elements of the fight against COVID-19 in this review, including monitoring, prevention, prediction, and diagnosis. We have shown how AI has changed epidemic surveillance and helped in inventing novel preventative strategies, diagnosing, and treating, albeit with ongoing limits. AI cannot be constructed overnight, but it may be combined with existing methods and technology to provide accurate and more effective response for future epidemics. This necessitates study and model development based on the aforementioned intelligences. We may also combine any two technologies to provide expected outcomes with additional values. Aggressive research is required to overcome AI limitations, so that it can be used to combat future pandemics.

References

[1] Alali, Y., Harrou, F., Sun, Y. A proficient approach to forecast COVID-19 spread via optimized dynamic machine learning models. Scientific Reports, 2022, 12(1), 2467.

[2] Alkhodari, M., Khandoker, A. H. Detection of COVID-19 in smartphone-based breathing recordings: A pre-screening deep learning tool. PLoS One, 2022, 17(1), e0262448.

[3] Asadzadeh, A., Mohammadzadeh, Z., Fathifar, Z., Jahangiri-Mirshekarlou, S., Rezaei-Hachesu, P. A framework for information technology-based management against COVID-19 in Iran. BMC Public Health, 2022, 22(1), 402.

[4] Basky, G., Vogel, L. Focus on technology: Surgical selfies, ransomware attacks, AI-assisted mental health care. Canadian Medical Association Journal, 2022, 194(1), E23–E25.

[5] Bauersachs, J., De Boer, R. A., Lindenfeld, J., Bozkurt, B. The year in cardiovascular medicine 2021: Heart failure and cardiomyopathies. European Heart Journal, 2022, 43(5), 367–376.

[6] Berlo, K., Xia, W., Zwillich, F., Gibbons, E., Gaudiuso, R., Ewusi-Annan, E., Chiklis, G. R., Melikechi, N. Laser induced breakdown spectroscopy for the rapid detection of SARS-CoV-2 immune response in plasma. Scientific Reports, 2022, 12(1), 1614.

[7] Cai, S., Chen, Y., Zhao, S., He, D., Li, Y., Xiong, N., Li, Z., Hu, S. Dynamic 3D radiomics analysis using artificial intelligence to assess the stage of COVID-19 on CT images. European Radiology, 2022.

[8] Brendlin, A. S., Mader, M., Faby, S., Schmidt, B., Othman, A. E., Gassenmaier, S., Nikolaou, K., Afat, S. AI lung segmentation and perfusion analysis of dual-energy CT can help to distinguish COVID-19 infiltrates from visually similar immunotherapy-related pneumonitis findings and can optimize radiological workflows. Tomography, 2021, 8(1), 22–32.

[9] Caren, G. J., Iskandar, D., Pitaloka, D. A. E., Abdulah, R., Suwantika, A. A. COVID-19 pandemic disruption on the management of tuberculosis treatment in Indonesia. Journal of Multidisciplinary Healthcare, 2022, 15, 175–183.

[10] Chakraborty, C., Sharma, A. R., Bhattacharya, M., Zayed, H., Lee, S. S. Understanding gene expression and transcriptome profiling of COVID-19: An initiative towards the mapping of protective immunity genes against SARS-CoV-2 infection. Frontiers in Immunology, 2021, 12, 724936.

[11] Desai, M. D., Tootooni, M. S., Bobay, K. L. Can prehospital data improve early identification of sepsis in emergency department? an integrative review of machine learning approaches. Applied Clinical Informatics, 2022, 13(1), 189–202.

[12] Dutta, A. K., Aljarallah, N. A., Abirami, T., Sundarrajan, M., Kadry, S., Nam, Y., Jeong, C. W. Optimal deep-learning-enabled intelligent decision support system for SARS-CoV-2 classification. Journal of Healthcare Engineering, 2022, 2022, 4130674.

[13] Fleuren, L. M., Dam, T. A., Tonutti, M., De Bruin, D. P., Lalisang, R. C. A., Gommers, D., Cremer, O. L., Bosman, R. J., Rigter, S., Wils, E. J., Frenzel, T., Dongelmans, D. A., de, J. R., Peters, M., Kamps, M. J. A., Ramnarain, D., Nowitzky, R., Nooteboom, F. G. C. A., de, R. W., Urlings-Strop, L. C., Smit, E. G. M., Mehagnoul-Schipper, D. J., Dormans, T., De Jager, C. P. C., Hendriks, S. H. A., Achterberg, S., Oostdijk, E., Reidinga, A. C., Festen-Spanjer, B., Brunnekreef, G. B., Cornet, A. D., Van den Tempel,

W., Boelens, A. D., Koetsier, P., Lens, J., Faber, H. J., Karakus, A., Entjes, R., de, J. P., Rettig, T. C. D., Arbous, S., Vonk, S. J. J., Fornasa, M., Machado, T., Houwert, T., Hovenkamp, H., Noorduijn, L. R., Quintarelli, D., Scholtemeijer, M. G., De Beer, A. A., Cina, G., Kantorik, A., de, R. T., Herter, W. E., Beudel, M., Girbes, A. R. J., Hoogendoorn, M., Thoral, P. J., Elbers, P. W. G. Predictors for extubation failure in COVID-19 patients using a machine learning approach. Critical Care, 2021, 25(1), 448.

[14] Garcia-Rudolph, A., Sauri, J., Cegarra, B., Opisso, E., Tormos, J. M., Frey, D., Madai, V. I., Bernabeu, M. The impact of COVID-19 on home, social, and productivity integration of people with chronic traumatic brain injury or stroke living in the community. Medicine (Baltimore), 2022, 101(8), e28695.

[15] Goel, T., Murugan, R., Mirjalili, S., Chakrabartty, D. K. Multi-COVID-Net: Multi-objective optimized network for COVID-19 diagnosis from chest X-ray images. Applied Soft Computing, 2022, 115, 108250.

[16] Guarnera, A., Santini, E., Podda, P. COVID-19 pneumonia and Lung Cancer: A challenge for the radiologist review of the main radiological features, differential diagnosis and overlapping pathologies. Tomography, 2022, 8(1), 513–528.

[17] Haq, A. U., Li, J. P., Ahmad, S., Khan, S., Alshara, M. A., Alotaibi, R. M. Diagnostic approach for accurate diagnosis of COVID-19 employing deep learning and transfer learning techniques through chest X-ray images clinical data in E-healthcare. Sensors (Basel), 2021, 21(24).

[18] Hemdan, E. E., El-Shafai, W., Sayed, A. CR19: A framework for preliminary detection of COVID-19 in cough audio signals using machine learning algorithms for automated medical diagnosis applications. Journal of Ambient Intelligence and Humanized Computing, 2022, 1–13.

[19] Hussain, S. A., Bassam, N. A., Zayegh, A., Ghawi, S. A. Prediction and evaluation of healthy and unhealthy status of COVID-19 patients using wearable device prototype data. MethodsX, 2022, 9, 101618.

[20] Jamshidi, E., Asgary, A., Tavakoli, N., Zali, A., Setareh, S., Esmaily, H., Jamaldini, S. H., Daaee, A., Babajani, A., Sendani Kashi, M. A., Jamshidi, M., Jamal, R. S., Mansouri, N. Using machine learning to predict mortality for COVID-19 patients on day 0 in the ICU. Frontiers in Digital Health, 2021, 3, 681608.

[21] Jung, C., Excoffier, J. B., Raphael-Rousseau, M., Salaun-Penquer, N., Ortala, M., Chouaid, C. Evolution of hospitalized patient characteristics through the first three COVID-19 waves in Paris area using machine learning analysis. PLoS One, 2022, 17(2), e0263266.

[22] Kamran, F., Tang, S., Otles, E., McEvoy, D. S., Saleh, S. N., Gong, J., Li, B. Y., Dutta, S., Liu, X., Medford, R. J., Valley, T. S., West, L. R., Singh, K., Blumberg, S., Donnelly, J. P., Shenoy, E. S., Ayanian, J. Z., Nallamothu, B. K., Sjoding, M. W., Wiens, J. Early identification of patients admitted to hospital for covid-19 at risk of clinical deterioration: Model development and multisite external validation study. British Medical Journal, 2022, 376, e068576.

[23] Kapoor, A., Kapoor, A., Mahajan, G. Use of artificial intelligence to triage patients with flu-like symptoms using imaging in non-COVID-19 hospitals during COVID-19 pandemic: An ongoing 8-month experience. Indian Journal of Radiology and Imaging, 2021, 31(4), 901–909.

[24] Ye, Y., Zhang, Q., Wei, X., Cao, Z., Yuan, H. Y., Zeng, D. D. Equitable access to COVID-19 vaccines makes a life-saving difference to all countries. Nature Human Behaviour, 2022, 6(2), 207–216.

[25] Larie, D., An, G., Cockrell, C. Preparing for the next COVID: Deep reinforcement learning trained artificial intelligence discovery of multi-modal immunomodulatory control of systemic inflammation in the absence of effective anti-microbials. BioRxiv, 2022.

[26] Li, Y., Chen, L., Chen, S., Liu, X. Delayed infliximab treatment affects the outcomes of patients with Crohn's disease during the COVID-19 epidemic in China: A propensity score-matched analysis. Frontiers in Medicine (Lausanne), 2021, 8, 819557.

[27] Lorca-Oro, C., Vila, J., Pleguezuelos, P., Vergara-Alert, J., Rodon, J., Majo, N., Lopez, S., Segales, J., Saldana-Buesa, F., Visa-Boladeras, M., Vea-Baro, A., Campistol, J. M., Abad, X. Rapid SARS-CoV-2 inactivation in a simulated hospital room using a mobile and autonomous robot emitting ultraviolet-C light. Journal of Infectious Diseases, 2022, 225(4), 587–592.

[28] Malik, A. A., Hussain, H., Maniar, R., Safdar, N., Mohiuddin, A., Riaz, N., Pasha, A., Khan, S., Kazmi, S. S. H., Kazmi, E., Khowaja, S. Integrated tuberculosis and COVID-19 activities in Karachi and Tuberculosis case notifications. Tropical Medicine and Infectious Disease, 2022, 7(1).
[29] Maldonado, P., Peng, A., Ouyang, D., Suckale, J., Ho, D. E. Science translation during the COVID-19 pandemic: An academic-public health partnership to assess capacity limits in California. American Journal of Public Health, 2022, 112(2), 308–315.
[30] Nwanosike, E. M., Conway, B. R., Merchant, H. A., Hasan, S. S. Potential applications and performance of machine learning techniques and algorithms in clinical practice: A systematic review. International Journal of Medical Informatics, 2022, 159, 104679.
[31] Prieto, K. Current forecast of COVID-19 in Mexico: A Bayesian and machine learning approaches. PLoS One, 2022, 17(1), e0259958.
[32] Roe, C., Lowe, M., Williams, B., Miller, C. Public perception of SARS-CoV-2 vaccinations on social media: Questionnaire and sentiment analysis. International Journal of Environmental Research and Public Health, 2021, 18(24).
[33] Sarabadani, S., Baruah, G., Fossat, Y., Jeon, J. Longitudinal changes of COVID-19 symptoms in social media: observational study. Journal of Medical Internet Research, 2022, 24(2), e33959.
[34] Singhal, L., Kour, I., Gupta, V. Diagnostic stewardship in times of Covid-19 pandemic. Infectious Disorders Drug Targets, 2022.
[35] Su, H., Zhao, D., Yu, F., Heidari, A. A., Zhang, Y., Chen, H., Li, C., Pan, J., Quan, S. Horizontal and vertical search artificial bee colony for image segmentation of COVID-19 X-ray images. Computers in Biology and Medicine, 2022, 142, 105181.
[36] Szaszi, B., Hajdu, N., Szecsi, P., Tipton, E., Aczel, B. A machine learning analysis of the relationship of demographics and social gathering attendance from 41 countries during pandemic. Scientific Reports, 2022, 12(1), 724.
[37] Turilli, E. S., Lualdi, M., Fasano, M. Looking at COVID-19 from a systems biology perspective. Biomolecules, 2022, 12(2).
[38] Wang, L., Davis, P. B., Kaelber, D. C., Volkow, N. D., Xu, R. Comparison of mRNA-1273 and BNT162b2 vaccines on breakthrough SARS-CoV-2 infections, hospitalizations, and death during the delta-predominant period. Journal of the American Medical Association, 2022, 327(7), 678–680.
[39] Wang, W., Chai, Z., Cooper, M. E., Zimmet, P. Z., Guo, H., Ding, J., Yang, F., Chen, X., Lin, X., Zhang, K., Zhong, Q., Li, Z., Zhang, P., Wu, Z., Guan, X., Zhang, L., He, K. High fasting blood glucose level with unknown prior history of diabetes is associated with high risk of severe adverse COVID-19 outcome. Frontiers in Endocrinology (Lausanne), 2021, 12, 791476.
[40] Xiong, Y., Ma, Y., Ruan, L., Li, D., Lu, C., Huang, L. Comparing different machine learning techniques for predicting COVID-19 severity. Infectious Diseases of Poverty, 2022, 11(1), 19.
[41] Yang, B., Bao, W., Wang, J. Active disease-related compound identification based on capsule network. Briefings in Bioinformatics, 2022, 23(1).
[42] Yang, F., Zhang, Q., Yuan, Z., Teng, S., Cui, L., Xue, F., Wei, L. Signaling potential therapeutic herbal medicine prescription for treating COVID-19 by collaborative filtering. Frontiers in Pharmacology, 2021, 12, 759479.
[43] Yang, Y., Chan, A. P. C., Shan, M., Gao, R., Bao, F., Lyu, S., Zhang, Q., Guan, J. Opportunities and challenges for construction health and safety technologies under the COVID-19 pandemic in Chinese construction projects. International Journal of Environmental Research and Public Health, 2021, 18(24).
[44] Ye, J., Song, Y., Liu, Y., Zhong, Y. Assessment of medical waste generation, associated environmental impact, and management issues after the outbreak of COVID-19: A case study of the Hubei Province in China. PLoS One, 2022, 17(1), e0259207.

Snigdha Sen*, Yukthi R Aithal

Evaluation of deep learning models for identification and prediction of new strains of COVID-19

Abstract: COVID-19 virus has caused an unembellished threat to mankind and industry over the last 2 years. Currently, when the entire world is reeling from the effects of the second wave of the pandemic, the third wave is in its beginning and is expected to be more deadly than earlier waves. Ever since the first Covid case was detected, the virus has undergone several mutations, with the delta plus variant, the delta variant, and the lambda variant being a few of the worst COVID-19 variants detected so far. During the last few months, there has been an exponential rise in the number of Omicron cases all over the world. Proper identification and detection of these new variants are vital in the current times. In this chapter, various deep learning (DL) and transfer learning models like convolutional neural network (CNN), Resnet50, VGGNet, and InceptionV3 have been explored that can help to forecast the spread and further mutations of the virus. The objective of the chapter is to study the performance details of all those algorithms comprehensively for prediction of Covid cases. As deep learning models are powerful in extracting complex features automatically without human effort, these models can formulate prevention strategies for the new strains of Covid.

1 Introduction

Since their existence, human beings have encountered and faced challenges caused by various health hazards due to the spread of infectious viruses. COVID-19 is a novel disease affected by the SARS-COV-2 virus that leads to respiratory problems when it infects a person. In Wuhan, China, in December 2019, the first COVID-19 case in humans was reported. It has since spread worldwide, overwhelming governments and health communities across the globe. Finally, the World Health Organization (WHO) announced this was a pandemic in the midweek of March 2020. Globally, as of 4:14 pm CET, December 29, 2021, there have been 281,808,270 confirmed cases of COVID-19, including 5,411,759 deaths reported to WHO.

Current evidence suggests that the disease is mostly spread during close contact and can also be spread by airborne transmission. From the time the first case was detected, the virus has undergone several mutations, with the delta plus variant, the delta

***Corresponding author: Snigdha Sen,** CSE, Global Academy of Technology, Bangalore, India
Yukthi R Aithal, CSE, Global Academy of Technology, Bangalore, India

https://doi.org/10.1515/9783110767681-013

variant, and the lambda variant being a few of the worst COVID-19 variants to be detected so far. Formerly known as a 2019 novel coronavirus [1], Covid-19 consists of a series of viruses with the scientific name Orthocoronavirinae or simply Coronavirinae that mostly affects human beings. After entering the human body, it causes major breathing trouble in patients; hence, ICTV termed it SARS-CoV-2. With the Covid virus, the first wave is severe and the initial stage impact is so huge that when the virus enters the human body, patients with a previous history of comorbidities mostly died rapidly; the number of death cases increased all over the world. This caused tremendous panic among people across the world. As the virus was rapidly transmitting and infecting the human body through coughing and sneezing, measures were taken to stop the spread of the virus quickly. The exponential rise of the infections among humans led WHO to declare it a pandemic in mid-March 2020.

Before SARS-CoV-2, two different species were causing fatal human diseases: The first one was SARS-CoV, which threatened society by causing severe acute respiratory syndrome (SARS); and the second was MERS-CoV, which causes Middle East respiratory ayndrome (MERS). Unlike SARS and MERS, the symptoms caused by COVID-19 are significantly high. At the same time, sometimes it propagates to people who do not show any symptoms. Such people are termed asymptomatic and the situation is more dangerous than with symptomatic patients in spreading the infection.

Human-to-human transmission has also been confirmed for SARS-CoV-2. Due to the recent occurrence of novel coronavirus pneumonia, the demand for artificial intelligence (AI) and its allied technologies is increasingly becoming popular. As the pandemic is spreading rapidly and RTPCR testing is taking quite a long time, there can be alternate image-based methods such as detection of Covid infection from chest x-ray images. Moreover, it is quite hard to differentiate normal infection from Covid infection through just X-rays. These limitations motivated us to engage in research and come up with experimental findings using AI and deep learning-based technologies to address this issue efficiently. This AI-based technique can be very useful as well as helpful in places where testing is very slow. It also offers pretty good accuracy that can be a boon to radiologists. Inspired by this, in this book chapter, we try to explore the effectiveness and pertinence of AI systems on deep learning (DL)-based methods to handle this situation better. CT scans and X-ray images are alternate powerful means to diagnose Covid 19 and provide early prediction. With the availability of huge datasets in the form of chest X-ray images, various DL algorithms are being applied to analyze that dataset more efficiently, quickly, and conveniently. Figure 1 discusses the first phase timeline of the Covid pandemic outbreak, and we show the complete transmission stage of the pandemic in Figure 2.

For the last few years, people are seeking the help of digital technologies in combating diseases. IoT, machine learning (ML), and DL – all have evolved as solution providers for critical issues faced by human beings. While everyone around the world is panicking about the pandemic, the responsibility lies on the computer science engineers, apart from doctors, to find a quicker solution for the same. Consequently, as

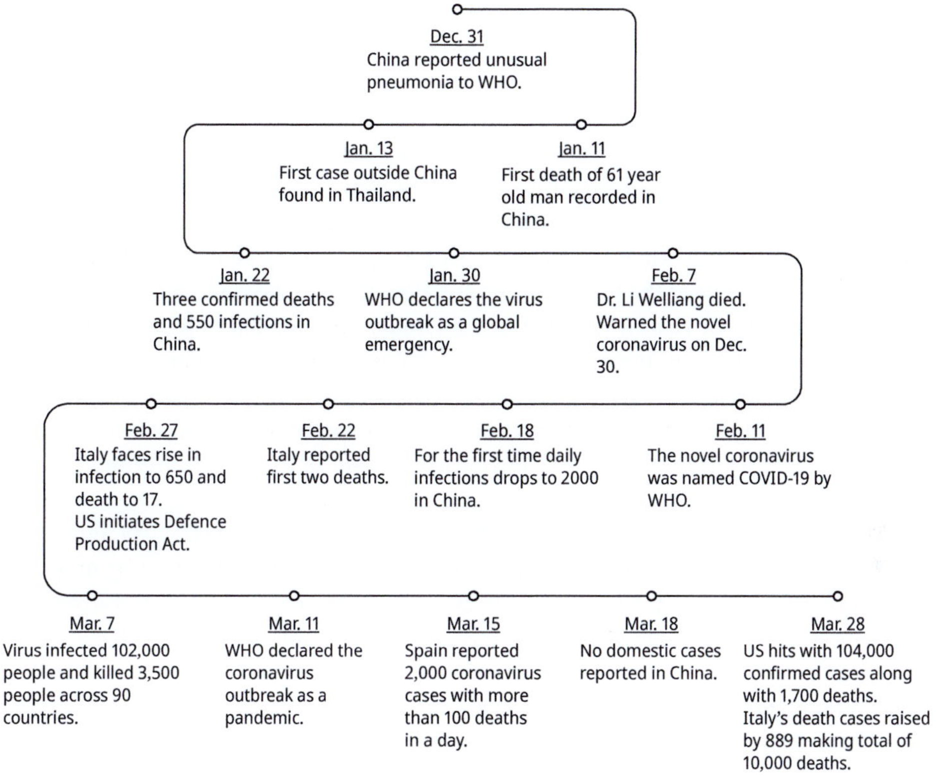

Figure 1: Initial timeline of Covid outbreak [2].

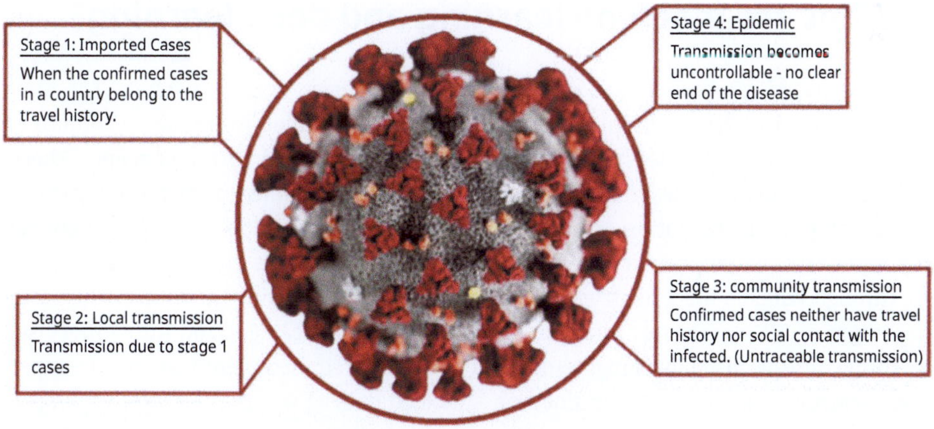

Figure 2: COVID-19: the complete transmission stages [2].

data science researchers, we tend to investigate how AI aided technologies and data analysis tools can help us to tackle and control this pandemic better. ML and DL are very powerful for data analysis and forecasting. Hence, the efficacy and usefulness of these tools should be explored as much as possible in detail to detect the disease early and take proper remedial steps to avoid further spread.

DL models can also be trained using protein structure data to calculate the prospective virus–host protein–protein interactions. Similar models have been successfully used in the past with HIV and H1N1, which significantly reduced the effort that was needed to represent the virus-host interaction, thereby expanding our knowledge of how the respective virus infects the human bodies and replicates in our cells. Some of the proposed DL-based methods are capable of accurately forecasting further mutations and their possible outcomes, based on the currently available datasets. Therefore, DL-based models play an important role in outcome prediction, which in turn provides a significant understanding of risk assessment of the infection from the new variants.

The remaining chapter is as follows. In Section 1.2, we give a brief idea about ML, DL, and transfer learning. Section 2 discusses the existing work reported by other researchers. In Section 3, we describe various Covid strains, and Section 4 discusses data sources. Section 5 explains the performance evaluation metrics of the classification models. In Section 6, we talk about experimental setup and implementation. Section 7 summarizes the results and analyzes the comparative performance of various algorithms experimented with so far. In Section 8, we present a few issues related to DL. Finally, we conclude with the prospective future scope.

2 What are machine learning and deep learning?

As we know, AI is a branch that is used to create intelligent agents or robots. The main objective of AI is that a computer system needs to be trained to act like a human or think like a human. The learning component of AI is provided by ML concepts. Therefore, the machine must learn from datasets. The machine will learn the hidden pattern, relationship, and association among the data, and try to develop a mapping between the input and the output variables in the dataset. Hence, ML is considered a subset of AI, through which a machine tries to learn and assist in predicting the future. The entire paradigm of ML consists of multiple algorithms that are categorized into supervised learning, unsupervised learning, semi-supervised, and reinforcement learning. In supervised learning, the machine is trained on a labeled dataset where the target variable is known, whereas in the unsupervised learning concept, the machine learns from an unlabeled dataset through clustering or finding similar patterns among datasets. In semi-supervised learning, the machine uses labeled as well as an unlabeled dataset. Finally, in the reinforcement learning process, the machine explores an unknown environment through several moves where it can be rewarded based on the correct move and punished for a wrong action.

Deep learning: Sometimes, when we need to manage and examine massive complex data, mainly in the form of images, traditional ML algorithms fail to provide satisfactory accuracy; it also fails to capture patterns from complex images and data. Therefore, DL has progressed as a subdivision of ML; it is capable of handling massive data that has a complex pattern. Multiple algorithms under DL have tremendous ability to extract features from images automatically without any human effort and labor, which has made DL a powerful and suitable choice in image analysis, classification, segmentation, and object detection. Even though DL is prevalent since 1960, its use was limited due to the scarcity of powerful systems and network bandwidth. In recent times, as computing processing power has increased and hardware resources have become cheaper, researchers and scientists started using more and deeper learning techniques for their work. Furthermore, the increasing speed of the internet is helping to generate more and more data in all industries and sectors. In most scenarios, DL shows more accurate performance than traditional ML approaches. It is observed that in the healthcare domain, sometimes DL excels doctors in predicting diseases. Thus, it is gaining popularity in the healthcare domain [3, 4] massively. DL performance is visible and dominant in other domains as well, such as in retail, IoT, Big data analysis, and in astronomical applications [5–7, 37]. The application of DL in Covid prediction is very promising as per recent studies over the last 2 years. In Figure 3, we present a diagram that shows how AI, ML, and DL are interrelated.

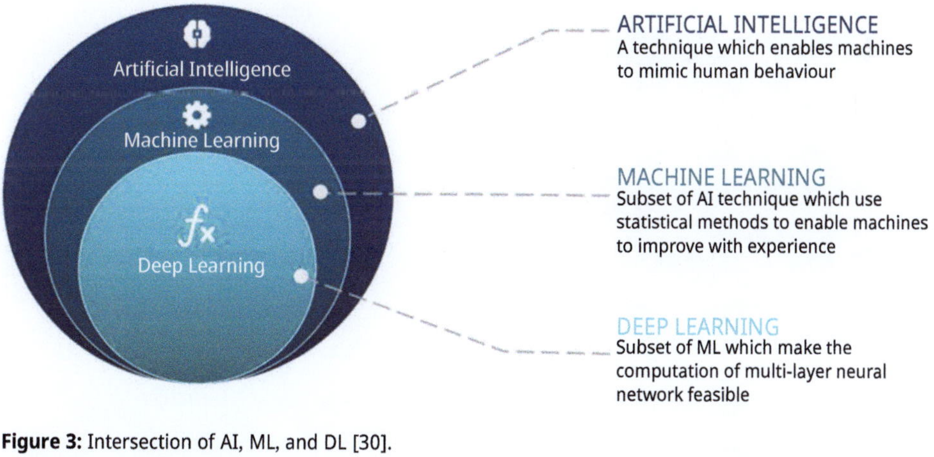

Figure 3: Intersection of AI, ML, and DL [30].

Transfer learning: Occasionally, some datasets in a specific domain are very limited. For instance, in the healthcare domain itself, we get very little data due to the scarcity of images on the disease. Furthermore, hospitals do not release datasets so as to maintain the confidentiality of patient information. Therefore, the application of the DL model does not provide acceptable results due to the non-availability of huge data. Transfer learning concepts become more useful in these scenarios. As the name suggests, it helps to transfer knowledge gained in one domain to another similar kind of domain and solve the issue there without much effort. The algorithms used here utilize pretrained algorithms and models, which are then applied to a new problem of a similar sort. The advantage here is that instead of training a new model from scratch, we can use the weights trained by another model that enhances reusability and reduces computation time and complexity [4]. Additionally, it offers enhanced performance. Transfer learning is used when we do not have much labeled data in that field and there exists a similar kind of model in another domain.

2.1 Popular deep learning algorithms

In this section, we elaborate few popular DL algorithms that could be useful for Covid prediction. Figure 4 describes the percentage of the convolutional neural network (CNN) model that has been applied in Covid data prediction.

2.1.1 Convolutional neural network (CNN)

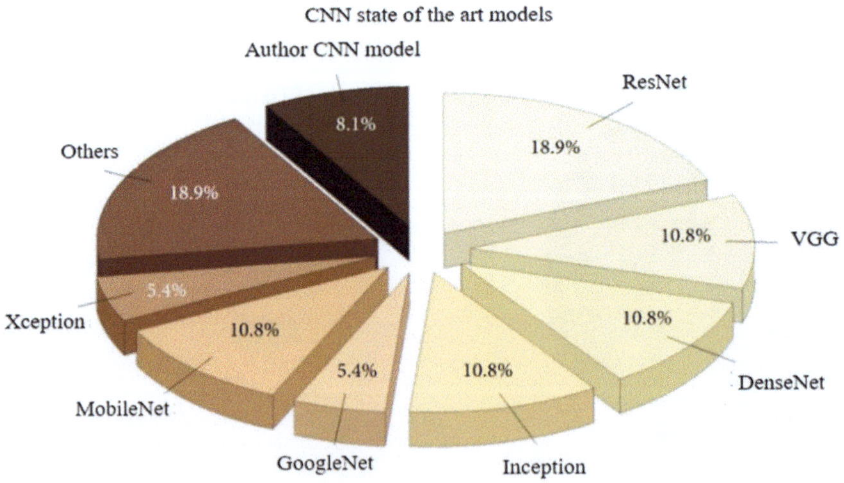

Figure 4: Usage of CNN models in Covid analysis [8].

A CNN is a special kind of neural network structure that specializes in image processing and classification. It is an efficient recognition algorithm mainly used in image processing, signal processing, and pattern recognition. CNN has powerful image processing capabilities, owing to the algorithm's two phases of functioning that try to replicate how a human brain goes about identifying an image:

- Feature extraction
- Classification

Modeling algorithms after the human brain is no small feat as it requires a thorough understanding of how we effortlessly process data daily. We detect and classify objects in our visual field by first extracting their features and then processing the object's spatial relations. Figure 5 depicts the typical structure of the CNN model.

The four main operations of CNN are:

- Convolution operation
- ReLu
- Pooling
- Classification

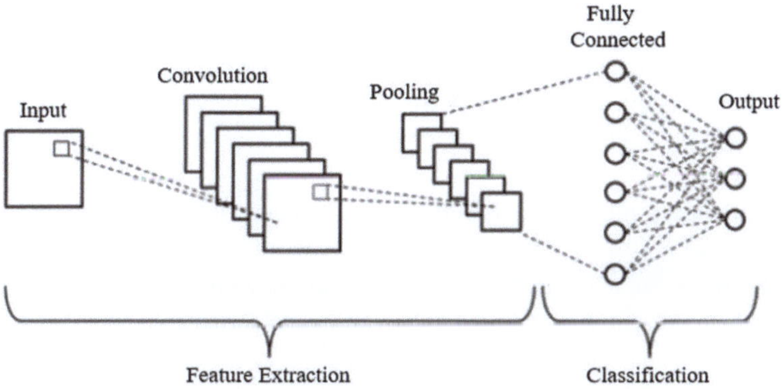

Figure 5: Typical structure of CNN model [9].

Let us discuss each operation in detail here.

2.1.1.1 Convolution

In mathematics, convolution can be defined as an operation between two functions that produces a third function that relates to how the shape of one is modified by the other. The input image, after being converted to pixel, is multiplied with the kernel to produce the feature map of reduced size, compared to the original image. In CNN, the convolution operation is employed on input image pixels using a filter to extract relevant features and produce a feature map. The process is described in Figure 6 [9].

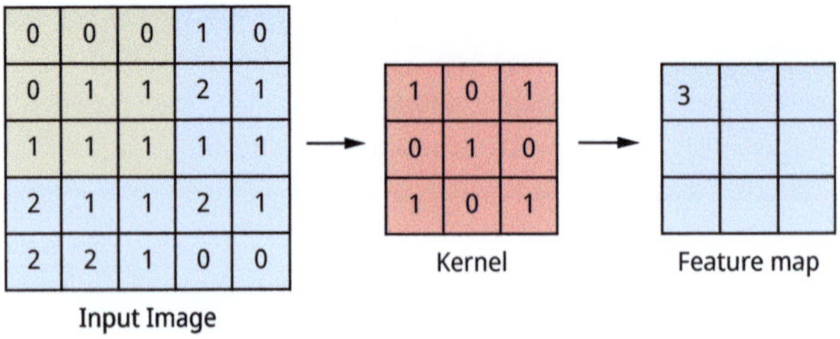

Figure 6: Convolution operation of CNN model [9].

2.1.1.2 ReLu

The result of the convolution operation is then subjected to Relu activation function. The rectified linear unit, popularly known as ReLu, is useful to address nonlinearity in a problem and helps to add non-linearity into the neural network.

2.1.1.3 Pooling

Pooling is performed after every convolution operation to reduce dimensionality. This operation helps in parameter reduction, which in turn helps shorten the training period. It also helps combat overfitting. In pooling, each feature map is down-sampled to reduce its height and width. Since pooling works independently on each feature map while down sampling, the depth remains intact. The majorly used pooling types are discussed in Figure 7.

- Max pooling: This is the most used one. Here, it considers the highest value in that pooling window.
- Average pooling: Here, the average value from the pooling window is considered.
- Min pooling: In this case, the least value is taken into consideration.

2.1.1.4 Classification

After multiple rounds of successive convolution, Relu, and Pooling, the next agenda is classification. The operations for feature extraction deal with 3D images represented as a matrix and subsequently, pixels with height, width, and depth. The output of the final pooling operation is then flattened and injected as an input to the next fully connected layers. Flattening is the process of simply arranging data configured to represent a 3D image into a 1D array. A fully connected network helps classify the data into various classes, that is, performs classification based on the extracted features

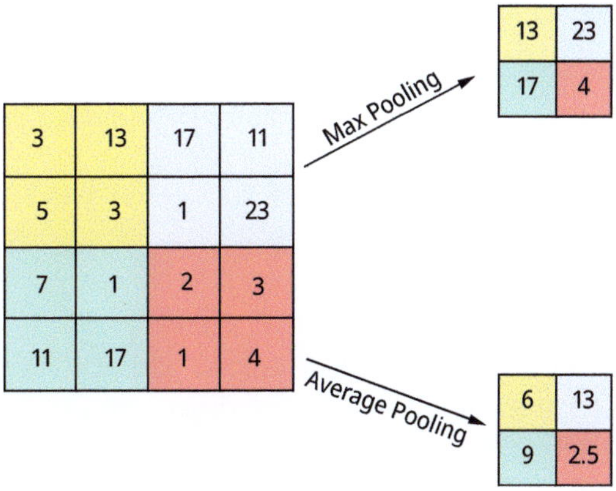

Figure 7: Pooling operation of CNN model [10].

Limitations: Although CNN is excellent in image processing, there are still some limitations. CNN is difficult to apply to large resolution images. When there are a lot of images to be handled, CNN does not show improved performance.

2.1.2 Alex Net

With the evolvement of many labeled image datasets such as ImageNet, the need for a deeper network is the need of the hour to efficiently process those datasets. ImageNet consists of 15 million high-resolution images. Alexnet is part of a pre-trained model used in computer vision, proposed in the year 2012. It majorly contains 5 max-pooling layers, with three fully connected layers. If we experiment by dropping any one of the CONV layers, performance will be degraded so much. Three different added advantages lie in Alexnet, such as the introduction of Relu, multiple Graphical Processing

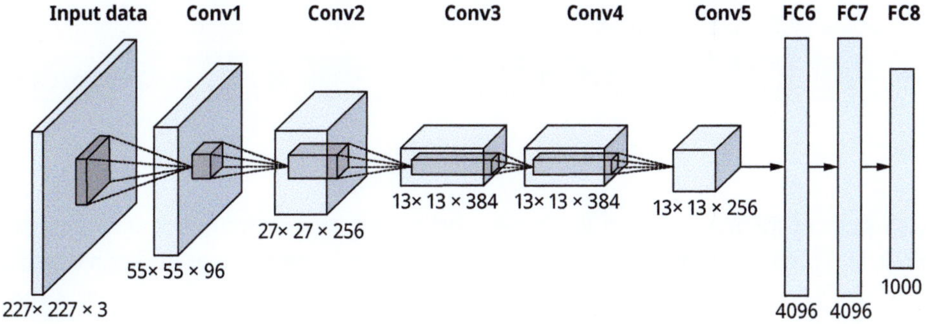

Figure 8: Framework of Alexnet model [31].

Unit (GPU), overlapping pooling, and dropout. It has potential use in object detection. Figure 8 describes the Framework of the Alexnet model.

Limitations: As there exists a lot of overlapping blocks, the memory requirement is high. Moreover, with color images, it is still not performing well.

2.1.3 ResNet

ResNet-50 and Resnet 152 are considered basics of transfer learning. As part of a very deeper architecture, with approximately 150 hidden layers, it is very powerful in an object detection task. The advantage of Resnet lies in skip connection. This skip connection helps to mitigate the effect of the vanishing gradient problem, which is a major challenge and an issue in training any DL network, by providing an alternate route. The benefit of the identity function ensures that higher layers will learn as well as lower layers. Figures 9 and 10 [11] depict the structure of the Restnet50 model and the skip connections, respectively.

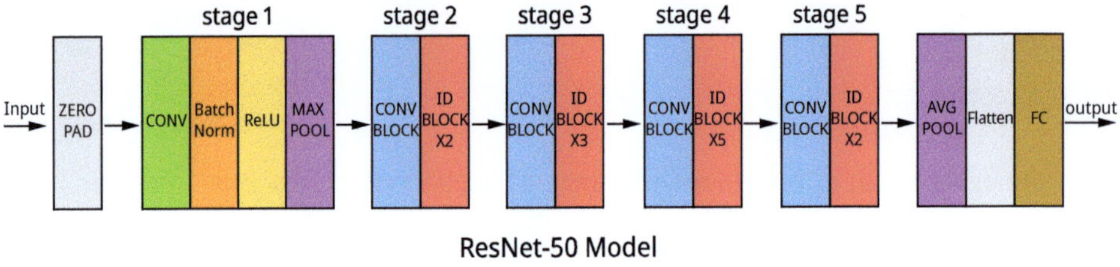

Figure 9: Framework of Restnet50 model [11].

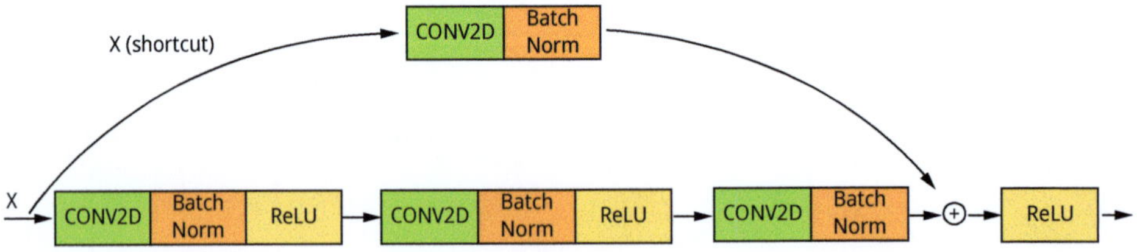

Figure 10: Framework of skip connection of ResNet model [11].

Each stage of the five stages in Restnet50 consists of a convolution block, identifies the block, and carries approximately 23 million trainable parameters. Keras library has made developer's life easier by providing suitable library packages to work with that algorithm and models.

Limitations: Major problem is a longer training time, as it is a deeper and more complex architecture.

2.1.4 Dense Net

Dense Nets simplify the connectivity pattern by ensuring maximum information flow. Here, each layer uses the feature map obtained from the previous layers. A single dense block contains batch normalization, Relu, and 3 × 3 convolutions. Dense net concatenates all feature maps instead of summing up as Resnet. It encourages feature reuse and reduces the number of parameters. Figure 11 depicts the structure of the Dense net model.

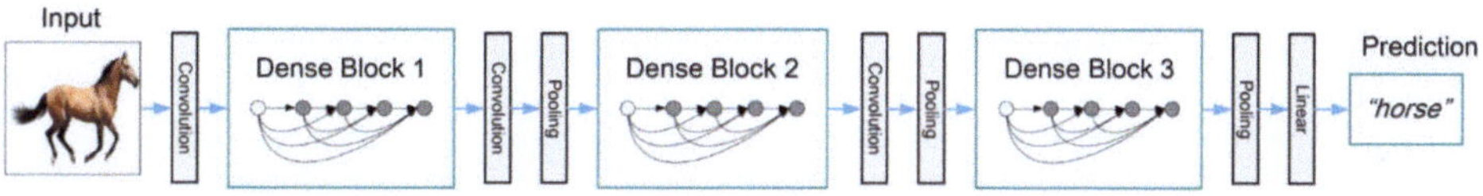

Figure 11: Framework of the Dense net model [32].

Limitations: Increased complexity of a model degrades computational efficiency as it leads to overfitting.

2.1.5 VGGNet

VGGNET is another variant of CNN that focuses on how deeper network architecture affects the performance of the model. It also uses a pre-trained ImageNet model. It comes in two categories – VGG 16 and 19. The model requires prolonged training time. Although they use a deep framework, the usage of a 3 × 3 kernel reduces total computational complexity. Contrary to vgg16, vgg19 has 16 layers for convolutional operations and three fully dense connected layers. Object localization and image classification are two major tasks performed by VGGNet. Figure 12 represents the structure of the VGGNet model.

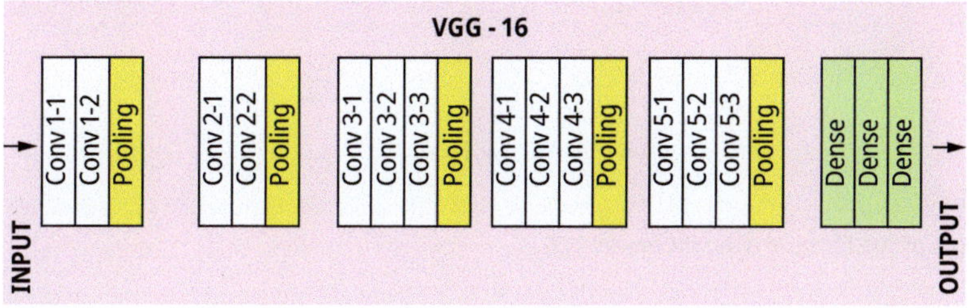

Figure 12: Framework of the VGGNet model [24].

Limitations: It is highly time-consuming to train. It suffers from the vanishing gradient problem and the network weights become comparatively huge.

2.1.6 UNet model

This model is primarily used for image segmentation. Segmentation deals with identifying multiple classes present in an image. Unet model has demonstrated effective performance in biomedical image segmentation when the intention of the analysis is not only to find out whether the disease is present or not but to find out the area of infection as well. Unet and capsule networks have combined power to address the issue of Covid as the capsule will be used for feature selection.

Limitations: Skip connections do not provide improved performance.

2.1.7 Deep capsule network

As discussed earlier, CNN has certain limitations. Although it is great in capturing important features from image pixels, according to Hinton, "The pooling operation used in CNN is a big mistake' as during pooling, much important information can be lost. Moreover, CNN needs a lot of data to learn properly, and spatial dimensions gradually decrease along with the layers. This is where the capsule network comes into existence. It uses 3D convolutional network using a dynamic routing algorithm. The main difference between a capsule and a neuron is that the capsule facilitates the output that has directions. For instance, when one image is rotated, the vector will also change its direction, where the neuron does not have that capability as it is a scalar entity. Capsule network is proficient to capture spatial useful information without losing data. The main component involved here is the dynamic routing algorithm. Figure 13 represents the structure of the capsule network model.

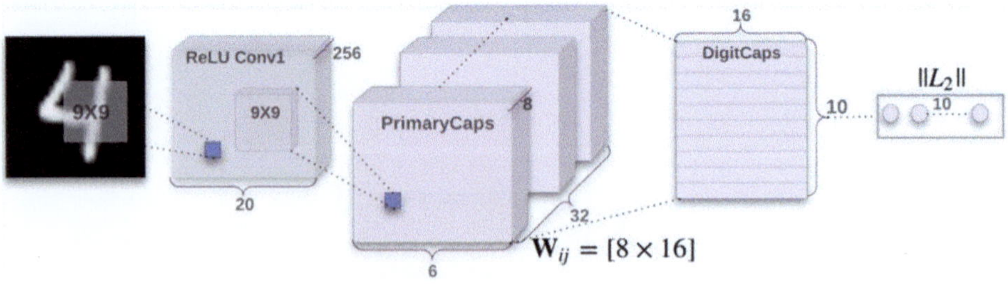

Figure 13: Framework of the Capsule network model [33].

A typical capsule net is structured as follows:

– Matrix multiplication: Input images are converted to vectors.

- Scalar weighting of the input: The current capsule output will be passed to the higher-level capsule, which will be determined in this phase.
- Dynamic routing algorithm: In this iterative process, information is transferred to various components.
- Squashing function: In this last phase, all inputs get converted to ≤1 vector while maintaining the direction.

Researchers have done Covid prediction with a deep capsule network [12]. As AI and its associated technologies help predict Covid from chest x-ray and CT scan images, some fusion-based methods such as CNN along with Capsulenet can be a powerful approach [13].

Limitations: Leads to more complexity; kind of slow because of dynamic routing, and has not yet been experimented on a large dataset.

2.1.8 LSTM

Long short-term memory (LSTM) is mainly utilized for sequential information processing. Starting from stock market prediction to Covid pattern sequence prediction, LSTM has shown notable performance. Sequence prediction is one of the hardest problems that require a special technique to address this issue, as it depends on previous data. A recurrent neural network is specifically designed for such a problem, but it has the shortcomings of short-term dependencies because of the problem raised by vanishing gradients. To overcome this issue, LSTM is introduced. The difference lies in LSTM, and RNN is the introduction of memory components. With the help of three

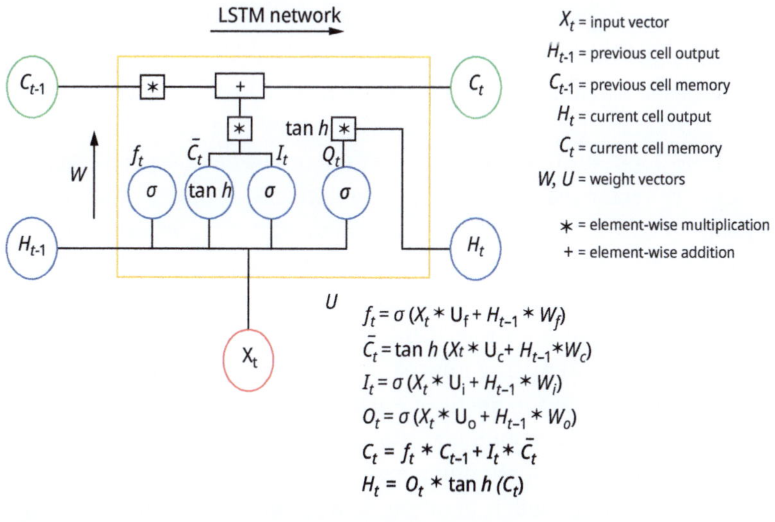

Figure 14: Framework of the LSTM network model [25, 26].

different gates such as a forget gate, an input gate, and an output gate, LSTM process a series of sequential data. Cell state and hidden state are used to transfer data to the next cell. A forget gate objective is to remove information that is not required to be passed to the next cell, whereas using an input gate, new information is added to the cell state. Figure 14 shows the composition of the LSTM network model.

Limitations: Training time is quite high and is very much susceptible to overfitting; requires more memory too. CNN_LSTM has limitations, for example, detection of small objects is quite difficult.

3 Background and related works

Big data, AI, and ML techniques and collaboration help expand our understanding of societal factors, individual-specific characteristics, and a variety of other factors that drive the spread of COVID 19. They can be instrumental in the accurate prediction of the emergence of epidemiological hotspots that can help in formulating the best measures and decisions for the smooth distribution of vaccines to the critical demographical segment. There exist multiple research studies that focus on and experiment with multiple ML and DL models for Covid forecasting. We have discussed a few significant studies here. In their research [14], Mellado B, et al. trained a DNN (Deep Neural Network) to distinguish two groups of data sets: More severe illness and less severe illness. This enabled them to understand the correlation between the fraction of the adult population of the Gauteng city and the reduction of severe illness amongst them. Their model outputted a dimensionless number between 0 and 1, with 0 indicating the highest risk of severe illness and vice versa, based on which the population was stratified. Their research helped to understand the importance of how continuous monitoring of the availability of vaccine can be done, and the usefulness and effectiveness of the vaccines in the near future.

Another such ML-based warning system developed by Yue Gao et al. enables mortality risk prediction (MRPCM) for COVID-19 [15]. This model is a kind of ensemble model consisting of four popular ML approaches – gradient boosted decision tree, Logistic regression, support vector machine, and neural network. It utilizes data in the EHRs (electronic health records) to identify patients based on their mortality risk during admission. Based on its output, a normalized probability ranging from 0 to 1, the patients infected with COVID 19 were classified into two categories: low risk if the probability was less than 0.6 and high risk if the probability was greater than 0.6. Their model was successful in predicting approximately 20 days in advance before physiological deterioration leads to the death of a patient infected with Covid-19. The model can help clinicians target those patients who are at a higher risk to succumb to the infection and thereby improve patient outcomes.

When relying on AI-based ML models to output predictions that could prove to be very crucial for the public, it is important to factor in the environmental and mobility factors that could influence the efficiency of such forecasting models. One such example is a study conducted by Rashed EA and Hirata A that investigated the variations in the accuracy of predictions of daily COVID-19 cases made by a deep LSTM neural network for six different districts in Japan, with the emergence of a new viral variant [16]. With the emergence of the Alpha variant (B.1.1.7), the surge is around 20–40% in the reported daily positive cases (DPC) and an increase of 20% in the effective reproductive number was noticed. When the neural network, trained with the data obtained from the early days of COVID-19, forecasted the number of potential infections for a given period, an underestimation in forecasting was observed within the period that included an upsurge in the number of reported infections due to the new viral variant. When the training data included data from the period in which the new variants were reported, the forecasting accuracy of the model increased gradually. The model needed approximately four weeks to learn and adjust the forecasting error. During a comparative study analysis between the ML-based predictions and the stated results, the authors reported a useful and effective means to measure the variation produced by newly identified viral variants that can be counted within the COVID-19 estimation models.

The spread of COVID-19 has shown how new zoonotic viruses have the potential to send ripples of disruption across the global health communities. Tracing the origins of these viruses can prove to be extremely challenging. Liam Brierley and Anna Fowler, in their research, have demonstrated the potential of combining ML algorithms with genetic resources to address the challenges faced in handling such emerging infectious diseases [17]. Using signatures within the viral genomes that are generated by long-term co-evolution, they showed that there is potential to uncover the animal hosts of a particular strain of the virus. They trained random forest models on genome compositional biases of spike protein (a protein that protrudes from the envelope of a viral surface that allows entry into host cells via attachment to cell receptors at the receptor-binding domain region) and whole-genome sequences to predict the parent animal hosts. When they applied random forest models to help classify human sequences of SARS-COV and MERS-COV, MERS-COV was predicted to be having camelid hosts whereas SARS-COV was predicted as having carnivore hosts. The predictions made by the model were found to be accurate as they were consistent with the respective known intermediate hosts of camels and palm civets.

The model predictions suggested that SAR-COV-2, the contributory virus species of COVID-19, has been hosted by bats, and supports the fact that bats are the main suspect of the COVID-19 pandemic. Their work is a demonstration of the successful implementation of an ML model to estimate the host origins of the novel coronavirus. This opens new avenues in research wherein ML algorithms can aid in addressing the challenges posed by emerging infectious diseases. Zain et al. have discussed a hybrid approach, consisting of the CNN-LSTM model, for Covid estimation. Their experimental results reported the minimum MAPE, RMSE, and RRMSE values on testing data, when compared to 17 baseline models. Combinations of the encoder–decoder CNN LSTM model boost efficiency in prediction [18]. Nagy Á et al. conducted a study wherein they made use of

6 Performance evaluator metrics

In ML, we mainly deal with two types of problems/tasks – one as a regression task where we try to predict continuous real-valued target variable and another one as classification, where we intend to find the discrete output in terms of yes/no, true/false, and so on. The purpose of our current study is to classify whether a particular X-ray image belongs to a Covid image or a non-Covid image so that early detection can be made. Every ML model needs to be evaluated to understand its performance. There exist a few metrics through which the ML model is generally evaluated. They are commonly known as performance evaluator metrics. As per the classification nature of our task, the model performance is judged based on the metrics of precision, recall, F_1-score, accuracy, and confusion matrix [23].

a) Precision: It helps determine what proportion of the said identification made by a model is correct, that is, precise:

$$\text{Precision} = \frac{\text{TP}}{\text{TP} + \text{FP}}$$

b) Recall: It quantifies the proportion of a said identification that was accurately predicted:

$$\text{Recall} = \frac{\text{TP}}{\text{TP} + \text{FN}}$$

c) F_1-score: This statistical measure combines precision and recall. It uses the harmonic mean of precision and recall. The closer the F_1-Score to 1.0, the better is the model's performance:

$$F_1\text{-score} = \frac{2}{\frac{1}{\text{Precision}} + \frac{1}{\text{Recall}}} = \frac{2 \times (\text{Precision} \times \text{Recall})}{\text{Precision} + \text{Recall}}$$

d) Confusion matrix: A confusion matrix described in Figure 15 exemplifies the assessment of a classification model in a matrix format. For binary classification, the matrix is in 2 × 2 format. This model intends to categorize images into two sets: Covid positive and Covid negative. The formula here is described for binary classification. The formula slightly varies for multi-class classification where more than one class is present in the dataset (green, blue, and yellow).

   True negative: When the actual label is negative and the estimated value from the model is also negative.
   True positive: When the actual label is positive and the model prediction is also positive.
   False positive: When the actual label is negative, but the model prediction is positive.
   false negative: When the actual label is positive, but the model prediction is negative.

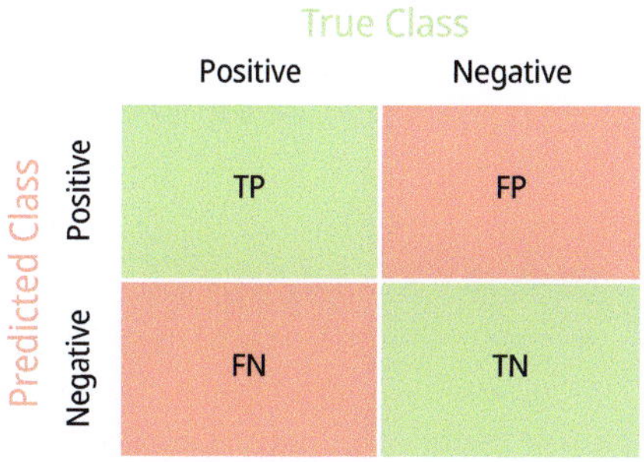

Figure 15: Confusion matrix [34].

e) ROC curve: It is also known as receiver operating characteristics. It tells the trade-off between the True positive rate and the False positive rate. It precisely indicates the classification accuracy of a model.

7 Experimental setup and implementation procedure

In this segment, we illustrate the performance of four algorithms we experimented with for this work. The entire work was implemented in Google Collaboratory, which is a cloud-based service and offers jupyter notebook interface for developing and building ML applications. Numerous python open-source libraries, such as Pandas, NumPy, Scikit Learn, Matplotlib, and Keras, have been used to develop and visualize the output of the model. Python is an open-source scripting language that offers multiple APIs to interact with DL models. The entire workflow is presented in the following block diagram in Figure 16.

7.1 CNN

The model takes in an input matrix of the dimension 150×150×3, representing an RGB image. The X-ray images undergo four rounds of successive convolution operation, Max-Pooling, and dropout, with a rate of 25%, before being flattened and fed into dense layers of orders 256, 126, and 1, respectively. Testing a patient for COVID-19 is a case of a binary classification problem and the CNN model being used is trained to make that classification between the lung X-ray image of a patient with and without COVID-19. At the last layer of the model, the use of the sigmoid activation function ensures that it gives a binary discrete output, which is used later as a positive or negative prediction.

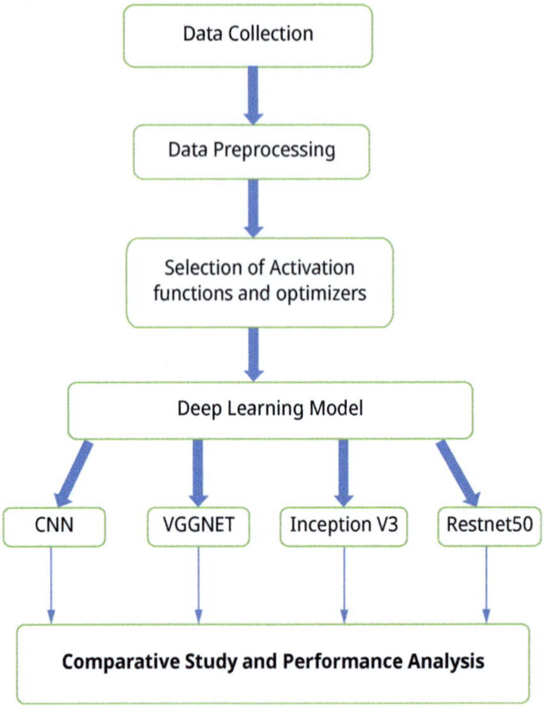

Figure 16: Proposed workflow.

When tested with sample images, the prediction of the model was found to be accurate. An instance of the model accurately classifying a COVID-19 patient's lung X-RAY image from that of a normal lung X-RAY image is shown in Figure 17.

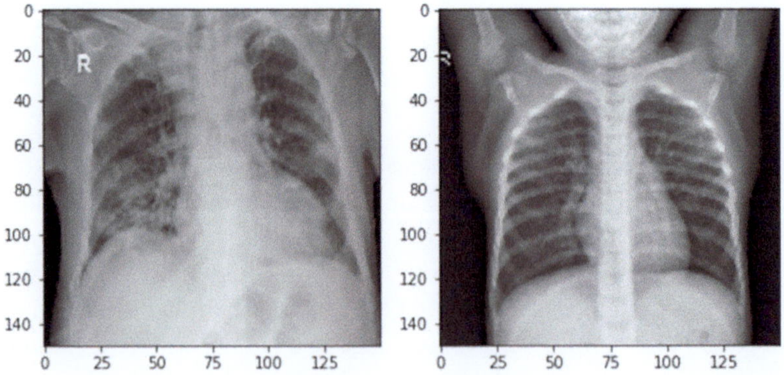

Figure 17: Output of the CNN algorithm correctly classifying Covid and non-Covid image.

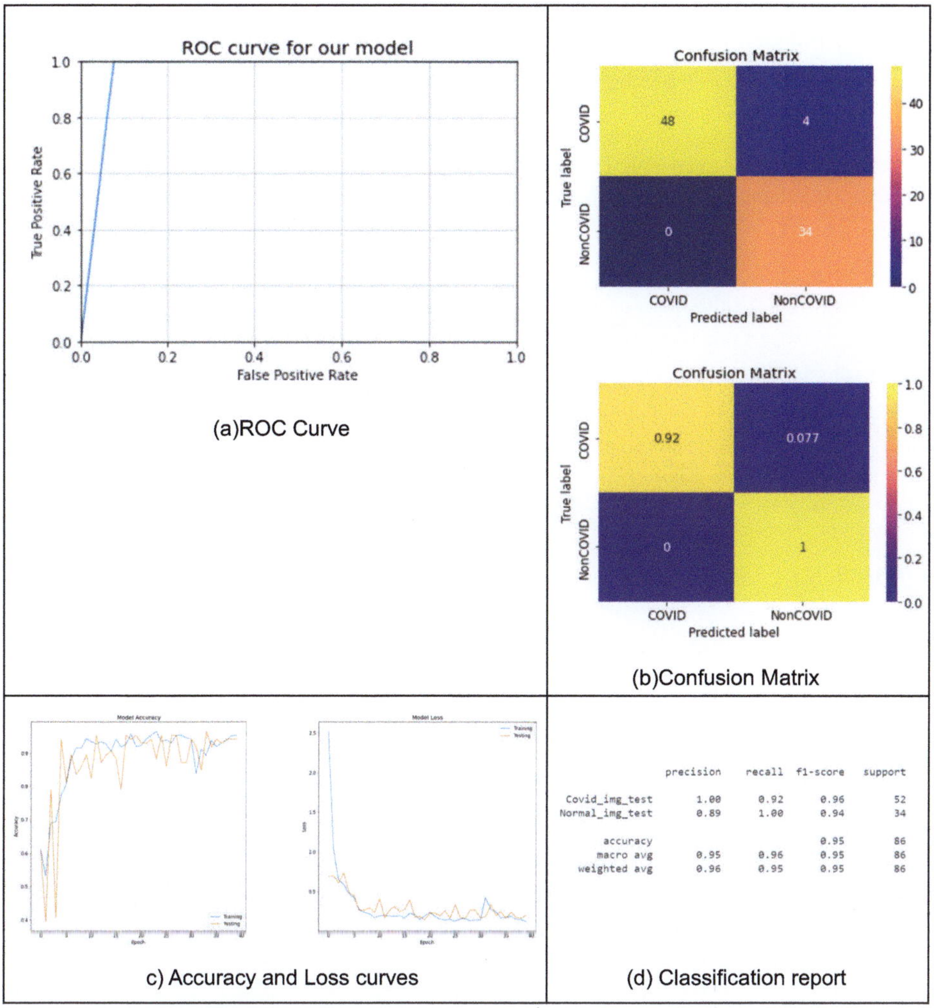

Figure 18: Performance results of CNN model.

The accuracy and the reliance of the model can be analyzed using the test dataset to obtain a classification report, a confusion matrix, and accuracy versus loss graphs for both the training samples and the test samples. Here, the model has been trained with a sample dataset containing 425 images over 40 epochs, with the batch size being set to 64. It was then tested with a dataset consisting of 86 images to obtain a classification report, a confusion matrix, a ROC curve, and a train versus test graph for both accuracy and loss. The results that detail the performance of the model are in Figure 18.

A confusion matrix helps to tabulate the assessment of any classification task model on test data where actual labels are already well known. This model intends to classify images into two sets: Covid positive and Covid negative. The *y*-axis of the confusion matrix characterizes the true label and the *x*-axis represents the predicted label. For the test data on which the above matrix is tabulated, the following conclusions about the model's predictions can be inferred:

Out of 52 positive cases, 48 of them were rightly diagnosed by this model as positive.
Out of 34 non-Covid cases, all were accurately diagnosed by the model as such.
Four Covid cases were misdiagnosed as negative. There were no cases of false positives.

7.1.1 Graphical analysis

The graphs in Figure 18(c) trace the train and validation (test) learning curves for accuracy and loss over 40 epochs. Although the overall performance of the model with respect to accuracy and loss does improve with each epoch, the noisy variations imply that the model needs more training. The model promises a good fit with more training.

7.2 VGGNET

Here, we have worked with VGGnet. The model has been trained with a dataset containing 425 images over 40 epochs, with the batch size being set to 64. It was then tested with a dataset consisting of 86 images. The performance analysis results are displayed in Figure 19.

The model tested 86 chest X-rays and classified them into two sets: COVID cases and non-COVID cases. The conclusions that can be derived from the confusion matrix generated for the test dataset are as follows:
- Total number of Covid cases successfully forecasted by model: 50
- Total number of non-Covid cases successfully forecasted by model: 34
- Total number of false Covid positives: 2
- Total number of false Covid negatives: 0

To assess the implementation ability of the model, let us look at the classification report generated for the test datasets chosen for this instance:
- Out of 86 chest X-rays, the number of occurrences of positive cases was 52.
- For COVID cases (represented by the class label 0): Let us look at the recall to determine what percentage of the positive cases was accurately diagnosed by the model. The model was successful in predicting 96% of the positive cases as positive. The recall being lower than the precision indicates that some positive cases were misdiagnosed by the model as negative.
- For non-COVID cases (represented by the class label 1): The model was accurate in predicting 100% of the non-Covid cases rightly as non-Covid.
- The overall exactness of the model is found to be 98% on the test dataset.

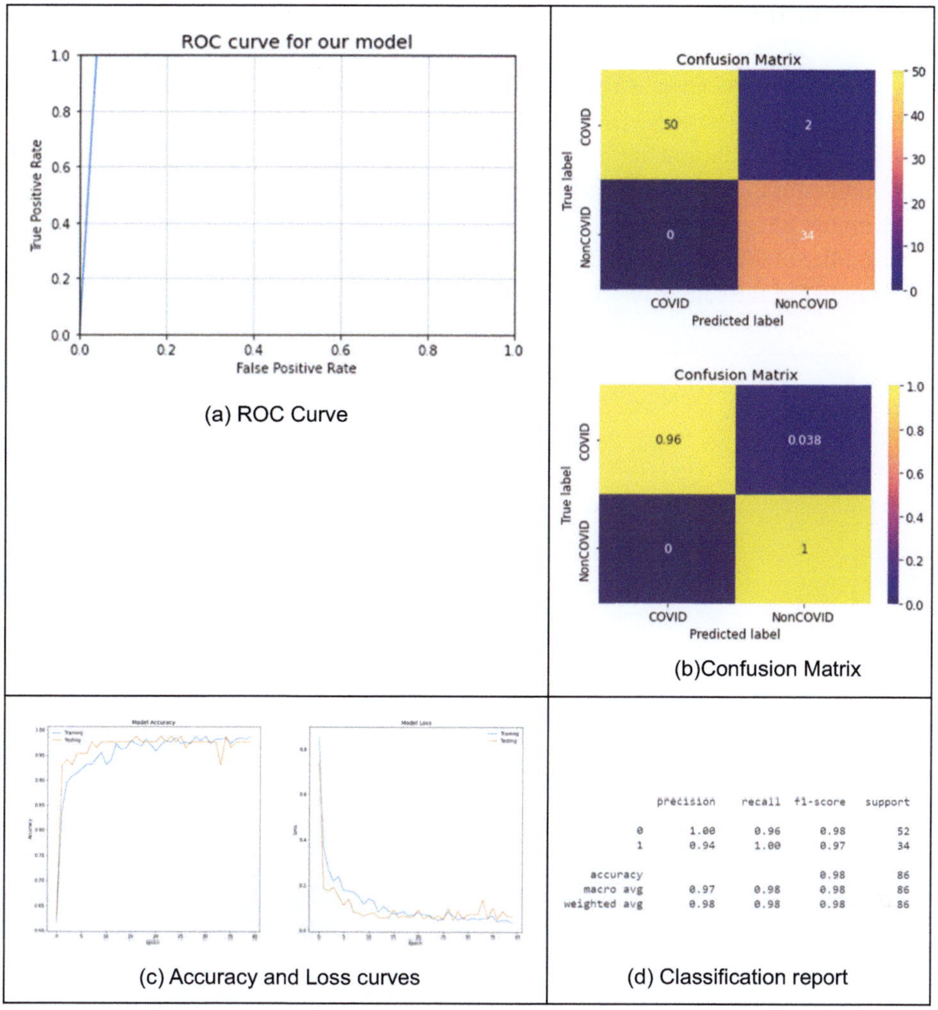

Figure 19: Implementation results of VGG Net.

7.2.1 Graphical analysis

The graphs in Figure 19(c) trace the train and validation (test) learning curves for accuracy and loss over 40 epochs. With each epoch, the accuracy seems to increase while the loss seems to decrease. While VGGnet shows the promise of a good fit, it would seem more time has to be devoted to training the model.

7.3 Inception V3

The model tested 86 chest X-rays and classified them into two sets: COVID cases and Non-COVID cases. The conclusions that can be derived from the confusion matrix generated for the test dataset are as follows:

- Number of Covid cases successfully forecasted by the model: 52
- Number of non-Covid cases successfully forecasted by the model: 34
- Number of false positives: 0
- Number of false negatives:0

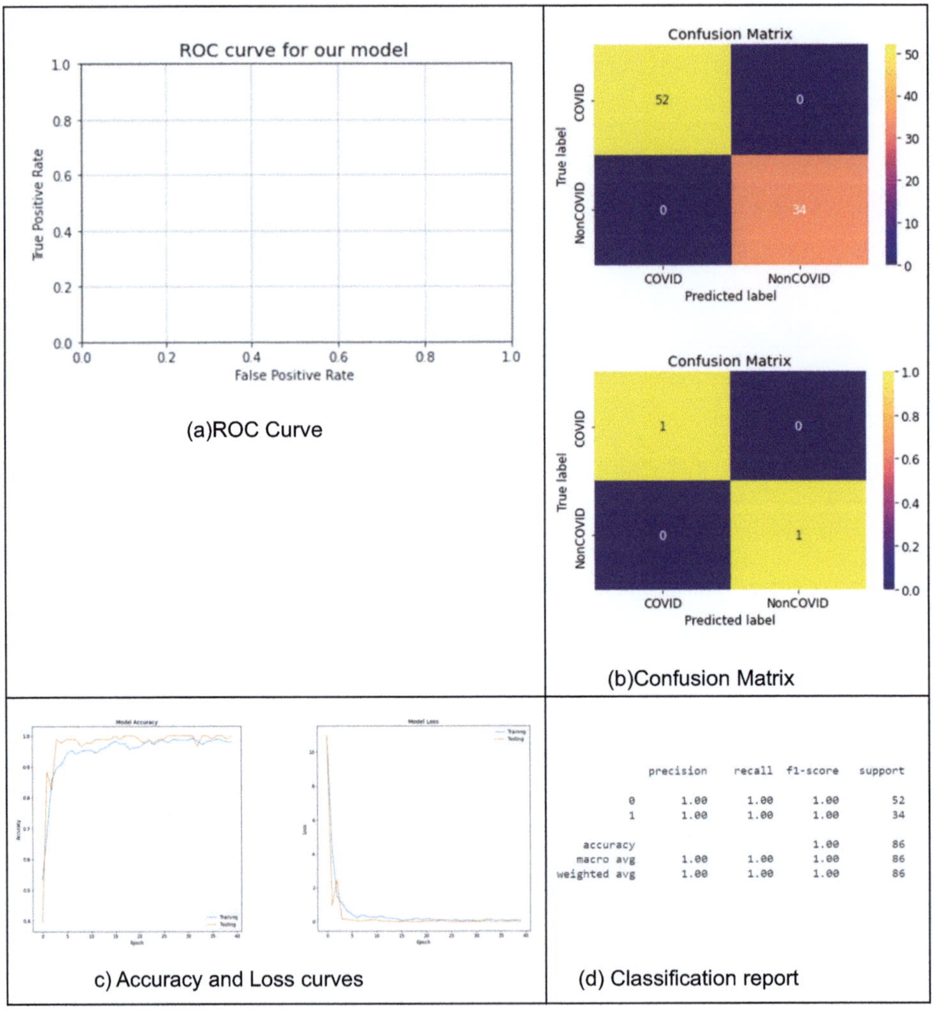

Figure 20: Implementation results of Inception V3.

The results are described in Figure 20.

To appraise the implementation ability of the model, let's look at the classification report generated for the test dataset chosen for this instance:

- Out of 86 chest X-rays, the number of occurrences of positive cases was 52.
- For COVID cases (represented by class label 0): The model was successful in predicting 100% of the positive cases as positive.
- For non-COVID cases (represented by class label 1): The model was accurate in predicting 100% of the non-Covid cases rightly as non-Covid.
- The overall exactness of the model is found to be 100% on the test dataset.

7.3.1 Graphical analysis

The graphs in Figure 20(c) trace the train and validation (test) learning curves for accuracy and loss over 40 epochs. The plots of both the learning curves demonstrate an example of a good fit.

7.4 Resnet 50

The model tested 86 chest X-rays and classified them into two sets: COVID cases and non-COVID cases. The conclusions that can be drawn from the confusion matrix generated for the test dataset are as follows:

- Sum of Covid cases successfully calculated by the model: 48
- Sum of non-Covid cases successfully calculated by the model: 32
- Sum of false positives: 2
- Sum of false negatives: 4

The results are described in Figure 21.

- To assess the implementation ability of the model and analyze its prediction accuracy, let us look at the classification report generated for the datasets chosen for this instance:
- Out of 86 chest X-rays, the number of occurrences of positive cases was 52.
- For COVID cases (represented by class label 0): The model was successful in predicting only 92% of the positive cases as positive. The recall being lower than the precision indicates that some positive cases were misdiagnosed by the model as negative.
- For non-COVID cases (represented by class label 1): The model was accurate in predicting only 94% of the non-Covid cases rightly as non-Covid. The higher recall compared to precision indicates that there were some false positives.
- The overall exactness of the model was found to be 93% on the test dataset.

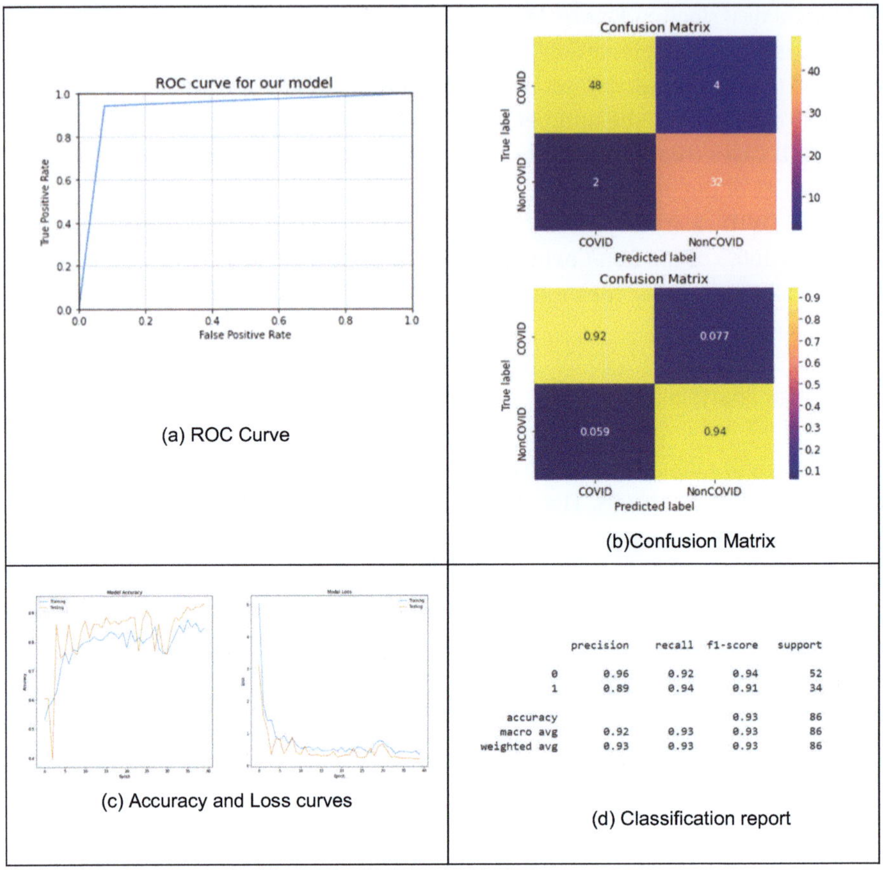

Figure 21: Performance results of Restnet model.

7.4.1 Graphical analysis

- The graphs in Figure 21(c) trace the train and validation (test) learning curves for accuracy and loss over 40 epochs. From the obtained curves, it is quite obvious that the training and validation curves of both accuracy and loss are noisy and barely coinciding. This implies that there is scope for improvement using the hyperparameter tuning method.

8 Results and discussion

As the primary intent of the experiment is to appraise the performance and significance of four algorithms and find the best among all, we tabulate the comprehensive result analysis of the algorithms.

Table 1: Comparative study of the algorithms.

Parameter	CNN	VGGNET	INCEPTION	RESNET
Training time (min)	46.89	197.32	**43.83**	48.41
AUC	0.9615	0.9808	**1**	0.9321
True positive rate/recall/sensitivity	92%	96%	**100%**	92%
Specificity	100%	100%	**100%**	94%
F_1-score (COVID positive class)	96%	98%	**100%**	94%
Accuracy	95%	98%	**100%**	93%

Analytical study of the performance of the algorithms

- Time: Time is an important parameter to factor into our decision-making process while choosing a model to suit our requirements. An accurate diagnosis at the right time can help improve a patient's prognosis. Out of the four models in consideration, Inception performed the best with respect to time.
- AUC: Area under the ROC curve is a distinguishing parameter that helps in choosing an optimal model of our choice. The closer the value of AUC is to one, the better is the performance of that model. In the above four cases, the AUC value obtained from the ROC curve for inception is one. This model functioned as a perfect classifier, that is, it was successful in differentiating all the positive Covid cases from the negative ones.
- TPR (true positive rate): When using a model in diagnosing a disease or an infection, we look to maximize the sensitivity, also called true positive rate or recall. This one is more crucial to diagnose as many of the positive cases as positive. Out of the above four models, Inception had zero cases of false negatives, which made it more ideal than the rest.
- Specificity [35]: From Table 1, it is observed that the sensitivity is lesser than the specificity for the same test data in the case of CNN, VGGNET, and Restnet50, indicating that the number of false negatives was more than the number of false positives, while Inception performs the best as there are zero cases of both false positives and false negatives, thereby acting as the best classifier in this context. This phenomenon is reflected in their respective ROC curves (see Figures 18–21(a)) which plots their TPR versus FPR at various threshold values. While AUC helps in providing an idea of the model's working as a classifier, the sensitivity versus specificity comparison

helps choose the best model for our area of application in which we aim to maximize the sensitivity as much as possible.
- F_1-score: In the above table, the F_1-score is represented as a percentage. Inception had the best F_1-score.
- Accuracy: Inception was the most accurate overall, while Resnet50 was the least accurate.

From the experiment above, we can conclude that inception V3 outperforms other algorithms in our classification model analysis. This work will support to provide readers with information about how image data can be fed into a DL model to formulate the learning task and finally come out with a prediction. The outcome of this experiment will surely help relevant authorities to decide on lockdown measures.

9 Limitations of deep learning

- A large amount of data is essential in DL. In many cases, especially in the medical domain, obtaining labeled data [36] is a major challenge. Furthermore, when using deeper architecture, it requires a lot of time to train, thereby needing a GPU-based system, which is an extra cost to users.
- DL works as a black box. Moreover, it works well on benchmarks dataset, but it fails miserably on real-life images.
- Huge training times leads to huge carbon emission, which certainly has an adversarial impact on the environment.
- It is more useful in classification problems rather than regression. It is vulnerable to adversarial inputs.

10 Conclusion

As Covid-19 continues to ravage governments and health communities worldwide, leaving a lasting impact, early prediction and detection can help in effectively drawing up strategies to curb this pandemic. In this chapter, we explored the effectiveness of different deep-learning-based models in accurately diagnosing Covid cases from chest X-ray images. Through a comparative study, we aimed to understand the capability of deep and transfer learning models, their limitations, and explored some of the possible solutions to address those limitations. Based on the experimental outcomes, proper strategies can be inculcated by doctors and clinicians, which in turn improves patient outcomes drastically and prevents the number of deaths through timely intervention. AI, ML, and, DL models help quicken the decision-making process by analyzing real-time data and images. These allied techniques help governments formulate and propose effective preventive strategies to combat the pandemic. Comparatively, in its beginning stages, advanced DL algorithms have a lot of scope in the medical field. With more experimentation with DL algorithms using the segmentation method on a large number of image samples, the future of such models looks to be bright in this field and we plan to extend our work in that direction. Despite their satisfactory performance, the huge time and data required to train these models pose a challenge to researchers and computer scientists alike.

References

[1] Sen, S., Thejas, B. K., Pranitha, B. L., Amrita, I. Analysis, Visualization and Prediction of COVID-19 Pandemic Spread Using Machine Learning. In: Innovations in Computer Science and Engineering. Lecture Notes in Networks and Systems, Saini, H. S., Sayal, R., Govardhan, A., Buyya, R. (eds.), Vol. 171, Singapore, Springer, 2021, https://doi.org/10.1007/978-981-33-4543-0_63.

[2] Punn, N. S., Sonbhadra, S. K., Agarwal, S. COVID-19 epidemic analysis using machine learning and deep learning algorithms. MedRxiv, 2020.

[3] Sen, S., Amrita, I. A transfer learning based approach for lung inflammation detection. In: International Conference on Emerging Applications of Information Technology. Singapore, Springer, 2021.

[4] Khasnis, N. S., Sen, S., Khasnis, S. S. A machine learning approach for sentiment analysis to nurture mental health amidst covid-19. In: Proceedings of the International Conference on Data Science, Machine Learning and Artificial Intelligence. 2021.

[5] Sandeep, V. Y., Sen, S., Santosh, K. Analyzing and processing of astronomical images using deep learning techniques. 2021 IEEE International Conference on Electronics, Computing and Communication Technologies (CONECCT). IEEE, 2021.

[6] Sen, S., et al. Astronomical big data processing using machine learning: A comprehensive review. Experimental Astronomy, 2022, 1–43.

[7] Sen, S., et al. Implementation of neural network regression model for faster redshift analysis on cloud-based spark platform. In: International Conference on Industrial, Engineering and Other Applications of Applied Intelligent Systems. Cham, Springer, 2021.

[8] Ghaderzadeh, M., Asadi, F. Deep learning in the detection and diagnosis of COVID-19 using radiology modalities: A systematic review. Journal of Healthcare Engineering, 2021, 2021.

[9] Ahamed, P., et al. Handwritten Arabic numerals recognition using convolutional neural network. Journal of Ambient Intelligence and Humanized Computing, 11(11), 2020, 5445–5457.

[10] Aljaafari, N. Ichthyoplankton classification tool using Generative Adversarial Networks and transfer learning. Dissertation, 2018.

[11] https://towardsdatascience.com/understanding-and-coding-a-resnet-in-keras-446d7ff84d33

[12] Darji, P. A., et al. Feature extraction with capsule network for the COVID-19 disease prediction though X-ray images. Materials Today: Proceedings, 2021.

[13] Wang, L., Lin, Z. Q., Wong, A. Covid-net: A tailored deep convolutional neural network design for detection of covid-19 cases from chest x-ray images. Scientific Reports, 2020, 10(1), 1–12.

[14] Mellado, B., Wu, J., Kong, J. D., Bragazzi, N. L., Asgary, A., Kawonga, M., Choma, N., Hayasi, K., Lieberman, B., Mathaha, T., Mbada, M., Ruan, X., Stevenson, F., Orbinski, J. Leveraging artificial intelligence and big data to optimize COVID-19 clinical public health and vaccination roll-out strategies in Africa. International Journal of Environmental Research and Public Health, 2021, 18(15), 7890. https://doi.org/10.3390/ijerph18157890

[15] Gao, Y., Cai, G. Y., Fang, W., et al. Machine learning based early warning system enables accurate mortality risk prediction for COVID-19. Nature Communications, 2020, 11(1), 5033. Published 2020 Oct 6. doi: 10.1038/s41467-020-18684-2.

[16] Rashed, E. A., Hirata, A. Infectivity upsurge by COVID-19 viral variants in Japan: Evidence from deep learning modeling. International Journal of Environmental Research and Public Health, 2021, 18(15), 7799. https://doi.org/10.3390/ijerph18157799

[17] Brierley, L., Fowler, A. Predicting the animal hosts of coronaviruses from compositional biases of spike protein and whole genome sequences through machine learning. PLoS Pathog, 2021 Apr 20, 17(4), e1009149. doi: 10.1371/journal.ppat.1009149. PMID: 33878118; PMCID: PMC8087038.

[18] Kumar, S., et al. Forecasting the spread of COVID-19 using LSTM network. BMC Bioinformatics, 22(6), 2021, 1–9.

[19] Kumar, R. L., et al. Recurrent neural network and reinforcement learning model for covid-19 prediction. Frontiers in Public Health, 2021, 9.

[20] Luo, J., et al. Time series prediction of COVID-19 transmission in America using LSTM and XGBoost algorithms. Results in Physics, 2021, 27, 104462.

[21] Kang, Y. Prediction models of COVID-19 based on SEIR and LSTM RNN. In: AIP Conference Proceedings. Vol. 2350. No. 1. AIP Publishing LLC, 2021.

[22] Masum, M., et al. r-LSTM: Time series forecasting for covid-19 confirmed cases with LSTMbased framework. In: 2020 IEEE International Conference on Big Data (Big Data). IEEE, 2020.

[23] Narin, A., Kaya, C., Pamuk, Z. Automatic detection of coronavirus disease (covid-19) using x-ray images and deep convolutional neural networks. Pattern Analysis and Applications, 2021, 24(3), 1207–1220.

[24] https://www.analyticsvidhya.com/blog/2021/06/build-vgg-net-from-scratch-with-python/.

[25] http://colah.github.io/posts/2015-08-Understanding-LSTMs/.

[26] Kafieh, R., et al. COVID-19 in Iran: Forecasting pandemic using deep learning. Computational and Mathematical Methods in Medicine, 2021, 2021.

[27] https://www.cdc.gov/coronavirus/2019-ncov/variants/variant-classifications.html.

[28] https://github.com/Jayanth9601/COVID-19_Detection_using_CNN/tree/main/Covid-19_Dataset/Covid-19_Dataset/Processed%20data.

[29] Á, N., Ligeti, B., Szebeni, J., Pongor, S., Gyrffy, B. COVIDOUTCOME-estimating COVID severity based on mutation signatures in the SARS-CoV-2 genome. Database (Oxford). 2021 May 8;2021:baab020. doi: 10.1093/database/baab020. PMID: 33963845; PMCID: PMC8106440.

[30] https://ospreydata.com/category/data-science/.

[31] Wang, S.-H., et al. Alcoholism identification based on an AlexNet transfer learning model. Frontiers in Psychiatry, 2019, 10, 205.

[32] Huang, G., et al. Densely connected convolutional networks. In: Proceedings of the IEEE conference on computer vision and pattern recognition. 2017.

[33] https://analyticsindiamag.com/understanding-capsule-net-with-its-implementation-in-computer-vision/.

[34] https://towardsdatascience.com/confusion-matrix-for-your-multi-class-machine-learning-model-ff9aa3bf7826.

[35] Trevethan, R. Sensitivity, specificity, and predictive values: Foundations, pliabilities, and pitfalls in research and practice. Frontiers in Public Health, 2017, 5, 307.

[36] https://medium.com/geekculture/the-challenges-recent-advances-and-future-of-deep-learning-d714304656b.

[37] Monisha, R., Sen, S., Davangeri, R. U., Sri Lakshmi, K. S., Dey, S. An approach toward design and implementation of distributed framework for astronomical big data processing. In: Intelligent Systems. Lecture Notes in Networks and Systems, Udgata, S. K., Sethi, S., Gao, X. Z. (eds.), Vol. 431, Singapore, Springer, 2022, https://doi.org/10.1007/978-981-19-0901-6_26.

Sougata Mazumder*, Rahul Deb Das, Snahasish Karmakar,
Madorina Paul Das, Prasun Ghosal

Role of IoT and drones in tackling COVID-19 and future pandemics: global use cases

Abstract: The role of technology in the fight against COVID-19 has been truly tremendous. Intelligent computing, complemented by the adoption of technology, has been the key to minimizing the pandemic's rippling effect by manifolds. At a time when the pandemic has affected millions of lives, it is essential for human kind to keep investing in technologies such as IoT, drones, etc. to combat the newer strains and the future pandemics. IoT has helped in the creation of smart frameworks and intelligent systems to respond to the ever-increasing COVID-19 cases in a much better way, whereas drones gave critical stakeholders an advantage over time and management constraints. During COVID-19, certain countries utilized drone services for disinfection, increased testing rates, speedy medical deliveries, etc. This chapter aims to discuss the role of IoT and drones to tackle COVID-19, from a global perspective. It highlights various use cases of leveraging drones and IoT in tackling COVID-19 effectively. An insight into this chapter will help tackle future pandemics or epidemics in a much convenient way. It will provide the readers a summary of the scenarios when technologies were leveraged and spark a field for future researchers to understand the gaps and improve the existing systems.

1 Introduction

COVID-19 has engulfed the entire world, claiming millions of lives in the last couple of years. While the effect of this pandemic could not be avoided entirely, leveraging technology helped us in restricting the spread to a large extent. Gradually, with the increasing innovations, it helped us not only in restricting the spread, but also in the fields of diagnosis, treatment and even logistic support.

This chapter aims to summarize the various global use cases related to leveraging of Internet of things (IoT) as a tool to tackle COVID-19. Scientists and innovators from across the world came up with amazing technologies to aid this pandemic. These were wearables, drones, robots, smartphone applications, etc. Each of them was leveraged to

***Corresponding author: Sougata Mazumder,** Indian Institute of Engineering Science and Technology, Shibpur, India
Snahasish Karmakar, Prasun Ghosal, Indian Institute of Engineering Science and Technology, Shibpur, India
Rahul Deb Das, IBM, Germany
Madorina Paul Das, University of Calcutta, India

https://doi.org/10.1515/9783110767681-014

help in social distancing, improving patient's healthcare, continuous monitoring, delivery of essential commodities, diagnosis, and treatment in a very cost-effective way. Broadly, these smart systems could help in the different phases of a pandemic, like early diagnosis, quarantine, and after recovery.

This chapter is informative in nature and discusses briefly about some IoT and drone use cases. This can give the readers an overview of the tools utilized for minimizing the effect of such a huge pandemic that devastates the lives of millions. This chapter has indeed proven how technology, with the help of healthcare, can save lives and prevent the spread of infections. In the future pandemics, such tools can be readily deployed at the initial phases to contain the widespread.

For the convenience of readers, this chapter has been divided into sections such as literature review, global use cases, conclusion, and references.

The literature review section highlights the various scenarios under which smart tools like IoT and drones has been utilized to mitigate the effects of COVID-19. The next section on global use cases discusses a total of 15 examples where such technologies were deployed. It contains illustrative figures to showcase the working mechanisms of some of the important cases. The conclusion section encompasses the final outcomes and narrative of the tools and use cases. To deep dive into the cases, references have been enlisted for the readers to have a detailed understanding of each case.

2 Literature review

A total of six epidemics have shaken the world in the past years, including the recent epidemic caused by SARS-CoV-2 virus, which is commonly known as COVID-19 [1].

An outbreak of COVID-19 was first identified in 2019 in Wuhan, China. It can cause mild to severe respiratory problems. In serious conditions, it causes death also. As per the World Health Organization, more than 43 crore people are infected now, while mortality exceeds 59 lakhs throughout the world. According to the World Health Organization, COVID-19 mainly spreads through droplets from an infected person when they sneeze, speak, or breathe. People can also get infected if they touch their nose, eyes, or mouth after touching any contaminated surface. To overcome the difficulties caused due to the pandemic, any alternative techniques should be evaluated to confront the new corona virus. Primarily, maintaining social distance, wearing masks, and getting vaccinated can help to manage the situation. The unavoidable need for social distancing has led to a surge in contactless delivery of different items.

All types of national resources like human, political, material, and financial have been mobilized in the fight against the COVID-19 pandemic on a very large scale across the globe [2]. Some countries have employed different smart technologies, which include cognitive robots, drones, sensor-based smart devices, and intelligent apps (applications), to manage and restrict the risk of COVID-19 pandemic [3].

IoT, robots, and drones were judiciously leveraged to tackle COVID-19. Manual collection of COVID-19 samples increased the chance of getting exposed to the virus for healthcare professionals, mostly. But the use of robots helped to minimize the risk of exposure, hasten sample collection, and increase the COVID-19 testing capacity. For example, checking body temperature at strategic points in public places were carried out by mobile robots integrated with automated cameras and a thermal sensor [4].

Drones, which play a dynamic role in the aviation industry, have also been used as a very special tool to fight this pandemic [5]. Nowadays, the use of drones in the professional world and during major crises, e.g., coronavirus is becoming more prevalent [6]. The usage of drone or airborne instruments is not new. This has been used in the past. For example, during the world wars and during other historical events, drones or airborne instruments have been used extensively. Although, drones are initially developed as an airborne weapons for survey and reconnaissance in the past (e.g., TDR-1 during World War II), over time, drones have been used for societal cause, humanitarian relief, in civil and construction industry, and for entertainment purposes. During World War I and World War II, airborne drones were used mainly for disruption of airspace above cities [7].

The widespread use of drones in the non-military field is increasing gradually to combat COVID-19. Drones are employed for cargo delivery, in search and rescue missions, and for disaster-response mapping [8, 9].

Drones by Dragonfly, equipped with latest technologies, enable the early detection of COVID 19 as well [10]. In terms of physical structure, there are primarily four types of drones available, e.g., multi-rotor, fixed wing, single rotor helicopter, and fixed wing hybrid VTOL. Different types of drones possess different flight capabilities, efficiencies, and payload capacities.

Multi rotor drones are capable of vertical take-off and landing and provide better cruise control and hovering ability. In fact, more the number of rotors, better is the hovering and the control it provides. The number of rotors can be 4, 6, or 8. However, as the number of rotors increase, the complexity of the drones also increases. This type of drone is often used for videography and photography. The main drawback of a multi-rotor drone is that they cannot fly for a long duration, as a fixed-wing drone.

A fixed-wing drone has two propellers on either side of its body and can fly long distances for over 16 h. This type of drone is generally used for tasks that require long flight distance travel, for example military surveillance, agriculture, or forest inspection, to name a few. One of the main drawbacks of this kind of drones is that they cannot take-off and land as easily as a multi rotor drone. A fixed-wing drone, due to its avionic property, cannot hover as easily as a multi rotor drone, either. This type of drone often requires a runway to take-off or land.

A single-rotor helicopter is a type of drone that acts like a multi-rotor drone in terms of take-off and landing. It can carry heavy payload. However, they are not as efficient as a multi-rotor drone. This type of drone is often used for surveying, 3D laser scanning and reconnaissance, and in situations where a heavy payload needs to be carried.

To take the middle ground, very recently, a specialized drone has been developed that can haul long distance like a fixed-wing drone and at the same time it can take-off and land vertically with better flight control. This type of hybrid drone is called a fixed-wing hybrid VTOL.

Usage of drone in policy execution, especially in a regulatory framework, to track public activities often needs approval from concerned authorities and government bodies. As drones can pose significant privacy concern and safety threats, there are lots of restrictions on using drones in the public sphere. However, it is seen that during any emergency, government makes changes in their regulations and adopts new technology. Integrating drones in monitoring public health and managing government regulations (e.g., social distancing, lockdown measure) involves changes in regulatory framework in different countries. For example, on March 23, 2020, the Italian Civilian Aviation Authority allowed the local police and the enforcement department to observe crowd movement during lockdown to ensure prevention of physical contacts and social distancing. On the same line, Portugal approved the usage of drone in the fight against COVID-19 in April–May 2020, followed by France [11]. Malaysian authorities implemented a drone-based monitoring system to observe and control public movement during COVID-19 [12]. In May 2020, in the USA, a consortium of commercial drone companies sought approval from the US Secretary of Transportation and the FAA Administrator to use drones for delivering packages to customers during the pandemic. This also helped in their last mile delivery problem, where traditional ground-based delivery vans could not reach [13].

In the context of the COVID-19 pandemic, based on the media reports and other available sources, the main uses of drones are broadly classified in three categories. These include: (a) lab sample pick-up, and delivery and transportation of medical supplies (in order to reduce the exposure to infection and to reduce the transportation time), (b) public place monitoring and guidance (especially during lockdown and quarantine), and (c) aerial spraying (to disinfect the potential contaminated areas) [14].

Several studies have been carried out by scientists to find out the efficacy of drones in managing COVID-19. Mbunge et al. [15] focused on the significant capacities of robots and drones to lighten the workload of front-line medical staff, particularly in sub-Saharan Africa [15]. The logistical problems with the drones that were being employed for delivery reasons were noted by Kunovjanek et al. In their study, they looked into how viral testing kits were distributed using drones to patients who might be infected . Their study was unique in that they employed already-existing drone infrastructure to carry out the assignment, reassembling drones owned and operated by various private and public bodies to distribute the necessary items, in the event of an emergency [16]. Poljak and Šterbene [17] conducted pilot studies where they used drones for transporting samples, vaccines, medicines, life-saving equipment, and organs [17].

Restas categorized six application areas where drone can be useful in the face of COVID-19 pandemic: (a) aerial surveillance with visual camera, (b) fever detection with thermal camera, (c) communication with loudspeakers or QR-coded flags, (d) general logistics applications to dispatch basic requirements and commodities, (e) medical logistics to dispatch medicine, drugs, defibrillators and collecting samples, and (f) special logistics for spraying disinfectants [18].

Aerial surveillance can typically take place over a small area or a large area that is limited to 10,000 sq. m. The selection of the size or the coverage of subjects is linked to the objective of the task. In the case of monitoring the traffic condition (especially during lockdown), the size could be larger. If it is to monitor public health, the size could be smaller. Currently, several cities are using drones to monitor crowds on the street, e.g., Budapest, Vilnius, and Istanbul, to name a few.

For fever detection, most countries are using thermal scanners and remote thermometers in all the public places. However, this could be made more efficient and safer by using drones with thermal scanners, especially in areas where personal contact is not possible or not recommended.

Generally, by using a thermal scanner aboard, a drone can detect the thermal anomaly and demarcate people with high temperatures. A further action can be taken to communicate with the person or the community, and recommend isolation until the febrile person recovers and shows normal temperature.

During the pandemic, many cities used loudspeakers onboard drones to announce and communicate various regulatory messages to the community. This could be towards a small group or a moderate group, or even a larger group of people.

Drones have been in use for logistic application before the pandemic. However, during the pandemic, the application has increased a lot. This helped in contactless delivery, solving last mile delivery problem, and specially to prevent exposure to the infection through physical contact. This approach has helped many communities, both in the urban and rural areas, during COVID-19. Although there is no reported literature on how drone operators optimize their route to minimize the fuel and maximize their efficiency and provide support to the people in need, some researchers and operators recently started exploring the optimization aspect in the light of the COVID-19 pandemic.

Drones have been a great tool to dispatch daily commodities as well as in collecting samples from symptomatic patients and dispatch that sample to the nearby laboratories. Once a person is detected to be positive, further medication and drugs could be delivered to that person through drones. In many cases, heavy duty drones delivered defibrillators to the patients.

Drones have been also used for spraying disinfectants to various communities. In fact, in the past, drones have been used for fertilizer and insecticide spraying over agricultural lands. The same approach is used for spraying disinfectant during COVID-19. Restas recommended that the droplet should be less than 300 mm, with an average droplet density of 200 pcs per square meters, with a 1.5 m flight altitude and at least 12% surface coverage, for an effective spraying operation [18].

Images taken by the drones often undergo image processing tasks and object detection through various artificial intelligence (AI) techniques, namely computer vision and various deep learning approaches. With the help of AI, corona virus infection can be addressed in a very creative way. Due to the unavailability of historical data, the COVID-19 training models for AI had difficulties. Robots and drones, outfitted with IoT devices, generate raw data that must be processed through computing in order to make it relevant and usable, without the involvement of humans [19]. Drones can be used to eliminate a very high percentage of contamination by minimizing human contact [20].

A majority of studies supported the use of unmanned aerial vehicle technology in healthcare by transporting blood samples and to help situations of out-of-hospital cardiac arrest [21–24].

According to data published by a research firm, Drone Analysis (2020) [25], in 2019, the U.S consumer drone fleet increased by a mere 6% in comparison to 2016. Drones have been in use in the e-commerce and logistics industries for parcel delivery before the pandemic. However, with the emergence of the pandemic, the commercial viability and potential use of such technology has increased significantly. Despite the negative aspect of COVID-19, it has a positive connotation for drone usage for the commercial sector. Wolf mentioned this pandemic period as a 'Golden Age' of drone delivery as various companies were using this opportunity to test the effectiveness of their drones at-scale, and in a real demanding situation [26].

Some countries, for example, Australia, used drones to fight COVID-19 by detecting whether someone had "doubtful" respiratory pattern or not [27]. Here, sensors were fixed to the drones to record the temperature, respiratory rate, pulse rate, and miscellaneous abnormalities. This was found very effective and useful too. Sanitization was monitored using a Terra drone by spraying disinfectant over large areas in China. This method was found effective in rural areas where scarcity of medical supply was seen [28].

Drones were mostly used for distributing medical and essential goods in contaminated areas, but in less densely populated or in mountain regions, it was a challenging task, especially for drones with limited flight altitude capability [29]. Sometimes, proper knowledge and training is needed for the health workers while dealing with these types of technologies. Despite few shortcomings, many countries were willing to adopt this type of technological support, which help nations to reduce gaps and work towards health coverage, while taking proper COVID-19-specific regulatory measures.

3 Global use cases

3.1 Case study 1

Proactive reaction to COVID-19 and increased rates of testing have been key to limit the spread. Limited response has resulted in higher rates of infection in countries such as USA [30]. On the contrary, countries such as South Korea adopted rapid monitoring and testing measures, leading to a successful tackling of this pandemic. It is often christened as syndromic monitoring system, which helps in gathering relevant information before interaction with a procedural healthcare process. This helped countries during COVID-19 to tactically reduce the transmission and detection rates. Taiwan is a great example of how by utilizing such big data, COVID-19 was tackled much proactively [31]. Even during the previous pandemics such as Ebola, rapid detection proved to be the correct way to control outbreaks in West Africa [32, 33].

Physiological data connected through connected devices are reliable to detect symptoms and control the spread of any disease. Parameters such as temperature, heart rates, etc. are crucial in response strategies [34]. Such physiologically grounded data from connected geolocated networks is helpful to enhance tracking and in the prediction of any outbreak, especially pandemics such as COVID-19 [35, 36]. Real-time syndromic data thus removes the constraint of time, offering stakeholders a buffer time to proactively respond to the situation [37].

In this case, we take the case of Kinsa, Inc., where geospatially connected smart thermometers helped identify anomalies of illness incidences [30].

The flowchart below (Figure 1) showcases how anomaly detection is done:

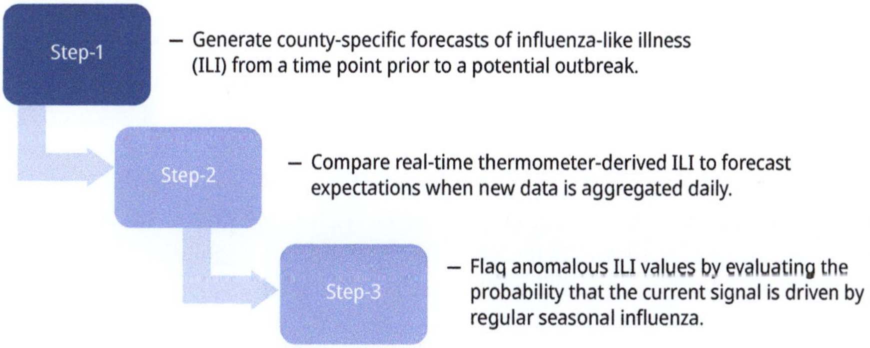

Figure 1: Steps in anomaly detection.

Kinsa manages a network of smart thermometers connected geospatially through smart-phones. Only those ILI values are flagged that exceed 97.5 percentile of the expected properties of influenza. Whenever a user records their temperature, the sensor network captures the data and the geolocation. Temperature is stored via Kinsa's Smartphone App, whereas location data is tracked on the basis of GPS Location or IP Addresses. Readings are anonymized and integrated to higher degree ILI (such as county and state) based on which, users with higher temperatures over a period of time are clustered. The recorded temperatures are used to create ILI signals, correlated with national ILI and region ILI by the Center for Disease Control and Prevention (CDC). It has been constructed strategically to identify anomalies at the granular level across cities. This analysis only considers counties with a minimum one case of COVID-19, since lack of cases could be attributed largely to testing and reporting, especially during a pandemic of this immense magnitude.

Catering to the varying patterns of seasonal flu transmission, population size and other factors, daily user data helps detect Local ILIs. This forecast considers the distinct but predictable intensity patterns, attributed to climate and population density of each city [38, 39].

Real-time implementation of Kinsa's solution yielded some interesting results. It was leveraged for Brooklyn, New York (NY), USA.
- March 1, 2020 (before large scale outbreaks at NY Metro Area): Forecast showcased divergence from influenza trajectories expected from the area.
- March 16, 2020 (school closures) and March 20, 2020 (stay-at-home order): Inflection back to declining ILI, owing to social distancing measures.
- More declining ILI trends observed in areas having 'Shelter-in-Place' order, such as Santa Clara, CA.

It suggested that social distancing has a direct impact on the estimates for proper identification of anomalies. Hence, on maintaining such measures, influenza transmissions could also be controlled, apart from COVID-19. To increase the sensitivity of the model and to include the effect of social distancing, reproduction rates for all days were reduced by 25%. This led to an increase in anomaly incidence. For Santa Clara County and Miami-Dada County, social distancing measures, such as school closures and shelter-in-place, were accounted for. This showed that real-time ILI values fell below anomalous levels, indicating a lesser rate of transmission. The authors also rightly mentioned how this 25% cannot be a perfect number, since policy adoption, implementation, execution, and adherence varies with place and situation. To increase the relevance of such anomaly detection methodology, social distancing measures could enhance the accuracy and refine results accordingly.

3.2 Case study 2

Coronavirus is a new form of virus that causes illness in both animals and individuals. It was first discovered in Wuhan in December 2019 and it spread in the world very rapidly. The virus was named "corona" because of the royal crown-shaped spike shell. The virus is very infectious and can easily pass from person to person [40–42].

The persons infected with corona show common symptoms like fever, dry cough, tiredness, running nose, and diarrhea, and feels pains and aches [43, 44]. However, most of the people do not show any symptoms; they are asymptomatic. About 80% of the people infected by COVID 19 recovered without getting any particular treatment, but it is severe with people having health disorders [45].

The health industry has also adopted IoT technologies. The primary goal of this study is to use a smart helmet, equipped with a Thermal Imaging System, to automatically detect the coronavirus using thermal images, with minimal human intervention. The thermal camera is incorporated inside the smart helmet, together with IoT technology, for real-time data collection, while the screening system is being monitored.

The system sends a notification if it detects a temperature more than the normal body temperature; the GPS helps in determining the present location of the person and sends a notification to the assigned mobile number through a GSM.

The project is based on Arduino IDE (Arduino Integrated development environment). It uses Java language. It also uses C and C++ languages. Proteus software helps in making real-time stimulation [46, 47]. Thermology is the best method for scanning individuals as well as large number of people. It helps in detecting the increased body temperature and the person to be isolated. AI helps in diagnosing COVID 19. Infervision software helps in automatically detecting the temperature through screening images and quickly diagnose, reducing human error.

GLH, Google Location history gives the detail information of all the places visited by the infected. GLH keeps record of each and every place. GLH helps in accessing the users' habit and mobility [48, 49].

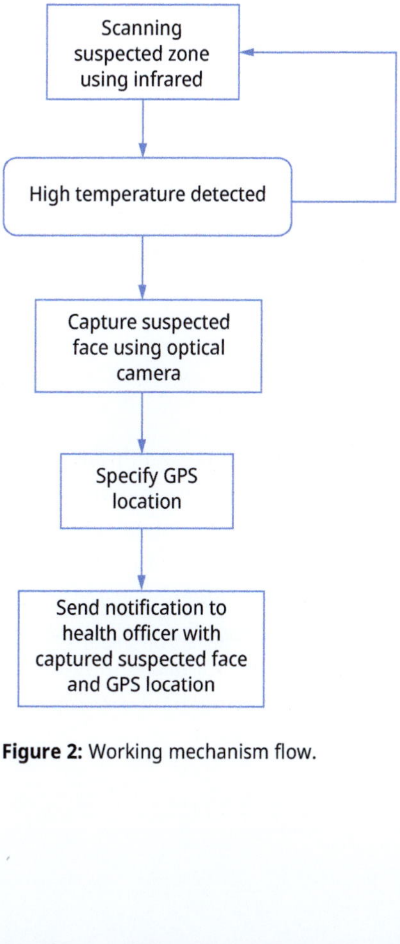

Figure 2: Working mechanism flow.

After getting all the information, like face, body temperature and GPS location by Arduino software, the micro-controller (NodeMcu) now spreads the information over the web so that everyone can access the information, and for this, an exterior server, called Blynk, was used. As soon as the camera detects a high temperature, the system sends it to the authorities and also to the health officer.

So, we have come to the conclusion that this innovative thermal imaging system will very much help the healthcare system in detecting coronavirus.

The working mechanism is given below in Figure 2:

3.3 Case study 3

The new form of coronavirus that infected a large number of people was also from the same group of virus, SARS. Infected people show symptoms similar to the previous one, like running nose, sore throat, body pain, fever, and diarrhea [50].

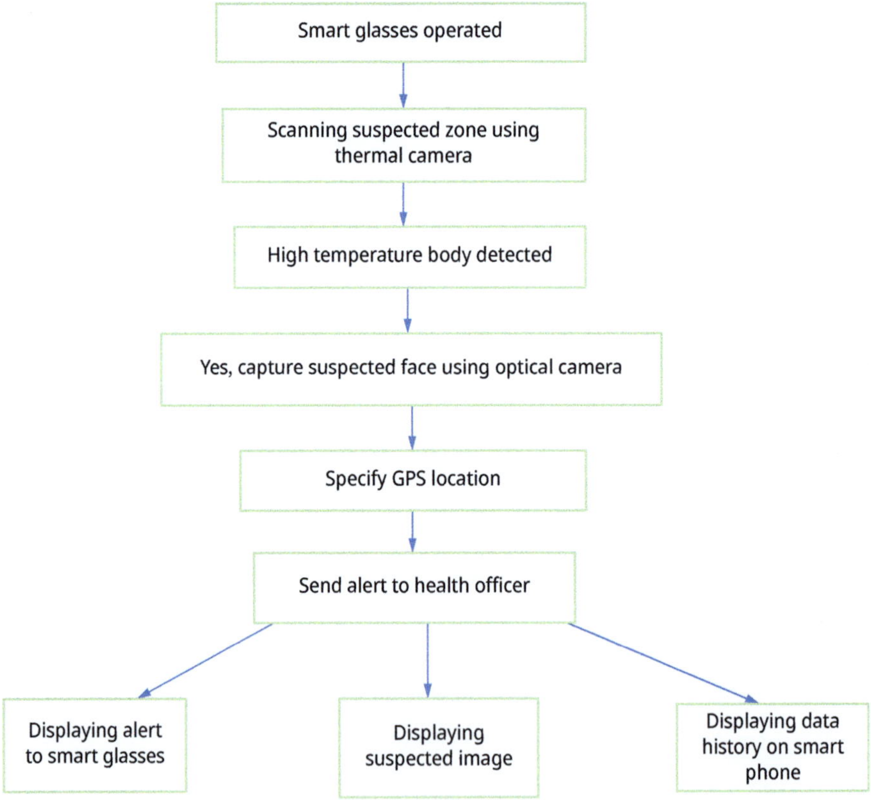

Figure 3: Working system mechanism.

The symptoms are very much mild in most people and the recovery rate is also more than 80%, but it is dangerous for people having serious health disorders. Lockdown was the only way to decrease the number of positive cases [51].

The health sector has become advanced with the introduction of IoT. It has played a great role in the medical sector. For example, smart sensors, telemedicine, medical equipment, clinical information systems, etc. are all applications of IoT [52].

For the quick detection of Covid 19, many new technologies have come based on IoT, like smart helmets, which have the capability to automatically detect the body temperature through a thermal imaging system [53].

A new form of device – smart glasses – has come to the market. It automatically detects the high temperature by thermal camera among the crowds and sends it to an officer. It can also tell the visited locations of the suspected cases through Google Location History (GLH) to provide authentic data, as part of the detection process [54–58]. The working system of smart glasses is given below in Figure 3:

Each and every information is linked with the Google user's account. The places visited by the infected person can be obtained through GLH (Google Location History). GLH is basically used for assessing the user's habit and user's mobility [59, 60]. This will make people aware beforehand, and prevent the spread of this infectious disease.

3.4 Case study 4

The Covid 19 pandemic caused by a newly discovered coronavirus has been spreading exponentially all around the world. It has completely changed the lifestyle of the people. A mask has become an important part of life. Till now, we have seen three phases of Covid 19 and the second phase was the worst. Most countries have imposed lockdown as it is the only option to prevent the spread of coronavirus. This coronavirus pandemic has led to economic crisis, unemployment, depression problems, etc. [61, 62]

Many new technologies have come in for the quick detection of Covid 19. One such innovative technology is an IoMT (Internet of Medical things)-enabled easy band.

Easy band basically contains a sensor that can detect the devices present within the range of 1–4 m (6–13 feet). It has three light signals, red, yellow, and green. Whenever a person wearing the easy band comes in contact with the other person, the device records each other's data and become available in the city or state. It vibrates if it comes within the range of 4 m. If it comes closer, yellow light changes to red light. This helps citizens to maintain social distance.

Easy band has a very complex mechanism system. It contains a power management unit, a Programmable System on Chip (PSoc), wireless stacks, sensors, vibrating motors, and an I/O unit [63].

Easy band contains sensors for contactless thermal profile. It has been seen that during Covid 19, people having health disorders like diabetes are mainly infected; so NIR (near-infrared) sensors from iGLU have been introduced, by which glucose can be monitored without the need for any blood sample [64].

In order to solve the privacy and security issues with easy band, lightweight blockchain and physical unclonable function can be incorporated in its system [65].

In easy band, communication is carried out through the BLE stack. BLEs are used in determining the distance between two devices, and the Wi-Fi unit, through TCP/IP connection, connects with the city server. The distance between the two bands is estimated through RSSI (Received Signal Strength Indicator). When two easy bands come in close contact with each other, the PSoC unit sends signal to both the bands. If the distance between two bands decreases, the color changes from green to yellow. If a person is detected positive, the city server will remove it from the graph and take appropriate action [66].

The IoMT-based easy band is a very advanced and innovative device for Covid detection. It is self-sensing and so, no human interaction is required. Easy band is very much advantageous over mobile apps as mobile apps may sometime not give appropriate information. If the bands are provided by government to all individuals, it would be much cheaper and affordable for the common people.

3.5 Case study 5

Robots are very much beneficial in the health sector. Though they are not commonplace of their cost, they can completely change the scenario of the healthcare system. Telerobotic systems can be made using liquid cleaning solutions and can be used during the admission and screening of patients.

The DaVinci surgical report by Intuitive has obtained popularity in hospitals all over the world. DaVinci is operated by a physician through a surgical console. However, the surgical console is placed in the same room as the patients. The main aim is to isolate the physician from the patients.

We know that in this Covid period, the demand for PPE has increased. Because of the nonavailability of PPEs, doctors and physician have to use a PPE for a longer period of time and reuse the PPE; these practices increase the chances of infection. In order to overcome this practice, Telerobots have come. It is very much helpful for frontline workers. The Telerobotic system allows workers to control the robot with the help of a remote. For example, if a physician needs to check the blood pressure, pulse, and body temperature, the physician can remotely check all these without coming in contact with the patients. So, a telerobotic system reduces the usage of PPE and also the risk of infection [67, 68].

The Telerobotic system can also be used in a normal healthcare system. It can be used to perform ultrasonography in pregnant women; similarly, many tests can be performed with the help of robots. Many major operations are also carried out with the help of the Telerobotic system. It prevents the spread of virus or any infection from one person to another [69].

3.6 Case study 6

John Putters first introduced the IoT (Internet of Things) buttons in hospitals. The IoT buttons are known as WandaQuick Touch. The IoT buttons sends signals to the management for cleaning operations in order to maintain public safety. The IoT buttons help to keep track of all the staff working in the hospitals during COVID 19. The technology enables the hospital management to keep track of all the cleaning activities, once at a time. Wanda Quick can be set up at any place without any infrastructure. The IoT buttons are battery operated and automatically connected to the LTE network. This device is gaining popularity in hospitals as it is affordable, easily installable, and user-friendly. The IoT buttons can be connected with mobile apps for easy tracking of a hospital's cleaning activities [70].

3.7 Case study 7

A new form of robots has come, known as autonomous robots, which help to kill coronavirus in hospitals. The best way to stop the spread of this virus is to break the chain of infection. The common preventive measures are washing our hands frequently, using sanitizers, and social distancing.

Nowadays, people avoid going to hospitals because of its dirty and unhygienic environment, and there is a high chance of infection; that is why autonomous robots have come in. UVD robots, a Danish robot making company, used to disinfect the patients' rooms and operating theatres in hospitals. UVD robots have powerful short wavelength ultraviolet-C (UVC) lights that produce enough energy to shred the DNA and RNA of microorganisms [71].

These robots are currently working in China. The first set of robots was introduced in Wuhan where the first covid case was reported. The target is to make it available in 2000 hospitals in China.

The technology used in autonomous robots is UV disinfecting technology. We have seen this technology mainly to disinfect water that causes damage to the skin and even to the eyes. It is quite costly to set up a UV disinfecting system in hospitals.

UVD robots consist of a mobile base containing multiple lidar sensors and an array of UV lamps mounted on the top. The robot is fully controlled by a computer. It scans the environment and the lidar automatically creates a digital map. With the help of this map, we can point out the places that need to be disinfected.

UVD robots use simultaneous localization and mapping (SLAM) for its navigation. It travels from the charging station through hallways and disinfects all the places automatically, and again returns back to the charging station. For safety, the UVD robots have sensors to detect motion and they automatically shut down when they come in close contact with a person [71].

3.8 Case study 8

The economy all over the world has been badly affected due to COVID19. Many people lost their jobs. Many companies have shut down completely. Work from home concept has been introduced, but it is not possible for all companies. Employees have to go to work to sustain their living.

Looking at their safety, Proximity Trace solution has been designed to maintain social distancing in the workplace. It consists of a compact device called a TraceTag, which is placed over the helmet of a worker [72].

Proximity Trace was designed in such a way that it gives signals or a reminder when a worker comes in contact with another. Contact tracing is the process of identifying a Covid-positive individual. Proximity trace helps to identify the person who has been in close contact with the tested positive individual.

Gateways are installed at entrances and exits. Trace Tags are mandatory for all workers and the Proximity Trace is well connected with the gateways and Trace Tags. It can be specially used at construction sites, in places of mining activities, etc. for the safety of the workers [73].

3.9 Case study 9

The physical health of a person can be indicated by their breathing rates and patterns, with irregular breathing patterns indicating more serious COVID-19 diseases. Therefore, breath monitoring is crucial in therapeutic settings. Traditional breathing measurements include the use of professional medical equipment and hospital visits. With the growth of IoT, breath monitoring is becoming relevant and omnipresent. New devices have come, like IoT sensors, camera, microphone, wave radar, and Wi-Fi, for monitoring breathing activities in detail.

BioWatch leverages devices such as accelerometer, supplemented with a gyroscope of wrist-mounted devices, such as smartwatches, to measure the heart and breathing rates. Within the fixed-end frequencies [0.13 Hz, 0.66 Hz], it uses data recorded by inertial sensors to extracts the breathing signal from wrist motion [74].

Using the self-training algorithms to recognize changes in wrist postures and breathing rates, the resilience and accuracy of bringing out breathing patterns from inertial sensors have been improved to a greater extent. To measure breathing rates during sleep, an accelerometer-based sleep monitor is deemed suitable. For more precise breathing estimation, it employs an advanced technique – the Kalman filter – to integrate the three axes acceleration data [75].

These days, more research has centered on the usage of radio frequency (RF) sensing strategies, primarily based totally on radar and Wi-Fi, to tune respiratory motions. Petkie et al. use Doppler radars with continuous-wave (CW), primarily to reduce the respiratory price at the Doppler-shifted meditated signals [76].

To identify breathing motions, Lai et al. discusses ultra-wideband (UWB) radar, which helps in tracking the breathing of several participants. However, UWB radar's transmission power has limits, reducing the signal-to-noise ratio and detecting range [77]. Recent research has used frequency-modulated continuous wave (FMCW) radars to provide reliable breathing monitoring, avoiding drawbacks of Doppler and UWB radars. Furthermore, the indoor propagation of the Wi-Fi signal such as reflection, scattering, etc. might get affected by breathing motions in the chest and abdomen, which makes it possible to capture breathing motions by analyzing the received Wi-Fi signals [78, 79].

Abdelnasser et al. initially propose UbiBreathe, a breathing estimator based on Wi-Fi, which calculates the breathing rates, depending upon the intensity values of the Wi-Fi signal. Liu et al. uses the amplitude fluctuations of the Wi-Fi channel state information (CSI), which is a measurement for breathing to estimate the breathing rates. Further research will use Wi-Fi CSI phase information to achieve accurate multi-subject breathing monitoring [80–83].

3.10 Case study 10

Blood oxygen saturation (SpO_2) helps in measuring the oxygen-carrying capacity of red blood cells. In general, a healthy person maintains a high level of blood oxygen regulation, which is around 95% or above. For patients, one of the indicators is declining blood SpO_2, and if the blood SpO_2 of a COVID-19 patient is less than 90%, additional treatments (e.g., supplementary oxygen) are required. Furthermore, a lot of research indicated that many patients not facing any discomfort or symptoms had lower levels of SpO_2 [84, 85].

Wieringa et al. proposed a new method involving the use of a camera, consisting of three contrasting wavelengths of LED light, for measuring blood SpO_2. However, a genuine system was not created to provide the measuring results in ambient light so as to detect a small range, i.e., around 97% to 99% of blood SpO_2. Kong et al. used two cameras. RGB camera is used by Guazzi et al. to detect the SpO_2 (over a large range, ranging from 80 to 100%) of subjects who are 1.5 m away. Shao et al. presented a new and low-cost methodology that is ideal for SpO_2 monitoring in home. This is done by measuring the SpO_2 by recording films of a patient's face [86–88].

3.11 Case study 11

The demand for Secufy's IoT Button to solve crucial use cases inside health organizations has resulted in a 100-fold increase in production in a short period of time [89].

The Secufy Button is being used in a variety of healthcare settings, including:

- A Secufy IoT Button is given to patients who test positive for COVID-19 and are discharged with minimal symptoms. When a patient presses the button, a message is sent to doctors via a predetermined communication channel if the patient's health worsens. By doing this, conventional phone helplines are not used.
- The Secufy Button is used in hospitals to provide a quick supplementary communications infrastructure for nurse-call systems.
- The Secufy Button can also be used as a tracker to verify that quarantine is followed or to alert family members if a senior relative has gone missing (and not returned).

The IoT button is simple and dependable, and it may be used to solve global critical care communication difficulties because it works everywhere in the world and is a cost-effective solution.

3.12 Case study 12

IoT in medicine is referred to as (IoMT). It assists in creating a large data analytics model that is focused on making decisions and connected to information technology in fields like communication, electronics, and medical. [90–93].

Doctors and specialists receive the automatically generated diagnoses and recommended courses of treatment for review. Using the nCapp assistant app on their cellphones, specialists and medical professionals can engage in the three-linkage IoT cloud plus platform, as needed [94, 95].

The steps for applying nCapp-assisted COVID-19 diagnosis and treatment system are:

1. The basic information of the patient is registered online.
2. After the patient is admitted, the page will display item-by-item questions, and the patient selects the response button to send the data back to the cloud online.
3. Diagnose with the use of AI. For user convenience, diagnostic suggestions are provided automatically.
4. Treatment with intelligent assistance. Treatment options are suggested, depending on the severity of the ailment.
5. Experts in the field, local relevant specialists, first-line experts, and clinicians are supplied with essential information.
6. Self-control-related information is supplied.
7. There is information regarding COVID-19 cases in the user's area.

Due to the fact that the nCapp wise assisted COVID-19 prognosis device gathers an enormous amount of scientific diagnostic data from COVID-19 patients, the data can also be clustered and analyzed using statistics, function engineering, and statistical techniques to gain a more informed distinction between suspected and suspicious cases in patients with a poor nucleic acid check result. The data can then be used for nCapp intelligent assisted treatment and diagnosis.

nCapp, which generates fast diagnoses, based on national recommendations, suggests that patients who satisfy the requirements be reported or transferred to the designated hospitals. To prevent missed diagnoses, these suspected patients should be monitored in the designated hospitals until a confirmed or an excluded diagnosis is made [96].

nCapp intelligent assisted treatment for COVID-19 suspicious patients. Patients who have an unsure epidemiological record and scientific manifestations, and CT scans that may be similar to COVID-19, however, are categorized as suspicious. In situations of healing challenges, docs can request the assistance of a cloud professional connection, which lets in them to talk with professionals or front-line skilled physicians over the internet. Suspected patients must be remoted and monitored for 14 days to ensure they are not misdiagnosed. The patient's frame temperature must be normal for more than three days, and breathing signs and symptoms must have considerably improved [97].

3.13 Case study 13

3.13.1 Usage of multi-rotor drones in supplying medical aids during COVID-19

Among the different types of drones, multi-rotor drones have been very useful in the fight against COVID-19 pandemic. More than 100 drones were used by China for surveillance purpose in many cities. This turned out to be a very convenient way to restrict viral transmission by alerting people whenever the distance between any two individuals was less than a specific value or if people were observed walking in public places without a mask. Besides identifying individuals who were not maintaining social distance or not wearing masks in public places, loudspeakers were used to broadcast these messages. The same strategy was followed in other regions, e.g., Spain, Turkey, Hungary, United Arab Emirates (UAE), and Kuwait [98].

Multi-rotor drones were also used in India with success during COVID-19. In the first trial, CSIR-National Aerospace Laboratories (NAL) in India developed a robust multi-rotor drone with 8 rotors. The drone was tested on 27th November 2021 by flying from CSIR-Indian Institute of Integrative Medicine (CSIR-IIIM) Jammu to Government Sub District Hospital in Marh. The drone can carry a moderate payload of 20 kg, with a flight time of up to 40 min. It is quite lightweight as it is made up of carbon fiber materials. The drone is equipped with an MEM-based autonomous guidance system. The drone is compliant with DGCA-NPNT protocols, geofencing, and 360-degree collision avoidance system. The drone was also successfully used to dispatch 50 sets of COVID-19 vaccines and syringes from Chandapura public health center from Electronics City in Bangalore. The entire flight took only 10 min to cover 7 km distance, which generally takes 40 min by car on a terrestrial path [99].

In an empirical study, Adwibowo showed a quadcopter can perform very effectively to dispatch medical aids to remote areas with rugged terrain, which are beyond the reach of walking or traveling by car [100]. The author selected an isolated village in a forest area in Southeast Asia. Adwibowo chose Baduy village in Banton province in Indonesia as the study area, which hosts a population of 10,486. The author experimented with different drone types, and showed that a quadcopter performed the best; it carried 500 vials of vaccines, with a 10 kg payload, over 2 km rugged trail in 3.13 min, which would have taken 1 h by 2 people to reach on the ground. In this experiment, the author showed that the same drone could carry 100 vials in 1.23–1.38 min and 250 vials in 1.57–1.66 min. The area has an irregular terrain, with a slope of 15–45°. Higher the slope, the more difficult it is to maneuver. Another challenge was to keep the vaccines in a cold environment, which involved a heavy cold carrier box to maintain the low temperature for a longer period of time (in this case, the box could maintain the low temperature for 72 h). Adwibowo discussed that while choosing the drone, it is important to focus on how much payload the drone can carry, its speed, and flight control.

3.14 Case study 14

3.14.1 Drones in health monitoring of people

Drones played a very significant role in measuring different health parameters and in improving health quality by early detection, especially during the COVID-19 pandemic. They provided great assistance in areas like sanitizing, monitoring, vigilance, and thermal scanning, at varying levels.

"Pandemic Drone" was developed by researchers from the Dragonfly Inc. and the University of South Australia (Canada based company) to detect and monitor people with infectious respiratory conditions. Computer vision system and a specialized sensor allowed the drones to measure heart rates, monitor temperatures, and respiratory rates, and also coughing and sneezing in public places like hospitals, airports, offices, and other group assembly scenarios.

Image-processing algorithms were validated by this partnership in 2017, which helped to detect human heart rate on a drone video. They have found that breathing rates and heart rates can be measured within ten meters of an individual using drones, and approximately within 50 meters, with fixed cameras of high frequency.

Moreover, another advanced algorithm was developed to interpret different human actions like sneezing and coughing [27].

Interestingly, this technology was originally developed for use in war zones, remote monitoring of heart rates among premature infants who were in incubators, and in natural disasters.

To combat the COVID-19 health catastrophe, Indian Robotics Solution (IRS) was successful in developing a real-time drone system, which was an aid in the situation, as it helped in monitoring, sanitizing, and controlling the COVID-19 pandemic, predominantly in Delhi, the National Capital Region (NCR) of India, and was named as thermal Corona combat drone (TCCD). In many areas of Delhi (NCR), this system helped in the identification of object and thermal scanning it. TCCD worked in a very interesting way. Without any explicit launching pad, the drone can take off vertically from the ground. At first, the most densely populated areas which need to be surveyed are identified, and clearances are obtained from the government. In those regions, the drone appeals to people to come out to their balconies. As soon as they come out, through a screening process, the temperature of the body is recorded one by one. This is done within a 20 ft. range of an individual. The alarm fitted on the drone beeps with an announcement over the loudspeaker if it detects the body temperature to be greater than 2 degrees Celsius than normal. After that, the person who has high temperature should recover, otherwise necessary official actions are taken for further health check-up for that individual.

In India, TCCD completed around scanning in 10 + areas having a large population per square kilometer, most being underprivileged areas, whose roads were in such poor condition that it was very difficult for individuals to reach there. By using the scanned images, sanitization of those areas was done within 7 days; approximately an area of 2 km radius was sanitized within just 10 min. After this success, IRS teams took the step to enlarge this experimentation further for a wider region with the help of proposed AI techniques and fast image processing. Electrostatic spray was used thereafter, which turned out to be a great help in obtaining more centric and overlapping droplets of sanitizer, and thus made this overall process more effective and minimized wastage [101].

3.15 Case study 15

3.15.1 Drones in indoor monitoring during COVID-19

Drones were used in indoor monitoring for COVID-19. In the case of indoor activity, low or nano altitude drones were used due to their various advantages [102, 103]. In the hospital's internal buildings, a drone's camera was fitted and the camera was programmed so as to examine subjects on the basis of certain movements as well as density. The basic assumption of the manual cleaning of the wards at regular intervals has been considered. So, this drone-based sanitization was made mandatory in populated areas.

Leveraging real time data, the hospital rooms equipped with such drones were operated to sanitize and medicate specific areas. The accuracy of the proposed simulation was found to be around 93% or higher [104].

4 Discussion

The use cases can be clustered on the basis of application phases, as shown in Table 1.

The COVID-19 phases can be segmented as follows:

Phase 1: Symptoms detection for early detection

Phase 2: Control and quarantine time

Phase 3: Post-recovery

Table 1: Phase-wise clustering of use cases.

Category	Use Case	Phase
Smart thermometer	Case 1	1
Smart helmet	Case 2	1
Smart glasses	Case 3	1
Easy band	Case 4	3
Tele robots	Case 5	2
Cloud buttons	Case 6	1
Autonomous robots	Case 7	2
Proximity trace	Case 8	3
Accelerometer band	Case 9	3
Smart camera	Case 10	1
Cloud buttons	Case 11	2
Smartphone application	Case 12	1
Multi-purpose drones	Case 13	1,2,3
Thermal imaging drones	Case 14	1
Nano-altitude drones	Case 15	2

5 Conclusion

COVID-19 pandemic impacted various aspects of our lives by influencing the socioeconomic regime, physical and psychological condition of people and on policy frameworks at different granularities. As social distancing has been deemed to be one of the primary solutions to prevent widespread pandemic, there has been an increasing gap in the society. By their very nature, drones have been useful tool to close this gap in our social realm, especially the gap between the individual or a community in need and the authority or the service provider.

This article highlights various aspects of drones – including the types of drones and usage of drones to combat COVID-19 around the world. In this chapter, we discussed different types of drones, their usage, short case studies, and implications on regulatory framework.

Various studies developed empirical studies to compare the performance of different types of drones in terms of their speed, weightlifting capacity, and vibration, which are key to aid delivery in a critical situation [100]. Overall, it is seen in most cases that multi-rotor drones seem to be very useful in COVID-19 critical cases to deliver aids, with better flight control and payload capacity.

Usage of drone to fight COVID-19 is widespread and was used by many countries [11]. While drones play a vital role in addressing the COVID-19 pandemic by monitoring social distancing, dispatching critical aid and medical samples, and spraying disinfectant, there are still several ethical and regulatory questions. For example, the Italian authority has allowed the Italian police and the enforcement department to use drones to track social distancing. Adherence to lockdown measures were monitored by authorities in Portugal, France, Malaysia, and the USA. However, in the wake of privacy concerns, the respective enforcement departments had to stop using drones for public monitoring. And much of the legal concerns come from mainly two reasons: (a) the individual is tracked without her consent and knowledge and (b) there is no definite rule on how long the footage containing personal information can be stored. Although drones have been used in various COVID-19 aids, there is now a growing consensus on the privacy aspect related to a proper regulatory practice of using drones during such critical times. For example, in the interest of privacy concerns, the Conseil d'Etat in France restricted drone usage to track public movement [13]. Similarly, after being criticized by the American Civil Liberties Union on grounds of privacy concerns, Westport police department were forced to restrict the use of drones for people-tracking under the COVID-19 regulations [105].

There have also been a few safety concerns raised related to drone usage. One imminent safety concern is the way drones are operated in airspace; they may collide with civilian airplanes flying at a low altitude. Another safety concern relates to delivering contraband and harmful products in the guise of COVID-19 aid. Although there exists a counter-drone technology with several legal and technological limitations [11], there are no definite rules and systems in place that can track such unsafe and unethical drones.

Despite drones being useful to combat the COVID-19 pandemic, it is yet to be understood if there is public acceptance of the new regulatory measures where drones have been integrated with existing authoritative systems. There is also a lack of widespread adoption of this technology in different communities due to varied level of public acceptance. In some cases, people may also raise objections with the newly introduced technology, resulting in low public acceptance and participation. We need active players and public participation in the drone technology to combat COVID-19 more effectively, especially in the emergence of changed policies to track social distancing and aid delivery using drones.

Such a change in regulatory protocols has taken place in the past during an emergency or in humanitarian situations [106]. But this change often results in collateral effect, either on our personal sphere or on socio-economic or physical or psychological regime. Generally, whenever a new technology is integrated into a regulatory framework, it often lacks public acceptance, and that is partly because of lack of knowledge and privacy concerns [107]. Monsees [108[has argued that one way of gaining public acceptance is to get the public more engaged and participative with the technology than just communicating the new technology [108]. As a matter of fact, the integration of drone with the regulatory framework in the context of COVID-19 can certainly bring value but at the same time it can jeopardize people's privacy and increase psychological stress, resulting in the lack of public acceptance. Thus, it is imperative to monitor and re-evaluate the current practice of drone usage and its implications on society, public health, law enforcement, and public regime on a continuous basis.

Despite some privacy and ethical concerns related to drones, it could be concluded that drones have been very useful to alleviate social gaps and deliver support and aids on timely basis during the COVID-19 pandemic. Drones also helped the concerned authorities and medical facilities to monitor and manage pandemic situations. Although modern drones can carry sufficient payload with better flight control, they still need to be improve in terms of architecture and engineering to increase their flight stability, landing, take off, and payload capacity. With increasing adoption and proven value, drone are gradually becoming an integral part of the regulatory framework and strategic policies in explicit and implicit ways, supporting the government and policy planners to be more technocratic. However, there should be a controlled usage of drone, with more public acceptance and public participation. A close collaboration between the government and public is required to win the battle of COVID-19 and similar challenges in the future.

References

[1] Restás, Á., Szalkai, I., Óvári, G. Drone application for spraying disinfection liquid fighting against the COVID-19 Pandemic – examining drone-related parameters influencing effectiveness. Drones, 2021, 5, 58. https://doi.org/10.3390/drones5030058.

[2] Martin, B. O., Lavallée, C., Silkoset, A. Drone use for COVID-19 related problems: Techno-solutionism and its societal implications. Global Policy,2021, 12(5), 603–612. https://doi.org/10.1111/1758-5899.13007.

[3] Khan, H., Kushwah, K. K., Singh, S., Urkude, H., Maurya, M. R., Sadasivuni, K. K. Smart technologies driven approaches to tackle COVID-19 pandemic: A review. 3 Biotech, 2021, 11, doi: 10.1007/S13205-020-02581-Y/FIGURES/1.

[4] Khamis, A., et al. AI and robotics in the fight against COVID-19 pandemic. In: Modeling, Control and Drug Development for COVID-19 Outbreak Prevention. Studies in Systems, Decision and Control, Azar, A. T., Hassanien, A. E. (eds.), Cham, Springer, 2022, 366, https://doi.org/10.1007/978-3-030-72834-2_3.

[5] Andrasto, T., et al. IOP **Conference** Series: **Earth** and **Environmental Science**, 2021, 700, 012012.

[6] Jalel, E. U. C. H. I. Do drones have a realistic place in a pandemic fight for delivering medical supplies in healthcare systems problems? Chinese Journal of Aeronautics, 2021, 34(2), 182–190. ISSN 1000–9361, https://doi.org/10.1016/j.cja.2020.06.006).

[7] Merkert, R., Bushell, J. Managing the drone revolution: A systematic literature review into the current use of airborne drones and future strategic directions for their effective control. Journal of Air Transport Management, 2020, 89, 101929. https://doi.org/10.1016/j.jairtraman.2020.101929.

[8] Cui, J. Q., Phang, S. K., Ang, K. Z., Wang, F., Dong, X., Ke, Y., . . . Chen, B. M. 2015 Drones for cooperative search and rescue in post-disaster situation. In: IEEE 7th international conference on cybernetics and intelligent systems (CIS) and IEEE conference on robotics, automation and mechatronics (RAM), IEEE, 2015, July, 167–174.

[9] Karaca, Y., Cicek, M., Tatli, O., Sahin, A., Pasli, S., Beser, M. F., Turedi, S. The potential use of unmanned aircraft systems (drones) in mountain search and rescue operations. The American Journal of Emergency Medicine, 2018, 36(4), 583–588.

[10] 5G edge patrol robots deployed in China to detect Covid-19 cases n.d. https://www.eenewseurope.com/news/5g-edge-patrol-robots-deployed-china-detect-a.covid-19-cases (accessed August 21, 2021).

[11] Martins, B. O., Lavallee, C., Silkoset, A. Drone use for COVID-19 related problems: Techno-solutionism and its societal implications. Global Policy, 2021, 13007. doi: 10.1111/1758-5898.

[12] Lewis, S. CORONAVIRUS: Malaysia to use Drones to control public movement. Commercial Drone Professional, 2020, 23 March 2020. Available from: https://www.commercialdroneprofessional.com/coronavirus-malaysia-to-use-drones-to-control-public-movement/, (accessed July 2021).

[13] Fouquet, H., Sebag, G. French Covid-19 Drones Grounded After Privacy Complaint, Bloomberg, 2020. https://www.bloomberg.com/news/articles/2020-05-18/paris-police-drones-banned-from-spying-on-virus-violators, Accessed July, 2021.

[14] How Drones Can Be Used to combat COVID-19, UNICEF for every child, https://www.unicef.org/supply/media/5286/file/%20Rapid-guidance-how-can-drones-help-in-COVID-19-response.pdf.pdf.

[15] Mbunge, E., Chitungo, I., Dzinamarira, T. Unbundling the significance of cognitive Robots and Drones deployed to tackle COVID-19 pandemic: A rapid review to unpack emerging opportunities to improve healthcare in sub-Saharan Africa. Cognitive Robotics, 2021, 1, 205–213.

[16] Kunovjanek, M., Wankmüller, C. Containing the COVID-19 pandemic with drones – Feasibility of a drone enabled back-up transport system. Transport Policy, 2021, 106, 141–152.

[17] Poljak, M., Šterbenc, A. Use of drones in clinical microbiology and infectious diseases: Current status, challenges and barriers. Clinical Microbiology and Infection, 2020, 26(4), 425–430.

[18] Restas, A. Drone applications fighting COVID-19 pandemic – Towards good practice. 2022, 6, 15.

[19] Jat, D. S., Singh, C. Artificial intelligence-enabled robotic drones for COVID-19 outbreak. In: Intelligent Systems and Methods to Combat Covid-19. Springer Briefs in Applied Sciences and Technology, Joshi, A., Dey, N., Santosh, K. (eds.), Singapore, Springer, 2020, https://doi.org/10.1007/978-981-15-6572-4_5

[20] Jalel, E. U. C. H. I. Do drones have a realistic place in a pandemic fight for delivering medical supplies in healthcare systems problems? Chinese Journal of Aeronautics, 2021, 34(2), 182–190. ISSN 1000–9361 https://doi.org/10.1016/j.cja.2020.06.006.

[21] Amukele, T. Current state of drones in healthcare: Challenges and opportunities. Journal of Applied Laboratory Medicine, 2019, 4(2), 296–298.

[22] Kim, S. H. Choice model-based analysis of consumer preference for drone delivery service. Journal of Air Transport Management, 2020, 84, 101785.

[23] Sánchez-García, J., García-Campos, J. M., Arzamendia, M., Reina, D. G., Toral, S. L., Gregor, D. A survey on unmanned aerial and aquatic vehicle multi-hop networks: Wireless communications, evaluation tools and applications. Computer Communications, 2018, 119, 43–65.

[24] Thiels, C. A., Aho, J. M., Zietlow, S. P., Jenkins, D. H. Use of unmanned aerial vehicles for medical product transport. Air Medical Journal, 2015, 34(2), 104–108.

[25] https://www.thedronegirl.com/2020/08/14/2019-drone-growth-slows/.

[26] Wolf, H. We're About to See the Golden Age of Drone Delivery – Here's Why. World Economic Forum, Forbes, 2020. Available online: https://www.weforum.org/agenda/2020/07/golden-age-drone-delivery-covid-19-coronavirus-pandemic-technology/ Accessed on 22 July 2021.

[27] Draganfly selected to globally integrate breakthrough health diagnosis technology immediately onto autonomous camera's and specialized drones to combat coronavirus (covid19) and future health emergencies. [Online]. Available: https://apnews.com/Globe%20Newswire/dc01344350423d7d64c99ebbe8fb7548.

[28] Drones and the coronavirus: How drones are helping containment efforts. [Online]. Available: https://uavcoach.com/drones-coronavirus/.

[29] Padula, W. V. Why only test symptomatic patients? Consider random screening for COVID-19. Applied Health Economics and Health Policy, 2020, 18(3), 333–334.

[30] Chamberlain, S. D., Singh, I., Ariza, C. A., Daitch, A. L., Philips, P. B., Dalziel, B. D. Real-time detection of COVID-19 epicenters within the United States using a network of smart thermometers. 2020, medRxiv.

[31] Wang, C. J., Ng, C. Y., Brook, R. H. Response to COVID-19 in Taiwan: Big data analytics, new technology, and proactive testing. JAMA, 2020, doi: 10.1001/jama.2020.3151

[32] McNamara, L. A., et al. Ebola surveillance – Guinea, Liberia, and Sierra Leone. MMWR Supplements, 2016, 65, https://www.cdc.gov/mmwr/volumes/65/su/su6503a6.htm.

[33] Nouvellet, P., Garske, T., Mills, H. L., Nedjati-Gilani, G., Hinsley, W., Blake, I. M., Van Kerkhove, M. D., Cori, A., Dorigatti, I., Jombart, T., Riley, S. The role of rapid diagnostics in managing Ebola epidemics. Nature, 2015, 528, 7580.

[34] Radin, J. M., Wineinger, N. E., Topol, E. J., Steinhubl, S. R. Harnessing wearable device data to improve state-level real-time surveillance of influenza-like illness in the USA: a population-based study. The Lancet Digital Health.

[35] Miller, A. C., Singh, I., Koehler, E., Polgreen, P. M. A smartphone-driven thermometer application for real-time population-and individual-level influenza surveillance. Clinical Infectious Diseases, 2018, 67, 388–397.

[36] Miller, A. C., Peterson, R. A., Singh, I., Pilewski, S., Polgreen, P. M. Improving state-level influenza surveillance by incorporating real-time smartphone-connected thermometer readings across different geographic domains. In: Open Forum Infectious Diseases, Oxford University Press, 2019.

[37] Yang, S., Santillana, M., Kou, S. C., Accurate estimation of influenza epidemics using Google search data and ARGO. In: Proceedings of the National Academy of Sciences 112, 1447 3–14478.

[38] Dalziel, B. D., Kissler, S., Gog, J. R., Viboud, C., Bjornstad, O. N., Metcalf, C. J. E., Grenfell, B. T. Urbanization and humidity shape the intensity of influenza epidemics in US cities. Science, 2018, 6410, 75–79.

[39] Dalziel, B. D., Pourbohloul, B., Ellner, S. P. Human mobility patterns predict divergent epidemic dynamics among cities. Proceedings of the Royal Society B: Biological Sciences, 2013, 280, 1766.

[40] Immunohistochemical and molecular detection of natural cases of bovine rotavirus and coronavirus infection causing enteritis in dairy calves. Microbial Pathogenesis. 2020, Jan; 138:103814. doi: 10.1016/j.micpath.2019.103814. Epub 2019 Oct 19.

[41] Xie, C., Jiang, L., Huang, G., Pu, H., Gong, B., Lin, H., Ma, S., Chen, X., Long, B., Si, G., Yu, H., Jiang, L., Yang, X., Shi, Y., Yang, Z. Comparison of different samples for 2019 novel coronavirus detection by nucleic acid amplification tests. International Journal of Infectious Diseases, 2020, 93, 264–267, doi: 10.1016/j.ijid.2020.02.050, Epub 2020 Feb 27.

[42] Shen, M., Zhou, Y., Ye, J., Al Maskri, A. A., Kang, Y., Zeng, S., Cai, S. Recent advances and perspectives nucleic acid detection for coronavirus. Journal of Pharmaceutical Analysis, 2020.
[43] Li, Q., Guan, X., Wu, P., Wang, X., Zhou, L., Tong, Y., Ren, R., Leung, K. S. M., Lau, E. H. Y., Wong, J. Y., Xing, X., Xiang, N., Wu, Y., Li, C., Chen, Q., Li, D., Liu, T., Zhao, J., Liu, M., Tu, W., Chen, C., Jin, L., Yang, R., Wang, Q., Zhou, S., Wang, R., Liu, H., Luo, Y., Liu, Y., Shao, G., Li, H., Tao, Z., Yang, Y., Deng, Z., Liu, B., Ma, Z., Zhang, Y., Shi, G., Lam, T. T. Y., Wu, J. T., Gao, G. F., Cowling, B. J., Yang, B., Leung, G. M., Feng, Z. Early transmission dynamics in Wuhan, China, of novel coronavirus-infected pneumonia. New England Journal of Medicine, 2020, 382(13), 1199–1207. doi: 10.1056/NEJMoa2001316, Epub 2020 Jan 29.
[44] Velavan, T. P., Meyer, C. G. The COVID-19 epidemic. Tropical Medicine and Infectious Disease, 2020, 25(3), 278–280. doi: 10.1111/tmi.13383, Epub 2020 Feb 16.
[45] Ludvigsson, J. F. Systematic review of COVID-19 in children shows milder cases and a better prognosis than adults. Acta Paediatrica, 2020, 109, 1088–1095. https://doi.org/10.1111/apa.15270.
[46] Jamal, A., et al. Large hall temperature monitoring portal. In: 2019 IEEE International Conference on Automatic Control and Intelligent Systems (I2CACIS), 2019, 62–67.
[47] Fong, S. L., Yung, D. C. W., Ahmed, F. Y. H., Jamal, A. 2019. Smart city bus application with quick response (QR) code payment. In: Proceedings of the 2019 8th International Conference on Software and Computer Applications (ICSCA '19). Association for Computing Machinery, New York, NY, USA, 248–252. doi: https://doi.org/10.1145/3316615.3316718.
[48] Ruktanonchai, N. W., Ruktanonchai, C. W., Floyd, J. R., Tatem, A. J. Using google location history data to quantify fine-scale human mobility. International Journal of Health Geographics, 2018, 17(1), 28. https://doi.org/10.1186/s12942-018-0150-z.
[49] Ruktanonchai, N. W., Ruktanonchai, C. W., Floyd, J. R., et al. Using google location history data to quantify fine-scale human mobility. International Journal of Health, 2018, 17(28), https://doi.org/10.1186/s12942-018-0150-z.
[50] Li, Q., Guan, X., Wu, P., Wang, X., Zhou, L., Tong, Y., Ren, R., Leung, K. S., Lau, E. H., Wong, J. Y., Velavan, T. P., Meyer, C. G. The COVID-19 epidemic. Tropical Medicine and Health, 2020, 25(3), 278–280.
[51] World Health Organization. Coronavirus disease (COVID-19): situation report 74, 2019 2020.
[52] Fong, S. L., Chin, D. W. Y., Ahmed, R. F. Y. H., Jamal, A., Smart city bus application with quick response (QR) code payment. In: ICSCA '19 Proceedings of the 2019 8th International Conference on Software and Computer Applications, Penang, Malaysia, 248–252, – February 19 – 21, 2019.
[53] Mohammed, M. N., Hazairin, N. A., Al-Zubaid, S., Sairah, A. K., Mustapha, S., Yusuf, E. Toward a novel design for coronavirus detection and diagnosis system using IoT-based drone technology. International Journal of Psychosocial Rehabilitation, 2020, 24(7), 2287–2295.
[54] Mustapha, S., Merican, M., Rediscovery of empathy in youth through an interactive virtual reality experience In: 2020 IEEE 16th International Colloquium on Signal Processing and its Applications (CSPA 2020), Langkawi, Kedah, Malaysia, HIG Hotel, 28–29 February 2020.
[55] Sumi, N., Moshnyaga, V. A novel face recognition for smart glasses. In: **Proceedings** – 2016 IEEE **Region 10 Symposium** TENSYMP, 2016, 115–118, 2016.
[56] Kumar, N. M., Kumar Singh, N., Peddiny, V. K. Wearable smart glass: Features, applications, current progress and challenges. In: Proceedings 2nd International Conference on Green Computing and Internet of Things, 2018, I, 577–582, 2018.
[57] Berger, A., Maly, F., Smart google glass solution used as education support tool. In: Proceedings – 2019 International Symposium on Educational Technology ISET 2019, 265–267, 2019.
[58] Viola, P., Jones, M., Rapid object detection using a boosted cascade of simple features. In: Proceedings of the IEEE Computer Society Conference on Computer Vision and Pattern Recognition, 1, 511–518, 2001.

[59] Sardianos, C., Varlamis, I., Bouras, G., Extracting user habits from google maps history logs. In: Proceedings of the **2018 IEEE/ACM International Conference** on **Advances in Social Networks Analysis** and **Mining**, ASONAM, 2018, 690–697, 2018.
[60] Ruktanonchai, N. W., Ruktanonchai, C. W., Floyd, J. R., Tatem, A. J. Using google location history data to quantify fine-scale human mobility. International Journal of Health, 2018, 17(1), 1–13.
[61] C. S. G. of the International Committee on Taxonomy of Viruses. The species severe acute respiratory syndrome-related coronavirus: Classifying 2019-nCoV and naming it SARS-CoV-2. Nature Microbiology, 2020, 5(4), 536–544.
[62] Zhang, S. X., Wang, Y., Rauch, A., Wei, F. Unprecedented disruption of lives and work: Health, distress and life satisfaction of working adults in China one month into the COVID-19 outbreak. Psychiatry Research, 2020, 288, 112958.
[63] Mohapatra, A. G., Keswani, B., Nanda, S., Ray, A., Khanna, A., Gupta, D., Keswani, P. precision local positioning mechanism in underground mining using IoT-enabled wifi platform. International Journal on Computers and Applications, 2020, 42(3), 266277.
[64] Jain, P., Joshi, A. M., Mohanty, S. P. iGLU: An intelligent device for accurate noninvasive blood glucose-level monitoring in smart healthcare. IEEE Consumer Electronics Magazine, 2020, 9(1), 35–42.
[65] Mohanty, S. P., Yanambaka, V. P., Kougianos, E., Puthal, D. PUF chain: Hardware-assisted blockchain for sustainable simultaneous device and data security in internet of everything (IoE). IEEE Consumer Electronics Magazine, 2020, 9(2), 8–16.
[66] Mohanty, S. P., Choppali, U., Kougianos, E. Everything you wanted to know about smart cities. IEEE Consumer Electronics Magazine, 2016, 5(3), 60–70.
[67] Agostini, M., Moja, L., Banzi, R., Pistotti, V., Tonin, P., Venneri, A., et al. Tele rehabilitation and recovery of motor function: A systematic review and meta-analysis. Journal of Telemedicine and Telecare, 2015, 21(4), 202–213. https://doi.org/10.1177/1357633X15572201, pMID: 25712109.
[68] Fong, J., Martinez, C., Tavakoli, M. Ways to learn a therapist's patient-specific intervention: Robotics-vs telerobotics-mediated hands-on teaching. In: 2019 International Conference on Robotics and Automation (ICRA); 2019. 870876
[69] Tao, R., Ocampo, R., Fong, J., Soleymani, A., Tavakoli, M. Modeling and emulating a physiotherapist's role in Robot-assisted rehabilitation. Advanced Intelligent Systems, 0(0), 1900181. https://onlinelibrary.wiley.com/doi/abs/10.1002/aisy.201900181.
[70] https://wandasolution.com/wanda-quick-touch/.
[71] Ackerman, E. (2020) Autonomous robots are helping kill coronavirus in hospitals. IEEE Spectrum
[72] Wearable technology in the time of COVID-19. 2020. https://www.constructiondive.com/spons/wearable-technology-in-the-time-of-covid-19/577217/. Accessed June 27, 2020.
[73] Proximity Trace. 2020. https://www.triaxtec.com/resource/fact-sheet/proximity-trace/. Accessed June 27, 2020.
[74] Hernandez, J., McDuff, D., Picard, R. W., Biowatch: Estimation of heart and breathing rates from wrist motions. In: 2015 9th International Conference on Pervasive Computing Technologies for Healthcare (PervasiveHealth), IEEE, 2015, 169–176.
[75] Sun, X., Qiu, L., Wu, Y., Tang, Y., Cao, G. Sleep monitor: Monitoring respiratory rate and body position during sleep using smartwatch. Proceedings of the ACM on Interactive, Mobile, Wearable and Ubiquitous Technologies, 1, 3, 1–22, 2017.
[76] Petkie, D. T., Benton, C., Bryan, E. Millimeter wave radar for remote measurement of vital signs. In: 2009 IEEE Radar Conference, IEEE, 2009, 1–3
[77] Lai, J. C. Y., Xu, Y., Gunawan, E., Chua, E. C.-P., Maskooki, A., Guan, Y. L., Low, K.-S., Soh, C. B., Poh, C.-L. Wireless sensing of human respiratory parameters by low-power ultra wide band impulse radio radar. IEEE Transactions on Instrumentation and Measurement, 2010, 60(3), 928–938.

[78] Wang, G., Munoz-Ferreras, J.-M., Gu, C., Li, C., GomezGarcia, R. Application of linear-frequency-modulated continuous-wave (LFMCW) radars for tracking of vital signs. IEEE Transactions on Microwave Theory and Techniques, 2014, 62(6), 1387–1399.
[79] Alizadeh, M., Shaker, G., De Almeida, J. C. M., Morita, P. P., Safavi-Naeini, S. Remote monitoring of human vital signs using mm wave FMCW radar. IEEE Access, 2019, 7, 54958–54968.
[80] Abdelnasser, H., Harras, K. A., Youssef, M., Ubibreathe: A ubiquitous non-invasive WiFi-based breathing estimator. In: Proceedings of the 16th ACM International Symposium on Mobile Ad Hoc Networking and Computing, 2015, 277–286
[81] Liu, J., Wang, Y., Chen, Y., Yang, J., Chen, X., Cheng, J., Tracking vital signs during sleep leveraging off-the-shelf WiFi. In: Proceedings of the 16th ACM International Symposium on Mobile Ad Hoc Networking and Computing, 2015, 267–276
[82] Wang, X., Yang, C., Mao, S. Tensorbeat: Tensor decomposition for monitoring multiperson breathing beats with commodity WiFi. ACM Transactions on Intelligent Systems and Technology (TIST), 2017, 9(1), 1–27.
[83] Phasebeat: Exploiting CSI phase data for vital sign monitoring with commodity WiFi devices. In: 2017 IEEE 37th International Conference on Distributed Computing Systems (ICDCS), IEEE, 2017, 1230–1239.
[84] Xie, J., Covassin, N., Fan, Z., Singh, P., Gao, W., Li, G., Kara, T., Somers, V. K., Association between hypoxemia and mortality in patients with COVID-19. In: Mayo Clinic Proceedings, Elsevier, 2020
[85] Pulse oximetry and COVID-19 (interim guidance). Minnesota Department of Health, 2020. [Online]. Available: https://www.health.state.mn.us/diseases/coronavirus/hcp/pulseoximetry.pdf)
[86] Kong, L., Zhao, Y., Dong, L., Jian, Y., Jin, X., Li, B., Feng, Y., Liu, M., Liu, X., Wu, H. Non-contact detection of oxygen saturation based on visible light imaging device using ambient light. Optics Express, 2013, 21(15), 17464–17471.
[87] Guazzi, A. R., Villarroel, M., Jorge, J., Daly, J., Frise, M. C., Robbins, P. A., Tarassenko, L. Non-contact measurement of oxygen saturation with an RGB camera. Biomedical Optics Express, 2015, 6(9), 3320–3338.
[88] Shao, D., Liu, C., Tsow, F., Yang, Y., Du, Z., Iriya, R., Yu, H., Tao, N. Noncontact monitoring of blood oxygen saturation using camera and dual-wavelength imaging system,". IEEE Transactions on Biomedical Engineering, 2015, 63(6), 1091–1098.
[89] https://www.med-technews.com/news/iot-alert-button-finds-new-uses-during-coronavirus-pandemic/. Accessed June 27, 2020.
[90] Song, Y. L., Jiang, J. J., Wang, D., et al. Prospect and application of Internet of Things technology for prevention of SARIs. Clinical eHealth., 2020, 3, 1–4.
[91] Chunxue, B. Practical Medical Internet of Things, Beijing, People's Medical Publishing House Co., LTD, 2014.
[92] Chunxue, B. Medical Internet of Things Grading Diagnosis Manual, Beijing, People's Medical Publishing House Co., LTD, 2015.
[93] Chunxue, B., Jianlong, Z. Medical Internet of Things, Beijing, Science Press, 2016.
[94] Internet of things-aided diagnosis and treatment of COVID-19 Chinese experts group of clinical of eHealth. Chinese experts consensus on the internet of things-aided diagnosis and treatment of COVID-19. Fudan University Journal of Medical Science, 2020, 47(2), 151–160.
[95] Li, D. 5G and intelligence medicine-how the next generation of wireless technology will reconstruct healthcare? Precision Clinical Medicine, 2019, 2(4), 205–208. Montang C, Becker B, gan C. The multipurpose application WeChat: A review on recent research. Frontiers in psychology. 2018, 9(2247).
[96] Internet of things-aided diagnosis and treatment of COVID-19 Chinese experts group of clinical of eHealth. Chinese experts consensus on the internet of things-aided diagnosis and treatment of COVID-19. Fudan University Journal of Medical Science, 2020, 47(2), 151–160.

[97] Shangai respiratory clinical quality control center. Shangai expert consensus for respiratory clinic quality control during epidemic 2019-nCoV time. Fudan University Journal of Medical Science, 2020, 47(2), 143–150.

[98] Drone technology: A new ally in the fight against COVID-19. https://www.mdlinx.com/internal-medicine/article/6767 Accessed 15 April 2020.

[99] Octocoptered: Bengaluru sees its first Covid vaccine delivery using a drone https://www.newindianexpress.com/cities/bengaluru/2021/nov/13/bengalurus-first-drone-delivered-covid-vaccines-2383208.html Accessed 26 February 2022.

[100] Adwibowo, A. (2021). Assessments of heavy lift UAV quadcopter drone to support COVID 19 vaccine cold chain delivery for indigenous people in remote areas in South East Asia, MedRxiv, doi: 10.1101/2021.01.09.21249494).

[101] Kumar, A., Sharma, K., Singh, H., Naugriya, S. G., Gill, S. S., Buyya, R. A drone-based networked system and methods for combating coronavirus disease (COVID-19) pandemic. Future Generations Computer Systems: FGCS, 2021, 115, 1–19. https://doi.org/10.1016/j.future.2020.08.046.

[102] Palossi, D., Loquercio, A., Conti, F., Flamand, E., Scaramuzza, D., Benini, L. A 64-mw dnn-based visual navigation engine for autonomous nano-drones. IEEE Internet of Things Journal, 2019, 6(5), 8357–8371.

[103] Motlagh, N. H., Taleb, T., Arouk, O. Low-altitude unmanned aerial vehicles-based internet of things services: Comprehensive survey and future perspectives. IEEE Internet of Things Journal, 2016, 3(6), 899–922.

[104] Kumar, A., Sharma, K., Singh, H., Naugriya, S. G., Gill, S. S., Buyya, R. A drone-based networked system and methods for combating coronavirus disease (COVID-19) pandemic. Future Generations Computer Systems: FGCS, 2021, 115, 1–19. https://doi.org/10.1016/j.future.2020.08.046).

[105] Blair, R. Connecticut Town Scraps Plan to Use Temperature Tracking Drones in Fight against Coronavirus. Hartford Courant, 2020. https://www.courant.com/coronavirus/hc-news-coronavirus-connecticut-drone-20200423-tiakrmg3erez7fpkpxk6ixkacy-story.html. Accessed July, 2021

[106] Calhoun, C. The Idea of Emergency: Humanitarian Action and Global (Dis)order, New York, Zone Books, 2010.

[107] Boucher, P. You wouldn't have your granny using them: Drawing boundaries between acceptable and unacceptable applications of civil drones. Science & Engineering Ethics, 2016, 22, 1391–1418.

[108] Monsees, L. Public relations: Theorizing the contestation of security technology. Security Dialogue, 2019, 50(6), 351–546.

Ravi Ranjan, Prerona Saha, Labhvam Kumar Sharma,
Soham Guhathakurata, Sayak Saha, Soumyadip Daripa,
Sagnick Biswas, Arpita Chakraborty, Jyoti Sekhar Banerjee*

Designing enhancements for App-based cab services to the commuters during COVID-19 era: a new normal solution on Indian scenario

Abstract: In the COVID-19-impacted world, life has almost come to a standstill. The primary reason is the social distancing constraints that have been imposed on cab bookings, local shops, and restaurants. Here, the authors provide a possible solution through a mobile application to integrate multiple features required by people to make themselves comfortable in these "new normal" conditions. The application provides the perfect solution for organizations like the Airport Authority of India or any similar organization to resume their business and thrive in this period. All the said facilities are separately provided by many companies that earn a huge profit, while the Airport Authority does not see profits. To trade-off all these things, the authors have deployed a solution that can give all the required support required by the commuters while travelling via airplane; at the same time, the Airport Authority also gets due profits by providing facilities to the commuters while maintaining social distancing amidst COVID-19 risk prediction.

1 Introduction

India would be the third largest domestic and the fastest growing civil aviation market in the world by 2024–25, and Bangalore with 65% national share is the largest aviation manufacturing hub of India, as per reports released by the International Air Transport Association (IATA) [1]. By 2026, the country's aviation industry is expected to rank third globally, according to the IATA. Only 13 of the 125 airports that the Airports Authority of India (AAI) controlled were cost-effective in 2016, despite the organization posting a net profit of more than INR 25 billion. The major key factors for not generating revenue are

***Corresponding author: Jyoti Sekhar Banerjee**, Department of Computer Science and Engineering (AI & ML), Bengal Institute of Technology, Kolkata, India
Ravi Ranjan, Prerona Saha, Labhvam Kumar Sharma, Soham Guhathakurata, Sayak Saha, Soumyadip Daripa, Department of Computer Science and Engineering, Bengal Institute of Technology, Kolkata, India
Sagnick Biswas, Arpita Chakraborty, Department of Electronics and Communication Engineering, Bengal Institute of Technology, Kolkata, India

https://doi.org/10.1515/9783110767681-015

the hassles involved while traveling via airplane – from booking a flight to (reaching an unknown place) destination and coming back. In such cases, cab booking services play a significant role in the mode of transportation.

In this COVID-19 era [2–4], it is difficult to not only plan a trip efficiently but also to make the trip safe and sound. While planning a trip, users have to take care of flight booking, cab booking, hotel booking, managing food, buying gifts, and other stuff. In the current system, users have to deal with different apps to do each of the tasks, like Flipkart to buy gifts, OLA/UBER for cab booking, TRIVAGO for hotel booking, etc. In easy terms, the overall process becomes very time-consuming. Also, all these activities do not ensure that the user is not infected by COVID-19 [5, 6] and that he/she will not get infected while pursuing these endeavors.

To avoid all this, the authors have come up with a single software-based application that has all these features integrated into it. It ensures that the user undergoes a rigorous health check-up through the application before accessing the privilege of a flight booking system where users can book the ticket for flights. The user gets to access all the features of the application only if the application deems the person safe from COVID-19. We have a cab booking feature where the user can book a cab to or from an airport. The passenger will undergo thermal scanning before boarding the cab. What makes our system unique is the involvement of IoT-based thermal scanner, which stores the record of the passenger's temperature and also alerts the app admins when the recorded temperature is high. The cabs scheduled in the near future can be cancelled until the cab driver gets allocated. The user will have to bear a fine for the cancellation. Moreover, the user will also get a hotel booking facility to book the required accommodation easily.

Another distinctive feature of this app is that it provides a marketplace for the local shops and restaurants in the airport. It will help airport authorities grow their business. Users can order food and gifts beforehand through this app, without even visiting the shops, and this will save their precious time. Using modern artificial intelligence (AI)-machine learning (ML) [7] tools, the user will get recommendations for meals and gifts based on their taste and order history. The meals and ordered products will be delivered to the cab allocated for them. With this approach, we are providing the user with a complete solution to make their vacation flexible and trouble-free, while maintaining social distancing.

The chapter is written as follows. The literature review is discussed in Section 2. App-Cab sector development in India is presented in Section 3. Section 4 displays an analysis of existing problems of the App-Cab system and their possible solutions. The majority of the algorithms that are employed in an App-Cab-based system are presented in Section 5. The current App-Cab features are presented in Section 6 and the framework's difficulties are discussed in Section 7. Section 8 depicts the proposed system model followed by the flow sequence of the mobile application in Section 9. Section 10 presents the implemented twofold mobile application followed by the applications of ML model in Section 11. Section 12 deals with the implemented key features concerning the existing App-Cab procedure. Finally, Section 13 concludes the chapter.

2 Related studies

In this chapter, two distinct features are assembled, i.e., COVID-19 [6] mobile app and App-Cab services with a few other related essential services. Thus, in the related study section, existing research of both fields are described.

In their research, authors have identified many flaws in present App-Cab systems and provided some better solutions [8]. The major flaw in the existing systems is the use of centralized servers [9]. If the server goes down, the company's booking system will break down, causing significant losses. Researchers advise deploying a decentralized server to solve this issue. Due to long-term use of offline cab booking methods, individuals are accustomed to haggling with the drivers. The present system does not take care of this feature. Some authors have recommended giving the customer the chance to negotiate before booking. Cab systems do not provide real-time demand updates in various locations. A few researchers have recommended real-time updates [10], and therefore cab availability is not a major concern. Due to few number of taxis, users are often compelled to travel in an unsuitable vehicle, which is inconvenient. Glaschenko et al. recommend assigning the desired cab, which is about to finish its ride, above less acceptable cabs. Uber has also suggested strengthening current security mechanisms by allowing users and drivers to record the whole trip's audio. All these elements will enhance the user's experience and make the ride safer with smooth mobile communication.

Several organizations, including the government and other agencies, are releasing mobile applications that provide vital information about the epidemic, like the number of incidences recorded, number of lives saved, number of fatalities to date, and so on. In this article, the authors have focused on smartphone applications presently in use in India, since our mobile app displays just the most relevant information for India.

Akhtar et al. [11] explain App-Based Shared Mobility in pre- and post-COVID times. The authors discuss App-Based Shared Mobility (ABSM) services in Bengaluru and their influence on urban travel patterns, behavior, and automobile ownership. These services produce city-level data that may be used to enhance citywide mobility. The shift in consumer demand from ownership to accessibility has permeated the transport industry via transportation network companies (TNCs).

The World Health Organization (WHO) [12] says that implementing the suggested changes in transport networks may protect individuals from COVID-19 while promoting economic recovery, as outlined in the WHO manifesto for healthy recovery from COVID-19. This guideline supports prescription 5 of the manifesto on healthy and livable cities. They may assist in achieving various social goals, including transit efficiency and safety, enhanced urban life, greenhouse gas emissions, lower air pollution, and more to enable an active lifestyle.

The objectives of investigating how the COVID-19 might affect the choice of transport mode and the desire to buy a vehicle were covered by Luan et al. [13]. The decrease in travel and the avoiding of contacting carpool drivers has surprised the ride-hailing services greatly. The majority of non-car owners would likely use this method of transportation for retailing and other recreational activities.

The many elements that influence a driver's behavior while booking an app-based taxi in India were described by Thapa et al. [14]. The market for app-based taxi services was described by Jain et al. [15] along with the marketing tactics used and the difficulties that still remain. It will also provide some clarification on the current regulatory environment and raise doubts about the market's viability in the face of the epidemic.

Numerous smartphone applications have been developed due to COVID-19 that include all the real-time qualities and also gather the geo-location and other required archival data to guarantee public safety and keep people away from the virus-afflicted people [6].

A substantial effort has been made by Microsoft Bing [16] to provide an online visualization of the current COVID-19 epidemic in order to improve data clarity and traceability. Their solution integrated an interactive map known as the Bing map that focused on the world map. The map came with their innovation of rendering the COVID-19 statistics (active cases, recovered, deaths, confirmed cases) of the particular country by hovering over the map. In certain countries like India, the Bing map even shows data at the local level with very great precision.

APOLLO, known as the largest pharmaceutical behemoth in India, implemented a scanner for the risk assessment of COVID-19 outbreak in India and has given it the name "covid.apollo247" [17]. The application reached a significant part of the country during the outbreak. This solution can deftly forecast the likelihood of risk (high, mid, low) using their underlying ML algorithms based on the parameters provided by their numerous patients.

A group of around 20 people (professors and students) from Mahindra Ecole Centrale have built an interactive dashboard with a seamless user experience and high-quality representation of real-time data [18]. The website shows real-time information on fatalities, cures, and infections in India; nevertheless, a few discrepancies while using their method are also noted. They have used several charts and graphs on their web page to help users visualize the data even at the district level. However, considering the magnitude of the virus, more accuracy is expected as regards their results.

Aarogya Setu is a project of the Indian government that connects COVID-19-related vital health services to the people of India using a mobile application [19]. Even though it was a mobile application, the statistics display panel used web views. The application implemented geo-tracking facility to follow the coronavirus-diagnosed population and create a cluster.

Related forms of mobile apps are often used by various countries to tackle COVID-19. The name of the mobile application with characteristics are given in Table 1.

3 App-Cab sector development in India

Table 2 shows a comparison between Ola [20] and Uber [21] based on a few features. As India is a heavily populated country, the writers of this chapter have mostly concentrated on the many facets of cab services in India. Transportation systems in metropolitan cities' have been transformed by cab services. India is a country with a low rate of automobile ownership, since owning a vehicle is expensive for city inhabitants. When online cab services launched their online cab booking program in the years 2013 to 2015, the country's mobility needs received a much-needed boost.

Table 1: Various COVID-19 mobile apps used in different countries with their characteristics.

Country	COVID-19 Mobile App	Characteristics
North Macedonia	StopKorona	Bluetooth is used
Singapore	TraceTogether	BlueTrace protocol is used
Germany	ITO	The application is supported by Android
Israel	Hamagen	GPS and Bluetooth are used
Poland	ProteGO	Presently unavailable
Czech Republic	eRouska	Bluetooth is used
Australia	CovidSafe	TraceTogether's Related Product

Table 2: Comparison between Ola and Uber.

Features	OLA	UBER
Pin Verification	Secured with OTP	OTP not required
Personal Wallet	OLA Money	Don't have any personal wallet. Payment through e-wallet, debit cards and credit cards
Ride Check	Not available	Latest trip recording facility launched by UBER for securing purposes
Subsidiary	Foodpanda	Uber Eats
Availability in cities	250 cities since 2020	700 cities since 2019
Number of Users in India	23.96 million MAU since 2019	8.5 million MAU (Monthly Active Users)
Share in Indian market	80% since 2016	50% since 2020
Number of drivers	2.5 million since 2020	3.9 million since 2019
Number of rides	1.5 million per day, since 2017	17 million per day, since 2019

Cabs are becoming an essential part of the link between public and private transportation. The most intriguing aspect is that firms are always looking for fresh possibilities to expand their businesses. The authors have limited the comparison of the two taxi services in this research to Uber and Ola since they are the two biggest players in India's ride-hailing sector (see Table 2).

4 Analysis of issues and potential solutions for the existing App-Cab system

4.1 Single point of failure

Server-centric approach is embraced in the cab service system. The database of the complete system is sent to the remote server. Sometimes, the centralized server fails when a significant number of people attempt to book a cab at the same time. The whole system will be rendered inoperable, as a result. There is a large amount of loss to the organization as a result of this annoyance for people. Single point of failure is the name given to it [9].

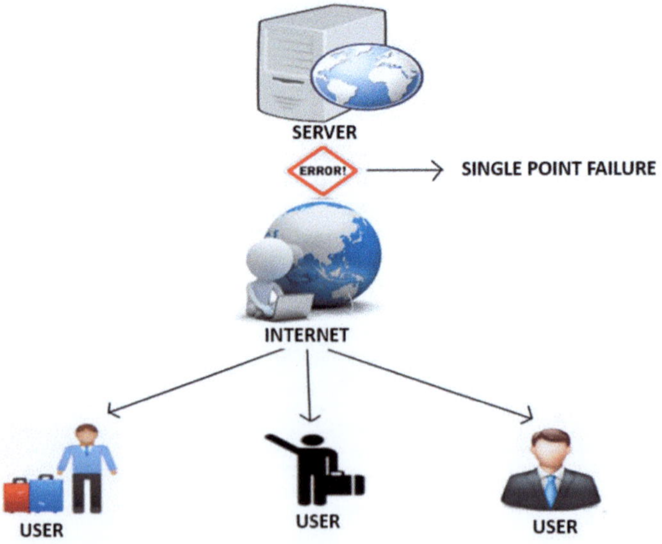

Figure 1: Single point of failure.

We can solve this issue by using a distributive strategy. Each unit of the system is broken down into smaller subsystems. In other words, it is a load balancer and does not cause any obstructions. There are two elements to the distributed system in VANETs [22]: de-blocking and taxi booking. The taxi de-blocking mechanism, on the other hand, guarantees that no two people hire the same cab at the same time. After allocating a taxi to a passenger, other taxis must be blocked from competing for the same customer. An online taxi booking system locates the closest driver and assigns him or her to a ride.

4.2 Negotiation problem

People are used to negotiating with offline taxi booking systems, before accepting a trip. However, the user and the driver are unable to negotiate over the fee before confirming the trip, when using the web application method. There is no room for negotiation on the final fare set by the system; neither the user nor the driver may change it.

Researchers have developed a negotiating feature [9] that will allow users to haggle over the fare in order to solve this issue. When a user searches for a taxi, the driver of the closest taxi will get a message inquiring if the taxi is available or not. The driver will respond to that message with the requested fare if he or she is available. The passenger will then be informed of the fare and asked for their chosen fare via the system. The system will then send the expected fare to the driver. The driver will then submit his last fare. The final fare that the driver has suggested will be disclosed to the passenger. The journey will be verified if the passenger accepts the total fare that the driver has suggested. The system will look for new drivers, if not.

4.3 Additional safety precautions

Travelers may take use of several safety elements in the current online car-hailing platforms. The cab drivers are not given any safety precautions. If a driver-related accident happens, they must report it right away, using the system.

The popular taxi service operator, Uber, has developed a function called audio recording in order to increase both the driver and passenger safety [23]. The audio recording of the journey may be started if the driver or the passengers experience any issues. Both of them will get a note after their journey, asking for their opinion. They can use the audio recording as support for their grievance. The recording will be kept in an encrypted manner in their ride history, if they choose not to submit it right away. It may be submitted later from the trip history by the passengers or the driver. However, they cannot play the audio recording on their gadget. They will only be able to decode that tape and take the appropriate steps, after submitting the feedback.

4.4 Taking action in the present moment

Traffic delays may force the driver to arrive at the pickup location substantially later than the ETA, i.e., Estimated Time of Arrival [24]. To save time, people prefer to book cabs online rather than via traditional methods. Even if a cab is booked online, the traveler will have a negative experience if they have to wait for the cab to come.

The system is built in such a way that it can react in real-time scenarios in order to address this problem. As seen in the previously cited Figure 2, Cab-1 is caught up in traffic; the driver will alert the server. The system will start scanning for nearby drivers as soon as it receives the notice. The system will provide it to the passenger if it finds one. Since the Cab-2 is available for rides and has just ended a ride close to the passenger's location, Cab-2 was assigned to the passenger by the system. The passenger's time will thus not be wasted.

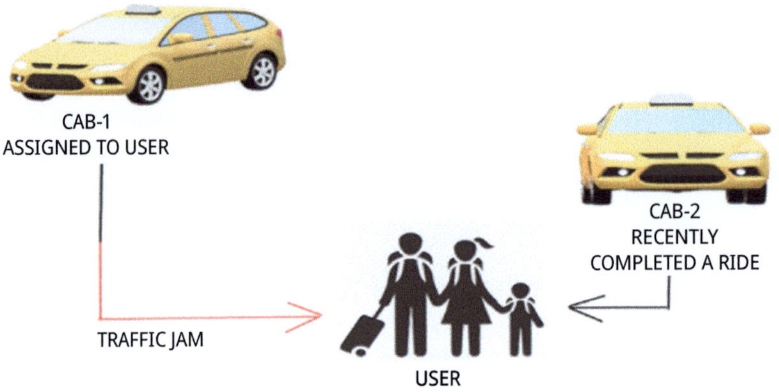

Figure 2: Taking action in the present moment.

4.5 Expanding the allocation of the cab

The driver's engagement in decision-making with the existing system is quite minimal. However, the cab driver is the one with high situational awareness and understanding. There are instances when there is a strong demand for taxis because of public gatherings or the movement of a VIP. But compared to the demand, not many taxis are available. Cabs, however, are freely accessible in certain other places where demand is lower.

The mentioned technique places the cab driver in a good position since they are the ones who are most familiar with the current circumstances. In order for the system to organize cabs from nearby, if the driver observes a crowd while driving or learns of a VIP arrival, the driver must notify any gatherings. Travelers will not have to wait very long, as a result.

4.6 Fleet utilization

Each potential passenger needs specifics met by the cab service they choose. The goal of the system is to match the user with the best possible solution that satisfies all of their needs as a traveler. However, there may be instances when the user's needs cannot be addressed by the already accessible choices. Then, the algorithm is compelled to pair the rider with a less desirable cab.

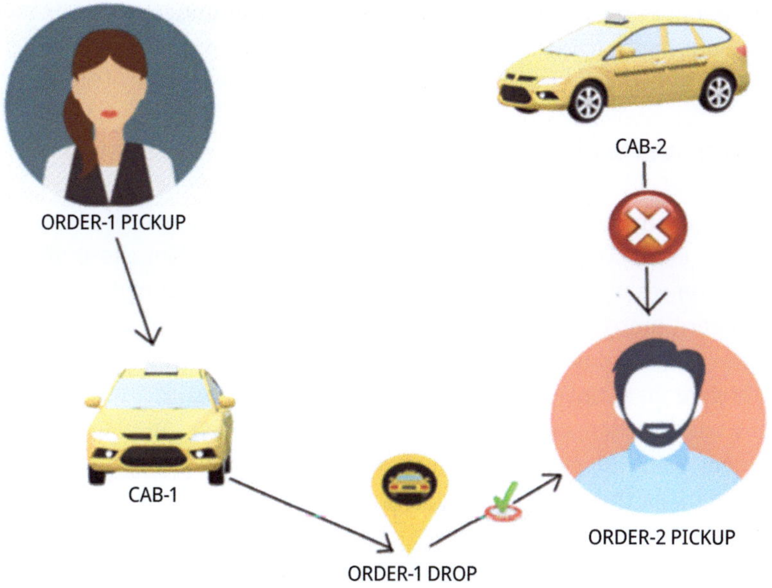

Figure 3: Fleet utilization.

The proposed approach uses fleet utilization to solve this challenge [10]. In Figure 3, the system searches for nearby cabs that meet user needs. The free Cab-2 does not meet all user needs. As no such taxi that matches needs is free, the system checks adjacent cabs ready to end their journeys to meet the user's needs. Cab-1 is almost done and meets all of the user's needs. The user gets Cab-1.

4.7 Dynamic order dispatch

In the present online cab system, drivers are assigned to customers in two ways. One technique allocates a driver depending on the user's selection. The driver has 20 sec to accept or decline the trip. If the initial driver declines, the service provider chooses another. Uber uses this technique. System assignment focuses on client choice. The system ignores the driver's decision. The driver-grabbing model is another technique.

The system advertises the user's request to neighboring drivers. The first driver to respond gets the ride. DIDI uses this strategy, which lets drivers to choose their transport. Neither method helps both the consumer and the driver.

The driver and passenger are both part of an online cab booking system. An ideal system should benefit both. Thus, the dynamic dispatch system [25] that combines the interests of both was created. Nearby drivers are grouped in sets by distance from the pickup point. The system broadcasts the user's ride request to the first set. The first driver to accept the ride gets it. If no one is available from that group, the service provider broadcasts the request to another set. The driver and passenger, both, receive benefits from this approach.

4.8 Identifying driver's cheating ways

The driver should not be the sole person making decisions about a journey. When all excursions are taken according to their own preferences, rather than those of the user, the user's preferences will be overlooked. The driver may attempt to deceive the system in order to earn more money. Despite the fact that they are just beginning a journey, they let the system know that they will be available in 10 min for the following journey. It will save them time when it is time to book their next excursion. However, commuters would face longer lines, as a result of this behavior. Another issue is that drivers frequently tell the system that they are heading home, which confuses the system. The drivers do this as they do not have to go far, and they can take free transportation back to their homes.

The aforementioned factors will result in an uneven distribution of drivers across all areas. There will not be enough cabs in certain areas if everyone wants to travel about their homes. Instead, the fleet may be allocated according to flow estimates, and the system should be kept up to date with driver schedules, in order to prevent the driver from making pointless demands [10].

5 Algorithms used mostly in online car-hailing platforms

5.1 Adaptive scheduling method

The main advantage of the new strategy is that it simply alters the portions of disruptive events that are already scheduled rather than completely rescheduling them [10]. The technique used for decision-making in dispersed events is multiagent technology [26]. It can deal with numerous complicated events with ease because of its distributive nature and object-oriented approach. In this method, various decision-making nodes cooperate with one another by sending messages to one another or compete with one another by using the same data space. The program is divided into independent components using the distributed paradigm. It delivers complicated problems to consumers in the most relatable way possible. In the system, customers are shown as agents. The system allocates a unique agent to compute each job. The most active agents, according to this method, are Order Allocation Managers. They maintain a list of available cabs and negotiate with vehicle brokers. Drivers function as reactive agents in this system. They only respond to orders from order agents and carry out the chosen course of action. Other agents include region loading managers and external event processors. When a new order is placed, the system immediately begins to look for the best vehicle and reserves a resource. The system typically needs 9 min to send a cab for urgent requests. The algorithm assigns a cab as soon as someone arranges a ride and continuously reassigns cabs when new, appropriate possibilities become available. When the driver must begin the trip in order to finish it, the system makes the ultimate choice. The usage of all object-oriented design features is enabled, thanks to the use of multiagent technology. The suggested method makes it extremely simple to optimize those schedules where it is difficult to use formalized algorithms, such as ant colonies algorithms or genetic algorithms, and it increases the productivity and development of the system. It cuts down on the time needed to set up real-time scheduling software. As a result, the total cost is also greatly reduced.

5.2 Distributive approach

Distribution method [9] consists of a number of independent parts. For the purpose of coordinating their shared objective, these units talk to one another. The MDTA, or Multiagent Taxi Dispatch Architecture, is used to implement user-bargaining functionalities. It makes use of the JADE, i.e., Java Agent Development Platform, a MultiAgent System (MAS)-based framework, for cab collection. JADE features a distributed architecture that is adaptable. This flexible nature makes it simple and lively to design, create, and test agents-based systems. With an add-on module, straightforward expansion is possible. The JADE framework was created using the Java language. Thus, it is simple to integrate with any Java development platform, including NetBeans, Eclipse, etc. Each agent on the platform receives a distinct name through the Agent Management System (AMS). The platform's AMS acts as the authority and has the ability to construct and destroy agents on distant containers. An agent requires another agent to fulfil his criteria in order to accomplish his objectives. The agent may discover such agents with the use of Yellow Pages services. The DF, i.e., Directory Facilitator provides these Yellow Pages services. JADE framework uses asynchronous message transmission. It takes advantage of FIPA-ACL message structure guidelines. The sender, list of recipients, communicative act (REQUEST, INFORM, PROPOSE, etc.), content language, and ontology are only a few of the fields included in message formats.

5.3 PDPTW method

The Vehicle Routing Problem with Time Window (VRPTW) algorithm is a well-known vehicle routing method that has been extended as the PDPTW, i.e., Pickup and Delivery Problem with Time Window algorithm [27]. PDPTW is an NP-hard algorithm. It was put in place to use several vehicles for collection and delivery along with time windows to tackle Singapore Taxi Advance Reservation (STAR) difficulties. A link-to-link shortest route method was included into the API application to find the shortest time path, using the PDPTW technique from source to destination. It makes use of automobiles all through the street market rather than from a central cab facility. Thus, it is now simpler for commuters to hail a cab at any time and from any location. Customers anticipate their cab to show up at the pickup location at the time they specify since they have reserved the cab in advance. A strict and highly limited time frame is being used by PDPTW. Users indicate the time point rather than the time frame when making an advance reservation so that consumers will not have to wait beyond the time they had planned for pickup. This strategy seeks to reduce two elements –the number of cars and the distance travelled. These two elements have the potential to significantly reduce the cost and fuel consumption of taxi operations. It primarily concentrates on the exchange and reallocate move procedures. The Construction phase and Improvement phase are the two phases of the PDPTW methodology. All the viable roots are first stored throughout the building process. In this stage, the "ad hoc" issue of taxi dispatching was solved using a temporal window insertion approach. Additionally, during the improvement phase, tabu search is used to enhance the current solution.

6 Existing features of an App-Cab

The existing online cab booking system has the following features.

1) User-friendly interface: The applications are hassle-free. In Ola/Uber, users can book a cab with just a few clicks. The user needs to sign up first. Then he will enter his pickup and destination location. According to his preferences (number of passengers, luggage carried), the user will select a suitable vehicle and confirm the ride.

2) Instant booking: This feature is used to provide an instant booking. In this feature, a cab is assigned to the user immediately after the booking is confirmed. At that very moment, cab details are shared with the user and the cab dispatched to the pickup location as soon as possible.

3) Advance booking: This feature helps the users to schedule a ride for future use. Sometimes due to heavy demand, the current booking system takes too long to find a ride, even if it fails to provide a cab during certain periods. To avoid this, users can book their cab in advance and make plans for touring, beforehand.

4) Cab sharing: Carpooling helps users share their rides with fellow users travelling to identical locations or locations en route to their destination. This feature provides a pocket-friendly trip to the users and it also helps the cab-driver to serve multiple customers at the same time.

5) GPS tracking: Once the user has booked a cab, he will be able to track the real-time location of the cab, and an estimated time of arrival will be provided to the user. It also helps the user track his real-time location during the entire trip.

6) Ride details: The detailed information of the booking is sent to the user when his booking is confirmed. Ride details include car number, car model, booking OTP, driver's name, driver's contact, etc. It helps the user to identify his cab easily.

7) Payment gateway: App-Cab allows both online and offline modes of transactions. The online mode of a transaction includes UPI and e-Wallet. Some cab services also offer their personal wallet (Ola Money) through which the user can make their payment. The users can choose the kind of payment method he wants and make their payments without any hassle.

8) Rewards and membership: This feature attracts a lot of users. Membership allows the users to avail of various exclusive offers. Users are rewarded with coupons that they can apply in the promo code section to avail the trip at a discounted fare.

9) Rental and outstation services: This feature is beneficial for the tourists. Users can hire a car for a particular distance or hours and add a particular number of halt stations in the way. The fare will be calculated on the basis of distance covered, and it can vary according to the travel time.

10) Rating and reviews: Rating and reviews help the system improve its services. Users can share their experience with the help of this feature. It also helps the user report any inconvenience that occurred during the journey.

11) Emergency contact: This feature is very crucial for the safety of the user. The user needs to add his preferred contacts in the emergency settings. If any mishap occurred during the ride, one can press the emergency button to share his ride details with the emergency contacts. They will get an alert with the real-time location of the user and take the necessary action for that situation.

7 Challenges in online car-hailing framework

Online cab services are in greater demand every day. However, at the same time as demand is rising, the problems that the taxi sector is facing are also rising. Here, we discuss about some of the difficulties that taxi booking services are facing and how it impacts the cab business.

- **Rising competition:** Each day, a slew of brand-new businesses floods the industry. Due to this, competition in the taxi sector is fierce. An industry cannot function without competition, and the taxi business is no exception. However, when a business loses consumers to rivals, the situation gets difficult. In order to succeed in today's cutthroat economy, they need to develop distinctive new capabilities. Each provider is making every effort to make his clients' trips pleasant. The providers may take a stand and triumph over this difficult position with the assistance of certain cutting-edge features, such as a further discounts, loyalty games, etc.
- **Dynamic pricing:** Dynamic pricing is one of the most unfavorable practices of online taxi reservation platforms [20]. When demand is great, there is always a dramatic price increase. Due to the large impact surge pricing has on demand growth, it may have favorable short-term effects. However, if we look at the long-term impact of surge pricing, the provider tends to lose clients. Nobody will choose a more expensive option for the same route. Customers would therefore believe that service providers prioritize generating money above offering high-quality services to their clients. Service providers must increase the availability of cabs in accordance with client demand, in order to reduce the rush during peak hours and offer customers excellent service without raising prices.
- **Searching for a ride takes too long:** To go anywhere, you may have to wait a while, especially if taxis are few. This might be quite inconvenient for the user in cases when he is in a rush. The customer stops making use of the service because of the poor experience they had. This may be avoided if taxi companies make more cabs available to their clients.
- **Discontinuation of ride without prior notice:** A poll cited by the Financial Express found that this occurs to consumers on an almost regular basis. If a driver accepts a ride request, they may have to wait forever to show up. It is not very uncommon for them to cancel the ride at the last minute, just before they are due to arrive at the pickup location. User cancellations made more than 10 min after the journey was booked incur a fee under the terms of most taxi reservation systems. The user is forced to pay an excessive fee for the driver's carelessness, even if they end up not using the service. The user is left bewildered and has a tough time locating a replacement vehicle quickly.

8 Proposed system model

In this chapter, the authors provide a possible solution through a mobile application named Vimaansathi to integrate multiple features like App-Cab, COVID-19 prediction, hotel booking, or purchasing necessary products separately via multiple apps required by the people to make themselves comfortable in these "new normal" conditions.

1. Hardware unit: The primary function of the hardware model is measuring the temperature of the passengers before they can board their cab and enter the airport. The added facility of this thermal scanning system is that it can store the data of a particular passenger on the cloud for the administration to take steps in critical conditions. This feature has been incorporated with the help of IoT [28–31]-based infrared thermal scanner that uses a barcode scanner to scan each user's unique code and store the data for every particular passenger. The hardware unit is a unibody structure resting the node MCU along with all the sensors, namely, OLED screen, infrared thermal sensor, 1D/2D code scanner, and battery. (See Figure 4)

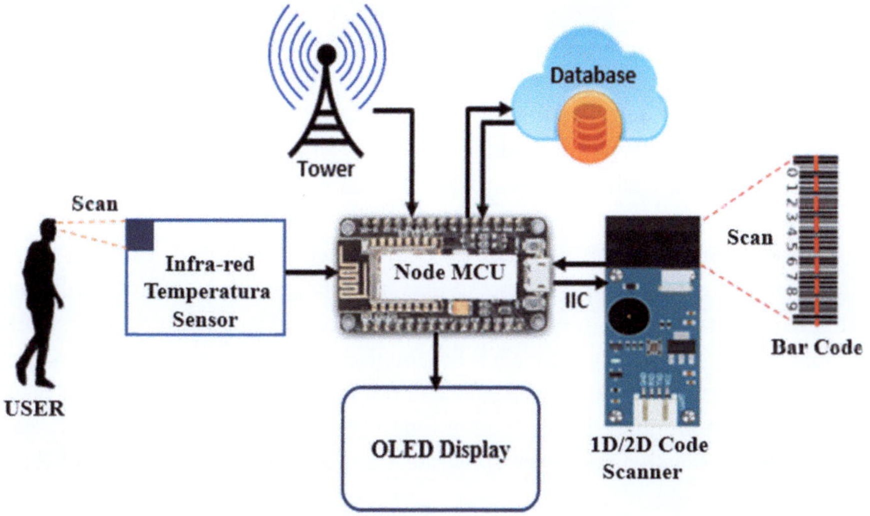

Figure 4: Proposed hardware architecture.

8.1 Working model

Thermal screening process:

1. The user needs to display his/her unique barcode to the screening official. This code will be available in the mobile application of the user.
2. The designated official should scan the barcode with the device.

3. The 1D/2D reader attached to the device reads the data and transmits it to the MCU (microcontroller unit) via wired IIC protocol.
4. The MCU communicates with the server-side cloud (via API) and fetches the user's information.
5. The basic information is displayed over the OLED screen attached to the device.
6. Then, the official needs to scan the user's body temperature by pointing the device toward the user's forehead (A distance of 5–20 cm must be maintained).
7. The infrared thermal sensor attached to the device measures the user's body temperature and displays the same in the OLED display and simultaneously uploads the data to the cloud.
8. The device resets to its initial state for the next screening.

8.2 Software architecture

Vimaansathi uses Amazon Web Services for processing and managing data. The key components of the system model of Vimaansathi include: tracking system (Figure 5(a)), database and caching (Figure 5(d)), processing unit (Figure 5(c)), and ML module (Figure 5(b)).

When a user enters the application, it faces the hosted zone (Route 53), which points to the load balancer. A load balancer is used to divide the traffic among various EC2 instances. An EC2 instance in Vimaansathi runs on Amazon Linux 2. Each EC2 instance runs a python server with a celery worker to manage synchronization. The synchronization is accomplished by the worker; it runs on the compute cloud and has a Redis server, which acts as a broker.

Vimansaathi stores data on Amazon RDS, which has PostgreSQL running on it and Database caching is done using Amazon Elastic Cache, making the accessibility of data faster when compared to other systems (Figure 5(d)). Figure 5(b) describes the machine learning module that uses AWS Personalize for recommendation System. The data is taken from the Amazon S3 bucket for training. AWS Personalize uses HRNN for recommendation systems. Apache Kafka (messaging system) is used to get real-time updates of the various systems, live location, and quality management (Figure 5(a)).

9 Flow sequence of the mobile application

Figure 6 depicts the flow sequence of the Vimaansathi application from the user's perspective. As soon as the user logs in with proper credentials, the application navigates to the chatbot section. The user is forced to answer the questions asked by the chatbots, which determines the COVID-19 risk of the user using an underlying support vector machine learning algorithm. If and only if the user carries a COVID-19 risk, the

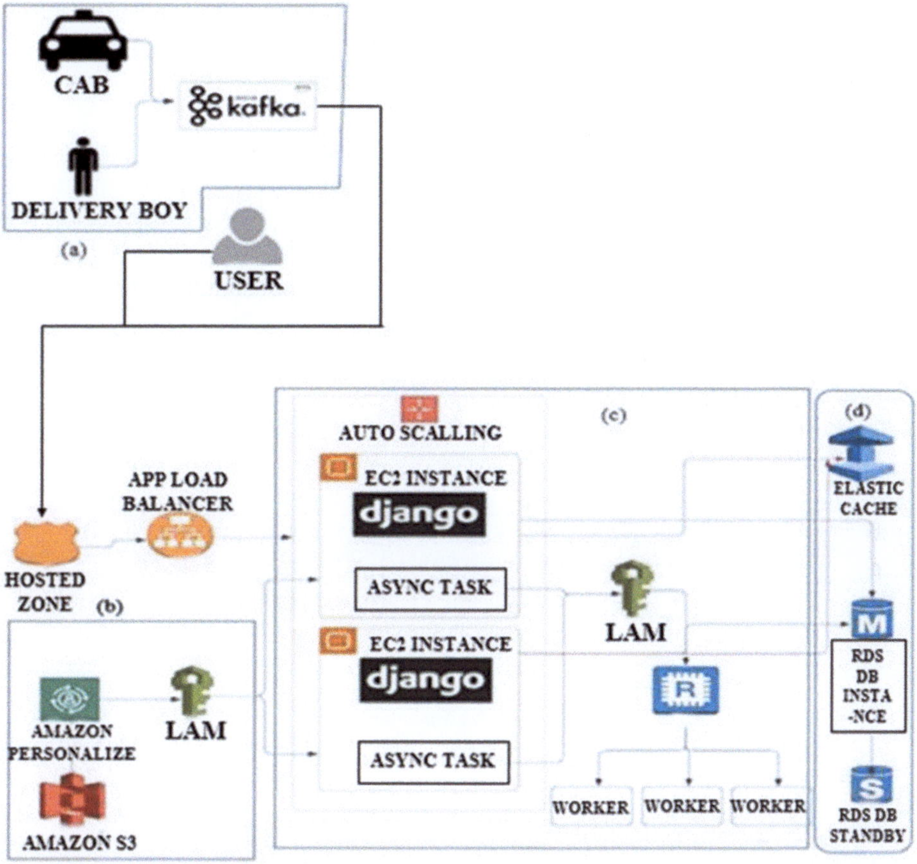

Figure 5: Software architecture.

features of the application become accessible; otherwise, the user is blocked from using the app for the next 7 days.

The user can book flight tickets from the application. Once the flight ticket gets booked, the application opens up different segments to the user. The user gets the facility of prebooking and normal booking of cabs to from the desired airport. The user can also check the shops and restaurants present in his visiting airport from the application. Vimaansathi provides the user with the luxury of buying items and ordering food from the visiting airport using the application, without being physically present there. The user can customize his/her delivery by asking the application to get the product delivered to the booked cab or can pick up the product from the store. The user also gets the benefit of booking hotels that are in the vicinity of the airport from our application. With fast QR code facility, the travelers enjoy fast check-in and check-out. To maintain social distancing protocols, the application has its own wallet to help the user pay online.

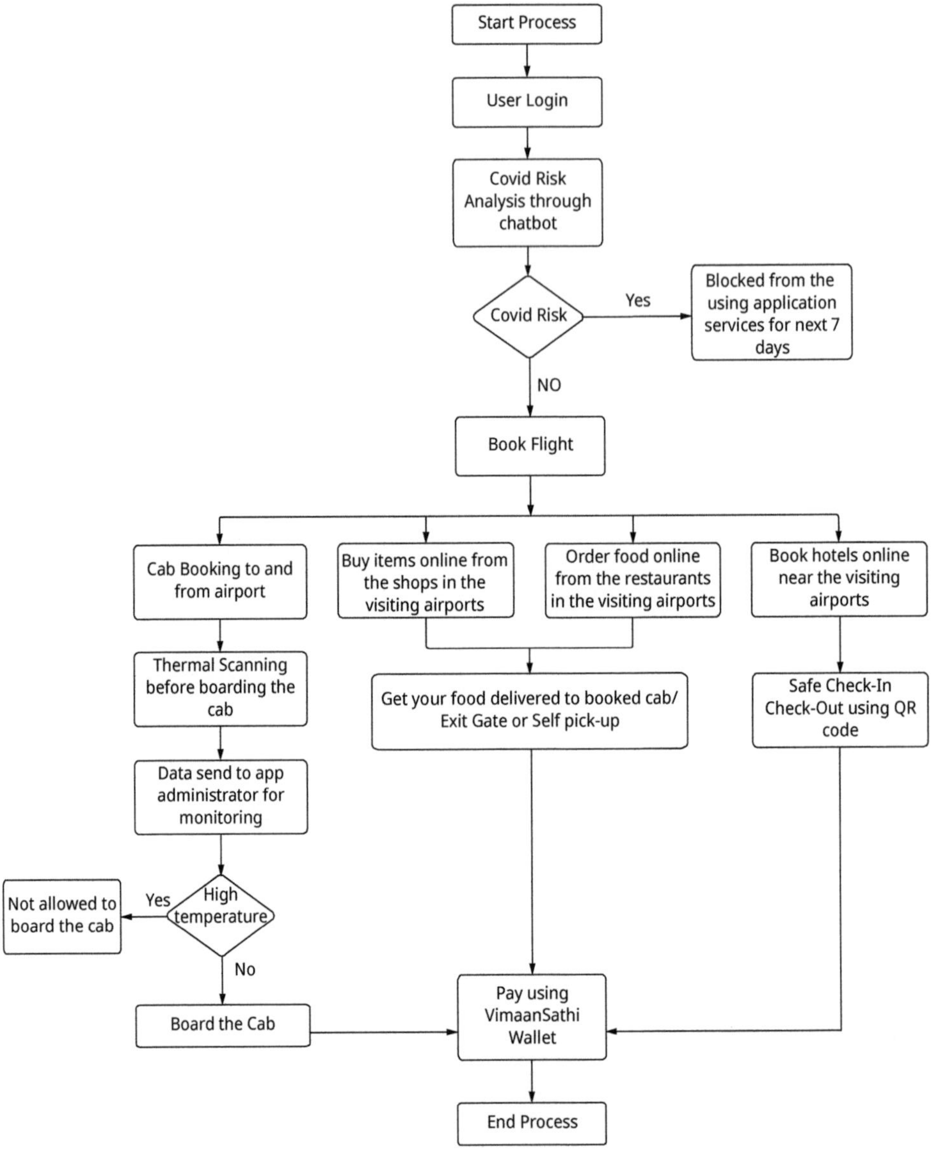

Figure 6: Proposed and implemented flow diagram of the mobile application.

10 Implemented twofold mobile application

User end:

1. Effortless login/signup: User Interface (UI) is a crucial part of an application. Better UI results in better user experience. It is observed that if users face any difficulty during signup, they automatically begin to avoid using that application. But if they find it easy to use, they will come back to that app. In the implemented system, users are asked to provide their basic details like user name, email-id, phone number, and password for signup. From the next time onward, users can simply log in using their id-password and navigate the app seamlessly.

2. Personal wallet: Our personal wallet termed as Vimaanpay provides a quick and reliable transaction for the users. Anything can be purchased and booked from our application using Vimaanpay.

3. Plan my trip: This feature will facilitate the customers to plan their trip in a sequential manner. Instead of visiting different sections for availing different facilities, they will be able to complete their bookings in a few simple steps. If the user wants to skip any section, he can do so with this application. It will save precious time and provide customized service (see Figure 7).

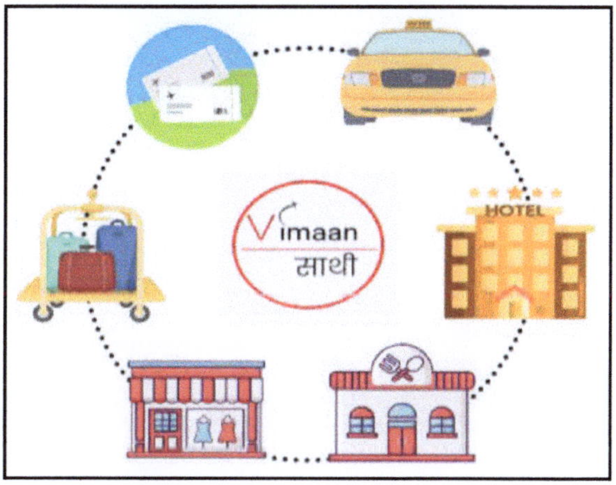

Figure 7: Plan my trip.

4. Service assistance Chatbot: Chatbots provide personalized interaction with the users by seamlessly resolving their initial queries. Earlier, the customers used to call the service agents for resolving issues related to report or order cancellation. But, using chatbots, the repeated queries can be easily resolved without even keeping the customer waiting. It will increase the productivity of the service agents as they will be focusing more on the major queries only. The chatbots will assist the customers in cancelling their orders. According to the standard cancellation policy, a certain percentage will be charged during a refund. The remaining balance will be credited to the wallet. Once the order is dispatched, it cannot be cancelled. If the customers want to report anything regarding the service, they can do it using this feature.

5. Premium membership: Premium membership provides access to avail additional services. The implemented system tracks the previous 60 days' records of a customer. According to their loyalty toward any particular airline, they will be rewarded with loyalty points. Using these loyalty points, the users can avail the premium features. This process will repeat every 60 days. The additional features provided to the customers are listed below.

- **Priority booking:** VIP customers will be provided top-notch services. Only the services having the highest rating will be recommended to the premium customers.
- **One-click trip:** Often, due to a hectic schedule, the users do not get time to do all the bookings properly. The implemented system provides a one-click booking facility for the premium members. This feature will offer premium customers an automated booking experience with just a single click. According to the previous purchases, it will automatically suggest a complete package to the user including flight booking, cab booking, hotel booking, ordering items, food ordering, luggage delivery, etc. It will save the users' time as they need not plan everything separately. The user can also make changes to the plan, if required (see Figure 8).

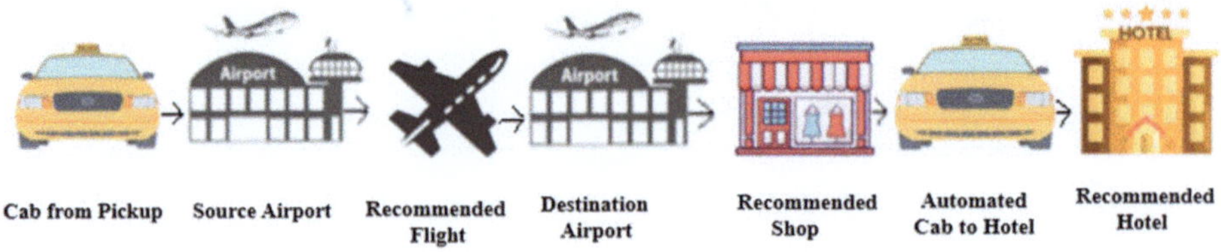
Cab from Pickup
Source Airport
Recommended Flight
Destination Airport
Recommended Shop
Automated Cab to Hotel
Recommended Hotel

Figure 8: One-click trip.

6. My orders: In this section, the user can see all his orders, which include current orders as well as previous orders.

7. Online feedback: Online feedback is the cornerstone of a sustainable customer-retailer relationship. It helps the users rate the services provided by, for example, restaurants. Along with the feedback, they can also add their suggestions, which will help the service providers to improve their services.

8. Cab booking: A few years back, it was very hard to imagine that we would be able to book a cab with just a few simple clicks. Instead of waiting for hours to get a ride, the cab can pick us from our doorstep and drop us at our destination. Our system is designed to be directed toward time saving and minimalism. The authors have discussed the entire cab booking feature, below (see Figure 9).

- **Enter pickup details:** First, the user needs to enter the pickup and destination location.

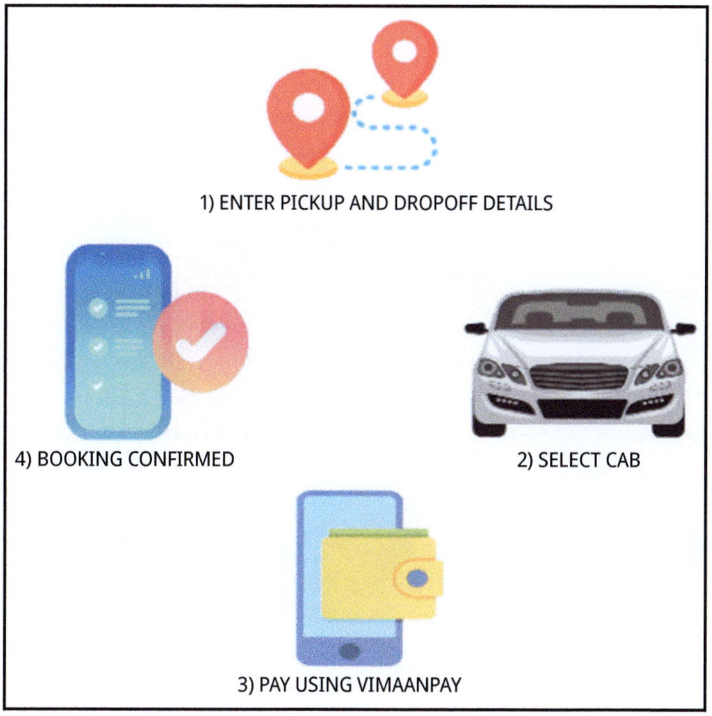

Figure 9: Booking the cab to airport.

- **Select cab:** After entering all the details, the user will get a display of a variety of modes of transportation. The implemented system provides the mini sedan, auto, and bike facility. The user has to select his preferred option.
- **Synchronize bookings:** The existing system does not provide cab services in a synchronized way. The cab drivers have to wait in the long queues of the airport to pick up the customers, which decreases their efficiency. To resolve these major issues, the implemented system has synchronized cab timing with the arrival of the flight. The cab will get a notification 20 min before the arrival of the flight, so that the person can reach the pickup location on time (see Figure 10).
- **Finding nearest ride:** Sometimes, due to long distances, the cabs take too much time to arrive at the pickup point. To minimize the estimated time of arrival, the implemented system starts looking for the nearby cabs and then assigns the nearest cab to the user.
- **QR scanning:** The existing systems use OTP to confirm the user before starting the ride. But the OTP does not provide complete security, so, in the implemented system, the user needs to scan the unique QR code before starting the ride. The QR code adds an extra layer of security to the trip.
- **Real-time tracking:** When there was no option for live tracking, users had to face a lot of uncertainty about the arrival of the cab. With the help of real-time

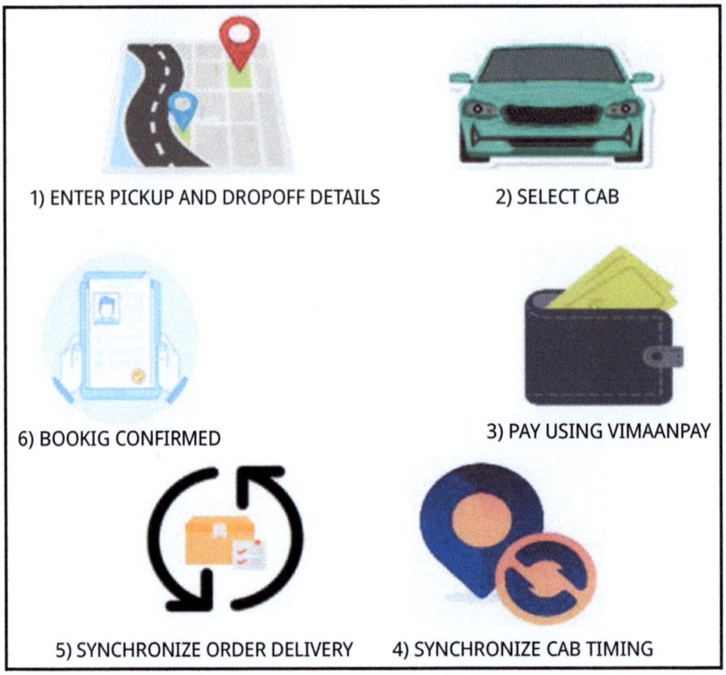

Figure 10: Booking the cab from airport.

tracking, it is possible to predict the ETA [22]. ETA provides unparalleled situational awareness to the users and allows them to make any scheduling adjustments, if required. Our system provides a real-time location tracking, where the user can track the driver's location after booking the cab. And, they can also track their entire journey with the help of a GPS tracker. Hence, if any problem arises during the ride, it can be quickly identified and dealt with (see Figure 11).

- **Reliable and transparent rides:** Transparency and reliability are the two key factors that help any system gain trust of the people. After booking a cab, from sharing the details until the payment, all the operations need to be transparent for both the driver end and user. After selecting the convenient mode of transportation, the user is provided with detailed information about the cab. It includes the driver's name, driver's contact, vehicle no, vehicle's name, the color of the vehicle, etc. At the same time, user's pick-up point, destination point, and contact details are also shared with the driver. After starting the ride, the GPS-enabled location tracking helps the user stay updated about his current location.
- **Utilization of fleet:** Each potential taxi passenger has certain needs that must be met before making a reservation. The purpose of the system is to provide the user with the most optimal choice that satisfies the traveler's needs. However, it is possible that the user's needs are not always addressed by the already accessible choices. When this occurs, the system is compelled to provide the user a less desirable cab (see Figure 3).

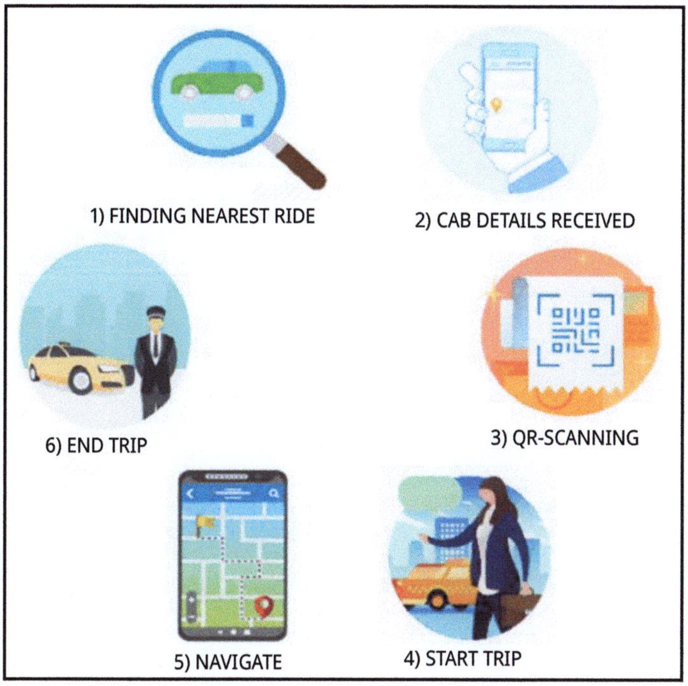
1) FINDING NEAREST RIDE
2) CAB DETAILS RECEIVED
3) QR-SCANNING
4) START TRIP
5) NAVIGATE
6) END TRIP

Figure 11: Entire cab booking process.

The proposed approach implements fleet utilization in an effort to solve this issue [9]. As shown in Figure 3, the system will first try to locate nearby taxis that are suitable for the user. Even if Cab-2 is free, it still does not meet all of the user's needs. Since there is no available taxi at that time, the app will look for ones close by that will be done with their current trips within a reasonable amount of time. The voyage in Cab-1 is almost over, and it has met all of the user's expectations. Thus, the system decides to provide the user Cab-1.

9. Shops and restaurants: Commuters having a tight schedule juggle so many things at the same time that it becomes onerous for them to spare some time to arrange their food or physically go shopping. Furthermore, to find a suitable shop after landing at an unknown place and standing in the long queues to get their required items leads to a significant wastage of their valuable time. In this scenario, e-commerce sites are winning customers' hearts with their flexibility and comfort factor. The implemented model provides an online marketplace for the local shops and restaurants of the airport. With the help of this app, users can order their essentials from the shops and restaurants located at the airport without even visiting the stores physically. The ordered items will be delivered directly to their cab, so they can get their essentials and grab a bite of their favorite food in their busy schedule. If the user has a sufficient amount of time, they can also opt for self-pickup. The online marketplace is far-reaching in

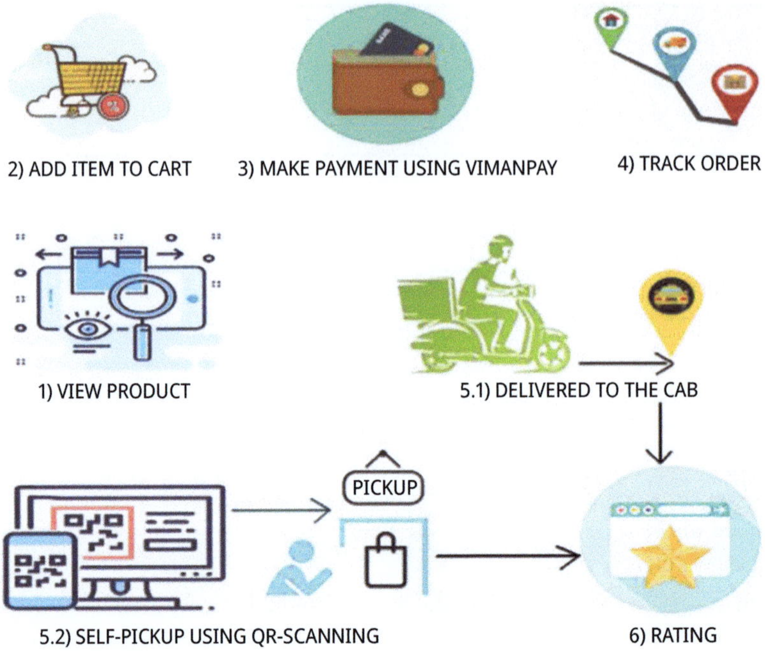

Figure 12: Food/order booking.

comparison to local advertisements. Internet accessibility helps millions of people to view the products at the same time, which will help the shop-owners grow their business by reaching out to a wider range of audiences (see Figure 12).

- **View product:** To expedite the navigation on the app, authorshave implemented filters based on the category of the available products. Thereis an option called "all products," where the user can browse allthe available products irrespective of the category. If the user is looking fora certain category of product, they can visit those by simply clicking on thatparticular category. After viewing any item, if the user wishes to visit thestore, they can easily do it by clicking the "visit store" optionavailable at the product detailsll show him all the products available at that particular store. It helps the shop and restaurant owners facilitate the user's experience and gain a broader audience to drive more sales.
- **Add to bag:** The shopping habits of commuters have drastically changed after the invention of online shopping sites. The number of street shops is gradually decreasing as the users prefer online shopping, which is more flexible, over the offline mode. The e-commerce sites are pleasuring users to sit on the couch and shop various products from their favorite shops without any hassle. Shopping cart acts as a coordinator between the payment gateway and the main application to make the transactions simple and straightforward. To increase the flexibility of the application and the transparency of transactions, authors have implemented a digital shopping cart. The users can add

their desired items to the cart so that they need not face any difficulties during checkout. Shopping cart improves the performance of the search engine and helps the application to handle a heavy user turnout. Another unique feature of this application is that heterogeneous orders can be clubbed together in this application. Users can simultaneously buy food and other items, at the same time, without separately paying for each product. They can simply pay the total amount with a single transaction. This will avoid any sort of confusion.

- **Order status:** Order status is a crucial feature of e-commerce sites. It helps the service providers gain their customer's trust by providing them the exact shipping details and tracking information of their order. The authors have implemented two types of delivery services. Either the user can opt for self-pick up or their parcel will be delivered to their allotted cab. For both available options for delivery, the item will be delivered only on the date of their journey.
- **Self-pickup:** If the user thinks he will have enough time after landing, he can choose the self pickup option while placing his/her orders. In the case of self pickup, the user will be provided the exact information when their order is accepted and packed. And, they have to collect their parcel from the shop within the allotted time.
- **Delivery to cab:** Commuters having a tight schedule might not get enough time for picking up their orders from the respective shops or restaurants. To make sure that despite having a busy schedule, the user gets his order delivered on time, the authors have implemented a delivery option. This option is available for only those who have booked a cab through Vimaansathi. In this feature, a delivery person will pick up the order from the respective shop or the restaurant and deliver it to the cab allotted for that particular user. The user can track his order after his order is confirmed. The user will be provided with all the information when his order is accepted and packed by the shop/restaurant. When the shop/restaurant assigns a delivery person to the order, the user will get the contact details of the delivery person assigned to his order.
- **Order delivery using QR code scanner:** In the existing system, most of the companies use OTP (one-time password) for user verification. However, an OTP does not provide fool proof security to the user. To enhance the security measures, the authors have implemented a system where dynamic QR code will be generated for each user. During delivery, the retailer will verify the user using this unique code. QR is an abbreviated form of Quick Response. We cannot read a QR code with the naked eye. The data transferred via QR code is fully encrypted. So, it adds extra security to the transaction.
- **Delivery to cab:** Before dispatching any order through a delivery person, the retailer scans the unique QR code generated for the delivery person. After scanning the QR code the retailer will be shown two options: one is "dispatched," while the other is "delivered." For delivery through the delivery person, he will click the "dispatched" button. When he clicks the button, a notification will be sent to the user that his order is out for delivery. After this process, the parcel will be handed over to the delivery person for delivery.

- **Self-pickup:** In the case of self pickup, the users directly collect their parcels from the respective shops/restaurants. During the time of pickup, the retailer will scan the unique QR code displayed on the users' application. Just after scanning that code, the retailer will click the "delivered" button and hand over the order to the user.
- **Map integration:** It is very difficult for the user as well as the delivery person to roam around the entire airport for finding a shop/restaurant. To solve this problem, the authors have integrated a floor map of the entire airport in the system. This map will help the user/delivery person to navigate to the exact location of the store. Thus, there will be no problem in locating the store.
- **Rating and review:** Online rating and reviews have become a trend that show no sign of going away. They help the service provider get a clear idea about their client's preference and help them improve their services according to the preference. Most of the time, it is observed that people prefer to check the reviews before trusting a site. A detailed review provides valuable insights to other users about the services provided by them.

10. Hotel booking: Online bookings have gone from being a risky proposition to becoming an essential part of everyday modern life. As online booking helps the users connect

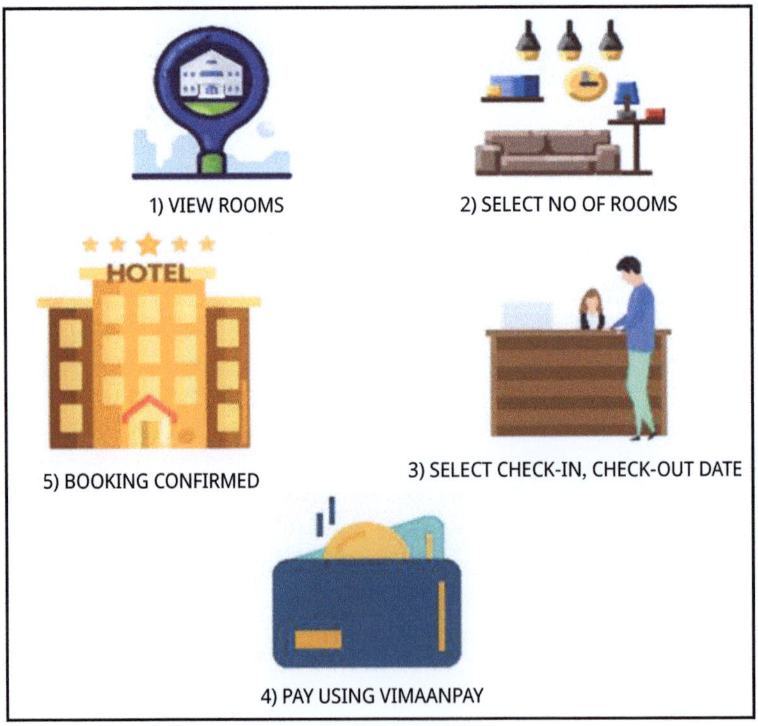

Figure 13: Booking procedure.

directly to the hotel, they need not bear the extra charges of the travel agencies. Users can make their bookings anytime without worrying about business hours. It allows exploring all the available deals and going for the best available deal, and that is why it has a far cheaper acquisition cost when compared to offline bookings (see Figure 13).

- **View rooms:** Here, users can view all the available rooms with the price and rating of each room. If the user wishes to view any store, he can do so by clicking the "visit store" option in the description section. It will display all the rooms available at that hotel. It will help the user get a clear idea about the services, and he will be able to choose the best room according to his budget.
- **Map interaction:** The frequency of visits decreases if the users face any difficulty reaching the hotel. Location is an important factor that helps the new customers find the hotel and the existing customers to visit again. The implemented system has a floor map that shows the current location of the hotel. Thus, it becomes easier for the commuters to reach the hotel.
- **Book rooms:** While viewing the rooms, if the user clicks one of the rooms, he will be shown the description of the facilities available in that room. After viewing the details, if the user wants to book the room, then he has to proceed by clicking the "continue booking" option. Then, he will be asked to enter the number of rooms required and his stay time. To complete the process, the user has to make the payment using Vimaanpay. Now, the user can access the booking from the all-order section.

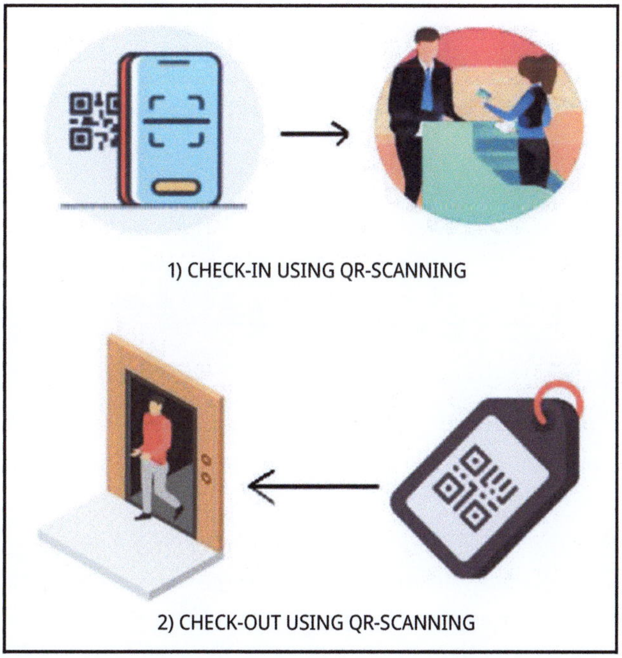

Figure 14: Check-in, checkout.

- **QR scanning:** To ensure a quick and secure experience, the authors have implemented QR-secure check-in and checkout for the hotels. When the users check in, they need to scan the unique QR code first. During the time of checkout too, they need to scan the unique QR code, before leaving the hotel (see Figure 14).

11. Flight booking: The implemented model aims to facilitate the commuters to make all their travel plans using the internet. The users can simply book their tickets at the best price, without visiting any travel agency or wasting a single penny on the extra hidden fees of the travel agencies. The flight booking procedure is mentioned below (see Figure 15).

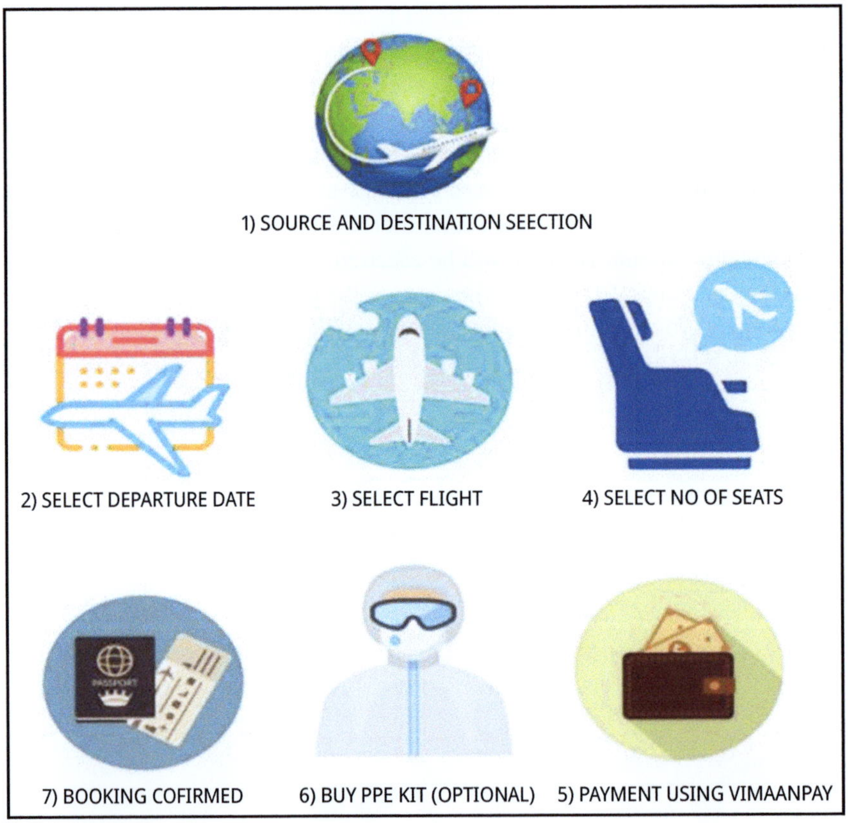
1) SOURCE AND DESTINATION SEECTION
2) SELECT DEPARTURE DATE
3) SELECT FLIGHT
4) SELECT NO OF SEATS
7) BOOKING COFIRMED
6) BUY PPE KIT (OPTIONAL)
5) PAYMENT USING VIMAANPAY

Figure 15: Flight booking.

- **Journey planner:** First, the user has to choose the source and destination. To avoid choosing the same place as destination and source, authors have implemented the system in such a way that it does not allow the user to choose the same place as source and destination. In the next step, the user has to select the date of their departure.

- **Selecting flight and number of seats**: After this, the user will be presented with a list containing all the airfares available for that route. The list will also have all details of the flight such as the airline company, number of seats available, duration of travel, traveling breakpoints, etc. Then, the user has to select the flight and number of seats he/she wants to book.
- **Booking confirmation:** After the selection of seats is complete, the user will be shown the total cost for the number of seats that he/she wishes to book. Now, the user has to make the payment. In order to make the payment transparent, the authors have implemented their own wallet. This helps the user bypass all the hassles of entering the card details. Using this wallet, users can make the payment in just a single click.
- **PPE purchase:** In the current pandemic situation, safety is the key to survival. During a journey, the user comes in contact with a lot of people, so he needs to maintain a safe distance and take proper precautions. In the implemented model, a PPE purchase option is available to ensure the safety of the user. If the user wishes to buy one, only then, he can opt for it. After completing the flight book-

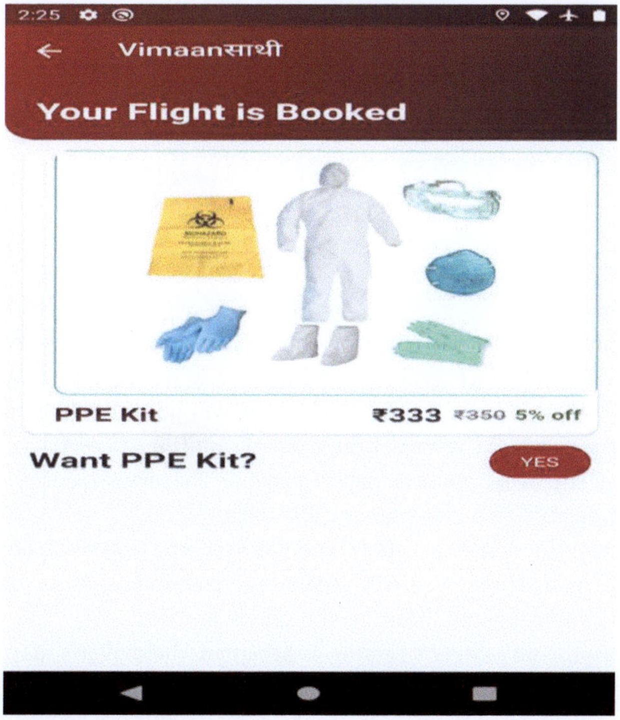

Figure 16: Screenshot of implemented "PPE purchase" feature.

ing, the user will be displayed an option for buying a PPE kit. If he orders one, it will be delivered to him before flight departure (see Figure 16).

Admin end:

1. Cab booking: The booking procedure is described in Figure 17.

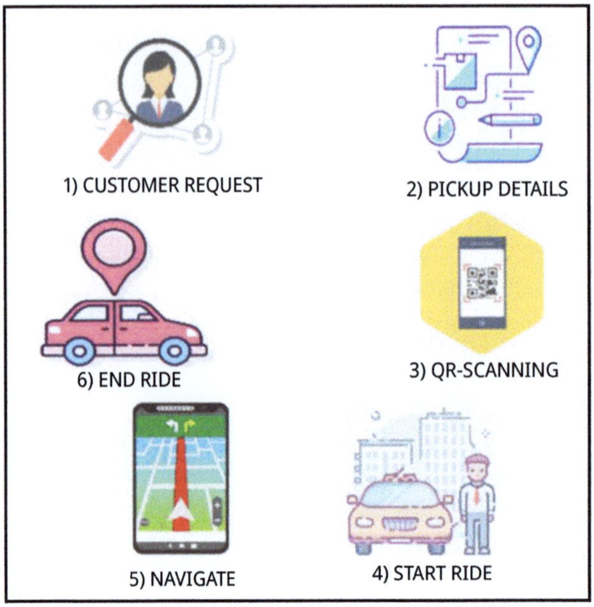

Figure 17: Order confirmation at admin end.

- **View customer request:** The cab driver has the luxury to select his current status, i.e., online or offline. Once the driver goes online, he/she will receive requests from the nearby passengers, one at a time. The driver will get time duration of 15 sec to accept the passenger. If the driver does not accept the passenger, a new request of another nearby passenger will again pop up. The whole process will continue until the driver accepts a passenger or goes offline.
- **Customer details:** Once the driver accepts the passenger, the app will redirect the driver to a new screen. The driver will receive the customer details, which include the customer's name, pickup location, and phone number.
- **Map integration:** Once the passenger's request is accepted, the driver's map will reflect a polyline from his/her current location to the passenger's pickup point. The driver can start navigation in the map provided, which will provide him with current location updates and shortest route to reach the passenger along with proper road assistance.

- **QR scanning:** After the driver reaches the pickup location, he/she needs to scan the QR code from the user. Once the scan is successful, the driver's map will be updated with a new polyline between the driver's current location and passenger's drop location. After the completion of the journey, the driver can press the "END RIDE" button to finish the journey.
- **Responding to live occurrences:** Due to delays in traffic, the driver may arrive at the pickup location much later than the ETA. Booking a cab online is preferred over using a traditional taxi service since it saves customers' time. If the consumer still needs to wait around for the cab to come after making an online reservation, that is not good.

The system is intended to respond to ongoing events in order to address this concern. The driver of Cab-1 will send a notification to the system, as shown in Figure 2 earlier, to inform it that the vehicle is now stalled in heavy traffic. As soon as the notification is received, the system will initiate a search for available drivers in the area. If the system locates a suitable one, it will be given to the user automatically. Since Cab-2 has just ended a ride in the area, it is now available for rides. Therefore, the customer is automatically placed in Cab-2. The user's time will no longer be squandered in this manner.

2. Shops and restaurants:

- **Profile:** Here, the shop owner can give detailed information about his profile. Including his shop name, name of the airport where it is situated, email-id, phone number, wallet balance, and the analytics of his shop.
  Add/update product: This feature provides shop owners the ability to add new products or update available products. The admin is presented with various options using which they can take care of the above. While adding/updating a product, the admin has to provide exhaustive information about the product. In the description section, the retailer has to provide a short description with a symbolic picture of that product. Then, he has to provide the category, stock, and the current status of that product to ensure whether the product is available or not. To keep track of the revenue gained from the sold products, he has to include the cost price, discount, and the selling price at which the product is available to the customers to buy after applying all discounts.
- **View product:** The seller can view all the products available in his shop. The products are displayed categorically, showcasing their image, name, price, and rating. By selecting an individual product, the retailer is navigated to the product details page, which meticulously describes the product.
- **Order status:** Order status has become increasingly crucial, as it removes a lot of pressure from the customer service team. If the customer is not updated with the current status of his order, he will call customer service more frequently, which will make the customer service team frustrated. The implemented application lets the retailer track the delivery status of all his orders from the app. This way,

the admin also gets to keep track of all the orders and they will be able to focus on the important queries of their customers.

- **Pending:** When the order is not accepted by the retailer, then the status of that order shows "pending."
- **Accepted:** Accepted status means that the order is accepted by the seller.
- **Packed:** Packed status indicates that the seller has packed the order.
- **Delivery person assignment:** If the user had opted for the order to be delivered by the delivery system, then a delivery person will be assigned to deliver the order. The user will be provided with all the necessary details of the delivery person (see Figure 18).

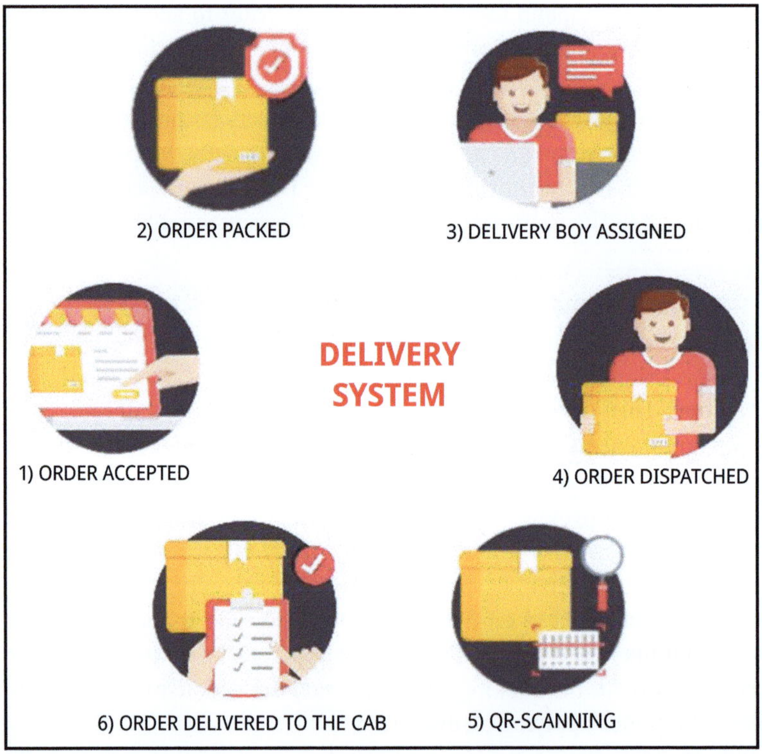

Figure 18: Delivery system.

- **Dispatched:** Once the delivery person collects the package from the shop, the parcel will be out for delivery. A notification will be sent to the user that his order is dispatched.
- **Delivered:** Now, if the user has opted for self pickup, then he/she has to go to the counter and scan a QR code, which will let the seller identify the package. After successfully scanning the QR code, the user will be allowed to collect his order (see Figure 19).

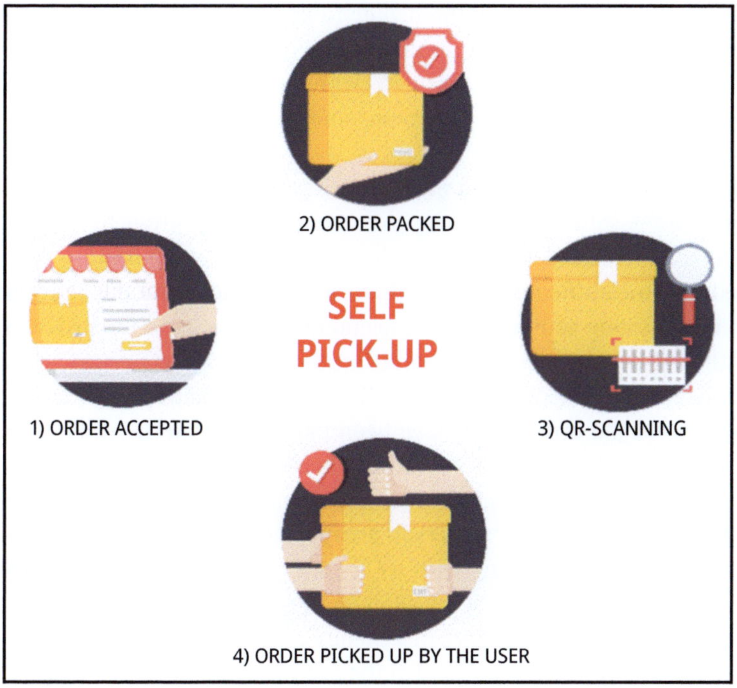

Figure 19: Self pickup.

- **Order history:** This section keeps track of all the previously delivered orders. Here, the retailer can check all the delivered orders with the unique order id and the details of the receiver.

3. Hotel booking:
- **Profile:** Admin profile helps the owner gain insight into his online store. The section displays the detailed information of the hotel, including the name of the restaurant, official mail address, phone number, and a floor map that indicates the exact location of the hotel. The admin profile shows a wallet balance, which displays the total amount present in the wallet and analytics, which is a graphical overview of the total revenue earned over time.
- **Add/update rooms:** The owner can add new rooms for booking or update the price or stock of the existing rooms. While adding a new room, the owner has to provide the pictures and description of that room, so that the user can have a better understanding of the room he is about to book. The seller can also change the current status of the rooms. If any room is not available for booking, he can change its status from “active” to “inactive.” The other rooms that are available for booking will show “active” as their current status.
- **View all rooms:** The hotel owner can view all the rooms available in his hotel.

- **Bookings:** Bookings section helps the owner to keep track of all his bookings. It will assist the owner in managing multiple bookings at the same time, without any confusion.
- **Current booking:** The list of booked rooms and checked-in rooms will be available in the recent bookings.
- **Booking history:** The list of rooms after checkout will be displayed in the booking history.

4. Delivery System: One of the most crucial features of this application is the delivery system. The delivery system provides the connection bridge between the products dispatched from the shops and restaurants and those same products received by the users in their booked cabs. The delivery system has three important phases, as follows:
- **Accept orders**: All the orders that have been packaged from the shops and restaurants enter the delivery pool. The orders become visible to delivery 20 min prior to the delivery time. The delivery person can accept any order of his choice.
- **Get the parcel:** After the delivery person accepts a certain order, he will be provided with the shop details along with a QR code. Not only that, he will also be provided with the exact location of the shop on the map to reach the shop without any hassle. Once the delivery person reaches the designated store, the store admin will scan the QR code and dispatch the product.
- **Deliver the product:** Once the product gets dispatched, the delivery person will get the details of the product that he is delivering along with the details of the cab, the delivery location, and the delivery time. The map provided in the app will display the current location of the cab along with the delivery point.

Government Officials:
1. Effortless login/signup: The User Interface (UI) is a very important part of an app. When the UI is better, the client experience is better. Users stop using an app if they have trouble signing up. But if it's easy to use, they will use that app again and again. In the system that has been put in place, users are asked to sign up by giving their user name, email address, phone number, and password. The next time a user wants to use the app, they can just sign in with their user ID and password and move around without any problems.

1. Flight Booking:
- **Add airport:** The admin is allowed to add new airports as required. To add a new airport, the admin has to provide the state where the airport is situated and the exact coordinates of the airport.
- **Add airline:** The admin is also allowed to add a new airline company. To add an airline, the admin is required to provide the start time, end time of that airline, and price of the tickets.

- **Add flight:** The admin is allowed to add a new flight. While adding a new flight, the admin has to provide necessary information regarding source-destination, arrival-departure time, and the number of seats available on that flight.
- **List of all Flights and airlines:** The admin has access to the list of the airlines and the list of all arriving and departing flights associated with our application. The admin can view the full list of airlines and the list of all arriving and departing flights when required.
- **Set frequency:** The admin can keep track of the flight frequency. While setting the frequency for a new flight, the admin has to provide flight ID, start date, end date, and the fare for that flight.

2. Feedback system: Feedback system helps the admin to analyze user's demand. Thus, they can reduce shopping cart abandonment by improving their services. Based on the feedback received from the users, if the services are not up to the mark, the appropriate authority will take necessary action.

3. Rent: If any shop or restaurant situated at the airport fails to gain the expected revenue from their business for a prolonged period, the authorities can increase their rent.

11 Applications of machine learning model

ML plays a crucial part in the proposed application. In different sections of the application, ML has been implemented to analyze large chunks of data and to predict certain outcomes. The fields of implementation are as follows:

1. Locating the closest cab: Before the advent of online cab services, passengers had to stand about for hours, wave their hands, and hope that a cab would eventually pull up. Many taxi drivers used to routinely refuse clients. With a high acceptance rate, app-based taxi-hailing systems seldom turn down a hail. AVLDS, i.e., Automatic Vehicle Location and Dispatch System [8] uses GPS to find the closest available vehicle and dispatch it to the user. The digital hail shows on the driver's mobile device whenever a client demands a cab. The driver will have 20 sec to consider the request (see Figure 20).

A human cannot possibly assign a cab, while taking into account the needs of each individual user. With ML, however [32], this is a breeze. Figure 20 describes the steps required to locate the closest taxi. As soon as the customer ordered a cab, the system began looking for available vehicles in the area. It located three available taxis in the area. Of the three available, Cab-2 has the shortest distance to travel to reach the designated pickup location. The user was therefore given access to Cab-2. When a user requests a ride, ML quickly returns results from a database containing information on thousands of drivers and riders. The KNN, or K-nearest neighbors method is

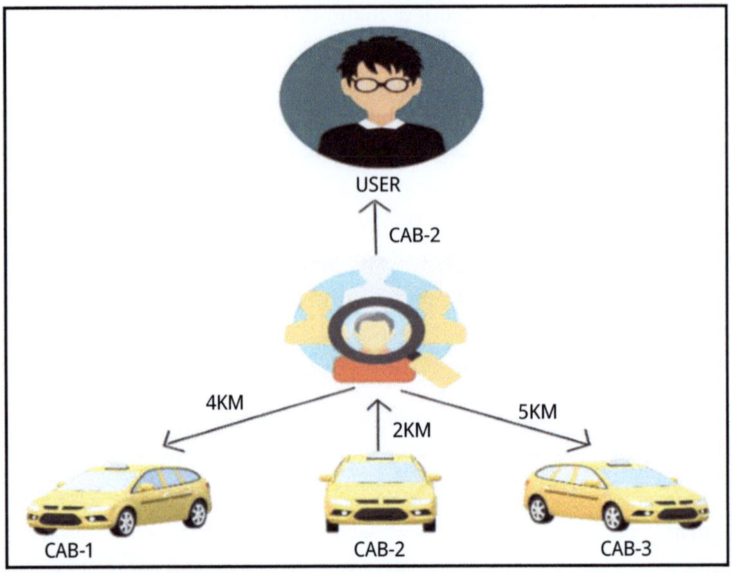

Figure 20: Finding the nearest ride.

often used by online cab systems to locate the nearest drivers and then perform a regression on them to determine which ones are the best possible matches.

2. COVID risk prediction: The risk predictor chatbot gathers 15 parameters from the user, using chat interactions. These parameters are then passed to the Support Vector Machine classifier (see Figure 21). The classifier classifies the risk among the three classes, i.e., no risk, mild risk, and high risk. Based on the prediction of the classifier, the chatbot displays the risk analysis to the user. Looking at how uncertain COVID-19 [33] prediction is, the classifier uses the "RBF" kernel for better prediction results.

The effects of these 15 factors on COVID-19 are detailed below:

1. **Age:** In coronavirus instances, older individuals had a higher mortality risk than younger individuals. The major cause of this trend is mostly attributable to the younger population's higher degree of immunity than the older population.
2. **Body temperature:** Body temperature is one of the most important COVID-19 symptoms [34–38]. Above 100°C is moderate fever, and 103°C is severe. Using sensors, the thermal scanner can quickly determine the user's body temperature.
3. **Dry cough:** A frequent indication of COVID-19 is a dry cough that does not produce phlegm or mucus [39–41].
4. **Tiredness:** Fatigue is the first symptom of COVID-19 disease [42].
5. **Chest pain:** A serious situation develops when chest discomfort is persistent and there are breathing difficulties.
6. **Nasal congestion:** This symptom should be taken seriously as it may be an indicator of coronavirus infection.

7. **Runny nose:** This is a fairly typical sign of a cold, but when combined with other symptoms such as high temperature and difficulty in breathing, a person may be expected to be in the initial phases of coronavirus infection.
8. **Sore throat:** It is a well-recognized feature of coronavirus infection. If you have a sore throat, you should visit a doctor.
9. **Diarrhea:** A coronavirus infection is common in patients with diarrhea.
10. **Breathing rate:** Over 30 breaths per minute indicates a life-threatening situation.
11. **Hypertension:** Those with hypertension at stage 1 (blood pressure of 140–159) are at lower risk of contracting the coronavirus than those with hypertension at stage 2. (160 and above blood pressure).
12. **Cardiovascular diseases:** Heart disease patients have a higher mortality rate [43].
13. **Diabetes:** This is one of the most important signs for assessing the likelihood of COVID-19 disease.
14. **Current smoker:** People who still smoke regularly are at a higher risk for developing acute respiratory illness syndrome.
15. **Recent proximity to someone who has a contagious illness of cold and fever:** Checking for this condition is crucial to determine where the coronavirus originated.

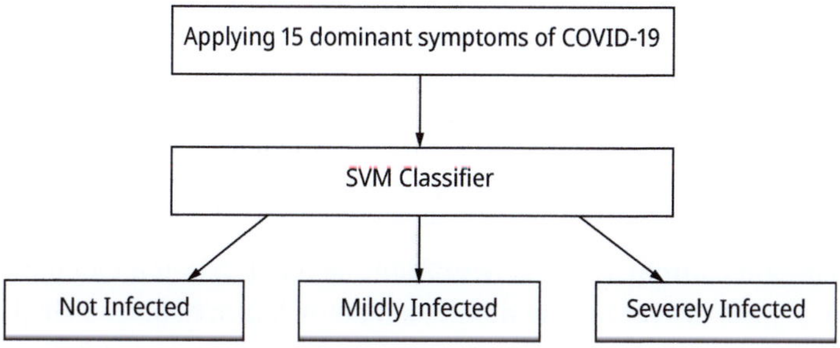

Figure 21: Schematic representation of the suggested approach for predicting COVID-19.

Figure 22 represents a test-arranged chatbot that helps users determine their health condition and the stage of risk (i.e., likelihood of being influenced by the coronavirus infections). This framework is outfitted with current AI-ML apparatuses, which allows it to decide the danger dependent on 15 subscriber inputs.

3. Cab fare estimation: Cab fare estimation is based on the four factors, which include the pickup time of the user, the distance of the journey, the type of cab booked (Sedan or Mini), and the availability of cab at that time in the surrounding area [44–46]. All these four factors are then fed to the Multiple Linear Regression model. The model uses a gradient descent approach to minimize errors and increase its accuracy. The regression model predicts the cab fare with an accuracy of 93%.

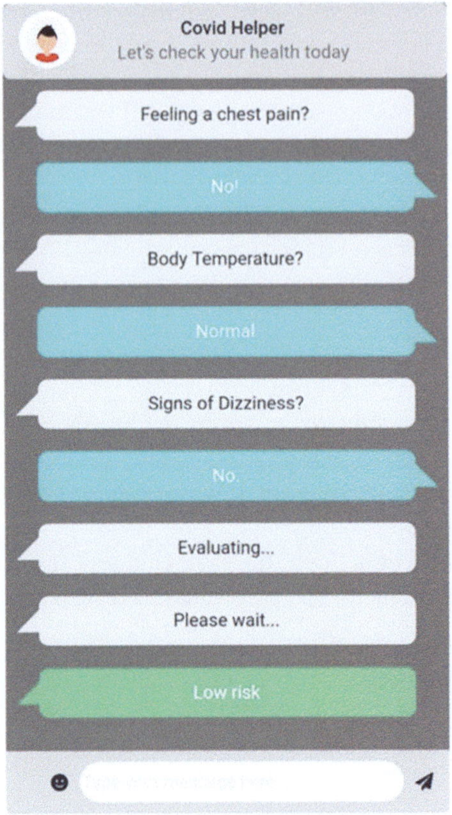

Figure 22: Test-oriented chatbot.

4. Customer reviews categorization: The reviews of the customer, based on an individual product, provide a great insight for the other customers. It also helps the shopkeepers identify the positive and negative points related to the item they are selling. Using Natural Language Processing, we are classifying the reviews into positive and negative and displaying them with different color shades for better identification for both the customer and seller. To begin with, each review that undergoes the classification process is turned into a simplified string without any unnecessary words present in the sentence. The reviews are then converted into the "Bag of Words" model. The model is then supplied to the Naïve Bayes classifier. The classifier calculates the probability of the review as positive or negative. Any review with a probability below 0.5 is deemed as a negative review and similarly, reviews with a probability above 0.5 are classified as a positive review. The model predicts with an accuracy of 73%.

5. Customized recommendation: The VIP users are provided with a customized complete journey package based on their previous bookings, orders, and interactions from our application. Using a hierarchical recurrent neural network, the VIP users are recommended a journey package. The significance of the model lies in the fact that it uses reinforcement learning but fetches the updated data of the user from the database to change its recommendations in course of time, based on the user's recent interactions and purchases.

6. Smart chat: It is crucial for the user and driver to be able to communicate throughout the journey. However, it is usually dangerous for the driver to respond while operating the taxi.

Drivers may easily react to typical queries with a single click using a chatbot that employs ML and natural language processing methods.

12 Implemented key features concerning existing App-Cab system

1. End-to-end solution: The proposed application provides an end-to-end solution. The users get the convenience of flight booking, cab booking, hotel booking, food ordering, and online shopping altogether, so they can tackle all their bookings with a single application.

2. Synchronized services: In the current system, if the user books a cab beforehand and the flight is delayed, the user has to cancel the previously booked cab and book a new cab after landing. Sometimes the user even has to pay extra charges for canceling the cab. As time is a very important factor, this can be hectic for many people. Our app provides synchronized services where the cab and order bookings of a user are automatically scheduled, based on the arrival time of the flight. Even if the flight is delayed, the cab and delivery are automatically rescheduled, based on the updated arrival time of the flight. This way, users do not have to worry about rescheduling their booking. As time is a very important factor for frequent travelers, this can be a major USP of our app.

3. Heterogeneous orders: In the current system, no two orders can be clubbed together. If the user wishes to buy anything from any shop and buy food from any restaurant, he has to pay separately for each order. This can be considered a major drawback, as it creates a lot of confusion. The implemented system has tried to resolve this issue. In the implemented application, the user can simultaneously shop from two different shops/restaurants in a single transaction. Hence, the users can easily manage their orders without any confusion.

4. Hassle-free delivery to the cab: In today's busy world, it is very difficult for the commuters to take out some time to go shopping, physically. If the user urgently needs to order anything for their journey, they might not get that item before departure. This major problem can be easily solved with our application. It will deliver the product directly to the allocated cab, before their departure time.

5. Privileged VIP features: Premium customers are offered the privileges of "Priority booking" and "One-click trip" features. Thus, they can avail the top-notch services without wasting their precious time.

6. Customized recommendation: Customized services are the key to better user experience. They help the user find the required item very easily. The implemented system has a customized recommendation facility, whereby users will be recommended the services according to their previous booking history.

13 Conclusion

Our proposed and developed mobile application can make life easier for commuters once put to use by organizations like the AAI or any similar organization. It will make the process of planning a journey much simpler and more time-saving. Starting from COVID-19 risk prediction, maintaining social distancing through QR code, booking flights, taking a cab to the airport, ordering food from the restaurants within the airport, and even booking hotels to stay in unknown places, all activities can be processed in one go with our application. Our application can have a significant impact on the daily lives of commuters traveling by airplanes regularly. The importance of this app is not only restricted to travelers but also beneficial to the shop owners, restaurants within the airport, and hotels in the vicinity of the airport. All these organizations enjoy the opportunity of attracting more customers through our apps, which can further increase their day-to-day income. All these services that are being provided by Vimaansathi are within the guidelines of social distancing protocols. The use of QR codes for check-in and checkout purposes in hotels and for receiving products from shops, along with the inbuilt Vimaansathi wallet, makes the entire process of the transactions smooth and elegant.

References

[1] https://www.iata.org/en/pressroom/pr/2018-09-04-02/ (Accessed on 2021).

[2] Guhathakurata, S., Saha, S., Kundu, S., Chakraborty, A., Banerjee, J. S. South Asian Countries are less fatal concerning COVID-19: A hybrid approach using machine learning and fuzzy AHP. In: Computational Intelligence Techniques for Combating COVID-19, 2021, 1–26.

[3] Guhathakurata, S., Kundu, S., Chakraborty, A., Banerjee, J. S., Novel, A. Approach to predict COVID-19 using support vector machine. In: Data Science for COVID-19, Academic Press, 2021, 351–364.

[4] Guhathakurata, S., Saha, S., Kundu, S., Chakraborty, A., Banerjee, J. S. A new approach to predict COVID-19 using artificial neural networks. In: Cyber-Physical Systems, Academic Press, 2020, 139–160. 2022.

[5] Guhathakurata, S., Saha, S., Kundu, S., Chakraborty, A., Banerjee, J. S. South Asian Countries are less fatal concerning COVID-19: A fact-finding procedure integrating machine learning & multiple criteria

decision making (MCDM) technique. Journal of The Institution of Engineers (India): Series B, 2021, 102(6), 1249–1263.
[6] Biswas, S., Sharma, L. K., Ranjan, R., Banerjee, J. S. Go-COVID: An Interactive Crossplatform Based Dashboard for Real-time Tracking of COVID-19 using Data Analytics. Journal of mechanics of continua and mathematical sciences, 2020, 15(6), 1–15.
[7] Saha, P., Guhathakurata, S., Saha, S., Chakraborty, A., Banerjee, J. S. Application of Machine Learning in App-Based Cab Booking System: A Survey on Indian Scenario. In: Applications of artificial intelligence in engineering, Springer, 2021, 483–497.
[8] Liao, Z. Real-time taxi dispatching using global positioning systems. Communications of the ACM, 2003, 46(5), 81–83.
[9] Nath, A., Khandelwal, A., Kanojia, A., Minocha, I., Niyogi, R. Design and implementation of an intelligent cab service system. In: 2017 Tenth International Conference on Contemporary Computing (IC3), IEEE, 2017, 1–6.
[10] Glaschenko, A., Ivaschenko, A., Rzevski, G., Skobelev, P. Multi-agent real time scheduling system for taxi companies. In: 8th International Conference on Autonomous Agents and Multiagent Systems (AAMAS 2009), Budapest, Hungary, 29–36), (2009, May).
[11] Akhtar, N., Kuriakose, P. N. Disruptive mobility in pre-and post-COVID times: App-Based shared mobility in Indian Cities – the case of Bengaluru. In: The Impact of the COVID-19 Pandemic on Green Societies, Cham, Springer, 2021, 57–91.
[12] World Health Organization. Supporting healthy urban transport and mobility in the context of COVID-19, 2020.
[13] Luan, S., Yang, Q., Jiang, Z., Wang, W. Exploring the impact of COVID-19 on individual's travel mode choice in China. Transport Policy, 2021, 106, 271–280.
[14] Thapa, G. Consumer Behaviour on Online Ride Hailing Apps In India. PalArch's Journal of Archaeology of Egypt/Egyptology, 2020, 17(12), 1176–1189.
[15] Jain, G. App-based cab services: Issues and challenges in the Indian context. Digital Marketing Outreach, 2022, 201–218.
[16] https://www.bing.com/covid.
[17] https://covid.apollo247.com/.
[18] https://covindia.com/.
[19] https://www.mygov.in/aarogya-setu-app/.
[20] https://expandedramblings.com/index.php/ola-statistics-facts/, (Accessed May 2020).
[21] https://expandedramblings.com/index.php/uber-statistics/, (Accessed May 2020).
[22] Sheu, J. P., Chang, G. Y., Chen, C. H. A distributed taxi hailing protocol in vehicular ad-hoc networks. In: IEEE 71st Vehicular Technology Conference, IEEE, 2010, 1–5. (2010, May).
[23] https://www.uber.com/en-IN/newsroom/new-safetyfeatures/#:~:text=We%20plan%20to%20pilot%20audio,time%20through%20the%20Safety%20Toolkit, (Accessed April 2020).
[24] Lam, H. T., Diaz-Aviles, E., Pascale, A., Gkoufas, Y., Chen, B. Grand Challenge: Real-time Destination and ETA Prediction for Maritime Traffic 2015.
[25] Duan, Y., Wang, N., Wu, J. Optimizing Order Dispatch for Ride-Sharing Systems. In: In 28th International Conference on Computer Communication and Networks (ICCCN). IEEE, 2019, 1–9, (2019, July).
[26] Awajan, A. An automated taxi booking and scheduling system. In: 8th EUROSIM Congress on Modelling and Simulation, IEEE, 2013, 502–505, (2013, September).
[27] Wang, H., Lee, D. H., Cheu, R. PDPTW based taxi dispatch modeling for booking service. In: Fifth International Conference on Natural Computation, Vol. 1, IEEE, 2009, 242–247, (2009, August).
[28] Pandey, I., Dutta, H. S., Banerjee, J. S. WBAN: A smart approach to next generation e-healthcare system. In: 3rd International Conference on Computing Methodologies and Communication (ICCMC), IEEE, 2019, 344–349, (2019, March).

[29] Paul, S., Chakraborty, A., Banerjee, J. S. The extent analysis based fuzzy AHP approach for relay selection in WBAN. In: Cognitive Informatics and Soft Computing, Springer, 2019, 331–341.

[30] Paul, S., Chakraborty, A., Banerjee, J. S. A fuzzy AHP-based relay node selection protocol for wireless body area networks (WBAN). In: 4th International Conference on Opto-Electronics and Applied Optics (Optronix), IEEE, 2017, 1–6, (2017, November).

[31] Roy, R., Dutta, S., Biswas, S., Banerjee, J. S.: Android things: A comprehensive solution from things to smart display and speaker. In: Proceedings of International Conference on IoT Inclusive Life (ICIIL 2019), NITTTR Chandigarh, India, Springer, 2020.

[32] Banerjee, J., Maiti, S., Chakraborty, S., Dutta, S., Chakraborty, A., Banerjee, J. S. Impact of machine learning in various network security applications. In: 3rd International Conference on Computing Methodologies and Communication (ICCMC). IEEE, 2019, 276–281, (2019, March).

[33] Huang, C., Wang, Y., Li, X., Ren, L., Zhao, J., Hu, Y., . . . Cheng, Z. Clinical features of patients infected with 2019 novel coronavirus in Wuhan, China. The Lancet, 2020, 395(10223), 497–506.

[34] WHO-China Joint Mission, Report of the WHO-China Joint Mission on Coronavirus Disease 2019 (COVID-19), https://www.who.int/docs/default-source/coronaviruse/who-china-joint-mission-on-covid-19-final-report.pdf, (accessed March 1, 2020).

[35] World Health Organization, Coronavirus disease 2019 (COVID-19) Situation Report – 47, https://www.who.int/docs/default-source/coronaviruse/situation-reports/20200307-sitrep-47-covid-19.pdf?sfvrsn=27c364a4_2, (accessed March 7, 2020).

[36] Wang, W., Tang, J., Wei, F. Updated understanding of the outbreak of 2019 novel coronavirus (2019-nCoV) in Wuhan, China. Journal of medical virology, 2020, 92(4), 441–447.

[37] Fang, L., Karakiulakis, G., Roth, M. Are patients with hypertension and diabetes mellitus at increased risk for COVID-19 infection?. The Lancet. Respiratory Medicine, 2020.

[38] Guan, W. J., Ni, Z. Y., Hu, Y., Liang, W. H., Ou, C. Q., He, J. X., . . . Du, B. Clinical characteristics of coronavirus disease 2019 in China. New England journal of medicine, 2020, 382(18), 1708–1720.

[39] Zu, Z. Y., Jiang, M. D., Xu, P. P., Chen, W., Ni, Q. Q., Lu, G. M., Zhang, L. J. Coronavirus disease 2019 (COVID-19): A perspective from China. Radiology, 200490, 2020.

[40] Chen, N., Zhou, M., Dong, X., Qu, J., Gong, F., Han, Y., . . . Yu, T. Epidemiological and clinical characteristics of 99 cases of 2019 novel coronavirus pneumonia in Wuhan, China: a descriptive study. The Lancet, 2020, 395(10223), 507–513.

[41] Zheng, Y. Y., Ma, Y. T., Zhang, J. Y., Xie, X. COVID-19 and the cardiovascular system. Nature Reviews Cardiology, 2020, 17(5), 259–260.

[42] Rothan, H. A., Byrareddy, S. N. The epidemiology and pathogenesis of coronavirus disease (COVID-19) outbreak. Journal of autoimmunity, 2020, 102433.

[43] The Epidemiological Characteristics of an Outbreak of 2019 Novel Coronavirus Diseases (COVID-19) – China, 2020.

[44] https://medium.com/analytics-vidhya/machine-learning-to-predict-taxi-fare-part-one-exploratory-analysis-6b7e6b1fbc78, (Accessed June 2020).

[45] https://medium.com/analytics-vidhya/machine-learning-to-predict-taxi-fare-part-two-predictive-modelling-f80461a8072e, (Accessed June 2020).

[46] https://www.mapsofindia.com/my-india/business/problems-faced-by-ola-and-uber-users, (Accessed June 2020).

Index

https://doi.org/10.1515/9783110767681-016

Bei Fragen zur Produktsicherheit wenden Sie sich bitte an:
If you have any questions regarding product safety,
please contact:

Walter de Gruyter GmbH
Genthiner Straße 13
10785 Berlin
productsafety@degruyterbrill.com